Clinics in Developmental Medicine No. 141/142

AN ATLAS OF NEONATAL BRAIN SONOGRAPHY

© 1997 Mac Keith Press
High Holborn House, 52–54 High Holborn, London WC1V 6RL

Senior Editor: Martin C.O. Bax
Editor: Pamela A. Davies
Managing Editor: Michael Pountney
Sub Editor: Pat Chappelle

Set in Times and Avant Garde on QuarkXPress

The views and opinions expressed herein are those of the authors and do not necessarily represent those of the publisher

First published in this edition 1997
Reprinted 2001
British Library Cataloguing-in-Publication data:
A catalogue record for this book is available from the British Library

ISSN: 0069 4835
ISBN: 1 898683 09 3

Printed by The Lavenham Press Ltd, Water Street, Lavenham, Suffolk
Mac Keith Press is supported by **Scope** (formerly The Spastics Society)

Clinics in Developmental Medicine No. 141-142

An Atlas
of Neonatal Brain
Sonography

PAUL GOVAERT
Gent University Hospital
Gent

LINDA S. DE VRIES
University of Utrecht
Utrecht

with contributions from
FREDERIK J.A. BEEK *and* FRANK VAN BEL – *University of Utrecht*

1997
Mac Keith Press

Distributed by 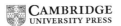 CAMBRIDGE
UNIVERSITY PRESS

AUTHORS' APPOINTMENTS

Paul Govaert, MD

Department of Neonatology, Gent University Hospital, Gent, Belgium

Linda S. de Vries, MD

Department of Neonatology, Wilhelmina Kinderziekenhuis, University of Utrecht, Utrecht, The Netherlands

Frederik J.A. Beek, MD

Department of Radiology, Wilhelmina Kinderziekenhuis, University of Utrecht, Utrecht, The Netherlands

Frank van Bel, MD

Department of Neonatology, Wilhelmina Kinderziekenhuis, University of Utrecht, Utrecht, The Netherlands

CONTENTS

Frank van Bel

    Technical aspects and quantification of cerebral blood flow velocity
    Identification and insonation of intracerebral vessels
    Neonatal cerebral blood velocity waveform patterns
    Research applications of (colour) Doppler ultrasound

PREFACE

Superficially, it might seem inappropriate to develop an atlas of neonatal brain sonography at a time when newer, more sophisticated techniques have promoted the 'decade of the brain'. However, since the first book on neonatal cranial ultrasound by Levene *et al*. (1985) and despite the widespread application and proven usefulness of bedside ultrasound scanning, there have in fact been very few publications in this field.

Thus with this book we have tried to produce a complete guide to ultrasonography of the central nervous system in the preterm and term newborn infant. Following an extensive look at normal neuroanatomy, there are sections covering not just haemorrhagic and ischaemic lesions but also brain tumours, congenital and neonatal infections and congenital anomalies, as well as brief discussions of 3D and colour sonography. In addition, we are most grateful to Erik Beek and Frank van Bel for their expert contributions on, respectively, sonography of the lower spinal canal and the cerebral Doppler examination. Because the book is intended for clinicians we have deliberately avoided tackling the more technical aspects. References have been left to the end of each section to make the reading as easy as possible.

We are aware that some disease patterns have been presented only in part or not at all, because we did not have appropriate pictures available or could not correctly interpret findings from the available literature. Quite often we put forward hypothetical diagnoses, knowing that we did not possess genuine proof. In such instances we quote the hypothetical nature of the statements, hoping such research will prove us wrong or occasionally right. The attentive reader will notice the emphasis put on patterns and their causes.

The numerous illustrations derive from many years of experience. Not all the sonography was performed by the authors, and thanks are given to Paula Eken, Karen Rademaker and Floris Groenendaal in Utrecht for performing many of these examinations at often odd hours. Our paediatric colleagues in both Gent and Utrecht have shared their knowledge with us unsparingly and we thank them for this.

Although treatment for neonatal brain disorders is still limited, the clinician's important task is to make a correct diagnosis so that s/he can discuss prognosis with the baby's parents in as informed a manner as possible. Cooperation with radiologists is essential when discussions about MRI or CT scanning for difficult clinical or sonographic problems are needed. And if babies die, it is vital to correlate the pathologist's findings with the neuroimaging pictures so that further progress in interpretation can be made.

We dedicate this atlas to paediatricians caring for sick newborn infants, and hope it will be of help to them in their work with the babies and their families.

REFERENCE

Levene, M.I., Williams, J.L., Fawer, C-L. (1985) *Ultrasound of the Infant Brain. Clinics in Developmental Medicine No. 92*. London: Spastics International Medical Publications.

PAUL GOVAERT, MD
LINDA S. DE VRIES, MD

SECTION I — NORMAL ANATOMY

I.1 SULCI AND GYRI

Sulci are echodense linear structures separating gyri. Most develop in a particular sequence well before the 28th week of gestation and constitute a good indicator for gestational age. Their echogenicity is brought about by the presence of collagen and blood vessels in the pia mater, contrasting with the watery brain parenchyma. Their anatomic presence precedes echographic visibility by two to six weeks (Table I.1 and Figs. I.1.a, I.1.b). Antenatal sonography clearly shows the interhemispheric fissure at the 12th week and the lateral fissure at the 19th week. The frontal parts of the cingulate, central and calcarine sulci show echographically shortly before the 26th week. The cingulate sulcus develops fully between the 28th and the 31st week, as well as the inferior temporal sulcus and the initial circular sulcus of the insula. The latter comes to full development with most ramifications of the cingulate sulcus and the tertiary sulci after the 31st week. The postcentral sulcus develops around the 30th week and constitutes a boundary with the postcentral gyrus. A 10 MHz ultrasound scanhead is recommended for evaluation of sulci and gyri along the convexity of the cerebrum (Fig. I.1.c).

Sagittal section (Fig. I.1.d)
Bordering the midline and above the level of the ventricles the following can be seen:
• the cingulate sulcus and the sulcus of the corpus callosum bordering the superior frontal gyrus, cingulate gyrus and corpus callosum;
• the craniocaudal course of the precentral sulcus, the cingulate sulcus and the parieto-occipital sulcus, which constitute a boundary with, respectively, the superior frontal gyrus, the paracentral lobule and the precuneus;
• the subparietal sulcus continues the course of the cingulate sulcus;
• the mesial end of the central sulcus, rostrally of the perpendicularly curved marginal and cingulate sulci; between the precentral sulcus and the cingulate sulcus there is the paracentral lobule;
• the calcarine sulcus forms a boundary with the cuneus and the medial occipitotemporal gyrus.

Parasagittal section (Fig. I.1.e)
Laterally in brain tissue one recognizes the insula, surrounded by the circular sulcus of the insula. The opercularization of the insula begins to show on a sonogram around the 28th gestational week and continues after 31 weeks. The different opercula are difficult to delineate with ultrasound. A dense line continues under the insula from front to back, constituting an upper boundary with the temporal lobe, the lateral sulcus.

Frontal section (Fig. I.1.f)
This section shows how the sulci penetrate the brain cortex over a short distance. The cingulate and corpus callosum sulci are perpendicular to the longitudinal cerebral fissure.

TABLE I.1
Anatomic development: gyri and sulci, corpus callosum, cerebellum

Week of gestation	
12	Emergence of sylvian fissure
	Genu and splenium of the corpus callosum recognizable
	Primary cerebellar fissure formed; dumbbell shaped cerebellum
16	Formation of the hippocampal gyrus; emergence of calcarine, parieto-occipital, cingulate and callosal sulci
	Cavum of the septum pellucidum recognizable, due to completion of callosal development
	Fourth ventricle covered by cerebellum
20	Parieto-occipital and calcarine sulci formed; emerging central sulcus
	Progressive rostrocaudal thickening of corpus callosum
24	Emergence of olfactory sulcus
28	Emergence of superior temporal sulcus and secondary sulci (parietal and temporal before frontal)
	Emergence of circular sulcus of the insula; opercularization complete around the 31st week
32	Branching of pre- and postcentral sulci; emergence of midtemporal sulci; emergence of superior frontal sulcus

Laterally in the brain parenchyma, on a level with the middle cranial fossa, one sees Y-shaped echodense lines. They are from the sylvian or lateral sulci. The extremities of the upward and downward branches of this Y correspond to the circular sulcus of the insula. Originally wide open, the insula closes later on (after the 31st week) (Fig. I.1.g). The lower arm of the sylvian sulcus is particularly long in frontal echosections whereas it is shorter at the level of the hippocampus. More ventrally the lateral sulcus constitutes the cranial boundary of the temporal lobe. The middle cerebral artery courses from medial to lateral in the lateral sulcus. The parahippocampal gyrus lies medial to the temporal horn of the lateral ventricle: this is the most medial gyrus of the temporal lobe, bordered by the collateral sulcus.

Axial section
The gyri recti are ventral to the optic chiasm. They are separated from each other by the longitudinal cerebral fissure, and laterally from the orbital gyri by the olfactory sulci.

REFERENCES

Bernard, C., Droullé, P., Didier, F., Gérard, H., Larroche, J.Cl., Plénat, F., Bomsel, F., Roland, J., Hoeffel, J.C. (1988) 'Aspects échographiques des sillons cérébraux à la période anté et péri-natale.' *Journal de Radiologie*, **69**, 521–532.
Feess-Higgins, A., Larroche, J-C. (1987) *Le Développement du Cerveau Foetal Humain. Atlas Anatomique.* Paris: Masson.
Huang, C-C. (1991) 'Sonographic cerebral sulcal development in premature newborns.' *Brain and Development*, **13**, 27–31.
Murphy, N.P., Rennie, J., Cooke, R.W.I. (1989) 'Cranial ultrasound assessment of gestational age in low birthweight infants.' *Archives of Disease in Childhood*, **64**, 569–572.
Slagle, T.A., Oliphant, M., Gross, S.J. (1989) 'Cingulate sulcus development in preterm infants.' *Pediatric Research*, **26**, 598–602.

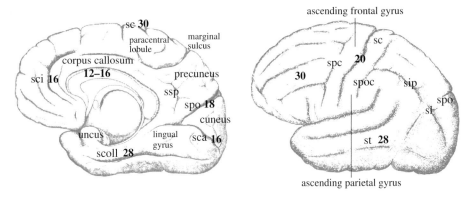

Fig. I.1.a. The main gyri and their first anatomic appearance (in weeks postconceptual age): sc = central sulcus; sca = calcarine sulcus; sci = cingulate sulcus; scoll = collateral sulcus; sip = intraparietal sulcus; sl = lateral sulcus; spc = precentral sulcus; spo = parieto-occipital sulcus; spoc = postcentral sulcus; ssp = subparietal sulcus; st = temporal sulcus. The central sulcus reaches the superior cerebral convexity around 30 weeks; the corpus callosum is completely shaped into its definitive form around 16 weeks. (Adapted by permission from Smith and van der Kooy 1985.)

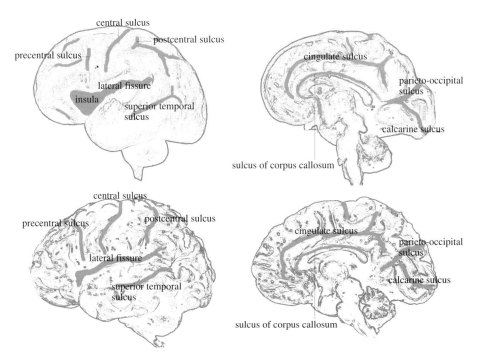

Fig. I.1.b. The primary sulci and fissures are highlighted on these drawings, adapted by permission from the atlas of Feess-Higgins and Larroche (1987); the top images are lateral *(left)* and mesial *(right)* views of the brain of an infant born at 28 weeks of gestation; the bottom ones are from an infant with a post-conceptional age of 37 weeks. Between 32 weeks and term the secondary and tertiary sulci appear; the gyral complexity at term resembles that of the adult.

3

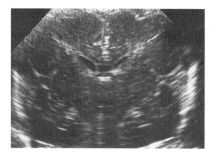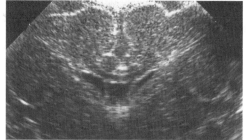

Fig. I.1.c. Coronal sonograms of a preterm infant (26 weeks gestation): *left*, 7.5 MHz; *right*, 10 MHz. Note how the 10 MHz scan increases definition in subfontanellar structures such as the parietal sulci.

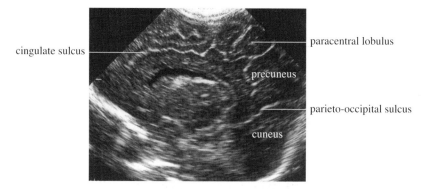

cingulate sulcus

paracentral lobulus

precuneus

parieto-occipital sulcus

cuneus

Fig. I.1.d. Parasagittal 7.5 MHz view of a healthy term infant. Recognition of the main mesial sulci and the areas they border is easy in a parasagittal plane near the midline.

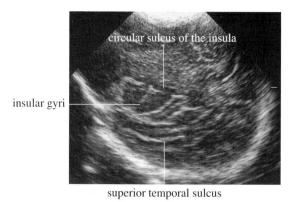

circular sulcus of the insula

insular gyri

superior temporal sulcus

Fig. I.1.e. Outward 7.5 MHz parasagittal view of a healthy term infant. A triangular shape filled with sulcal reflections and bordered by the circular sulcus of the insula at its upper margin represents the insula; underneath the insula at least one of the temporal sulci can be seen.

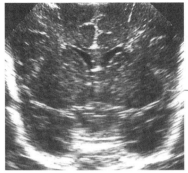

recumbent Y of the lateral fissure and insular gyri; the lower limb of this Y is prolonged towards the midline and contains the horizontal part of the middle cerebral artery

in front of the foramen of Monro

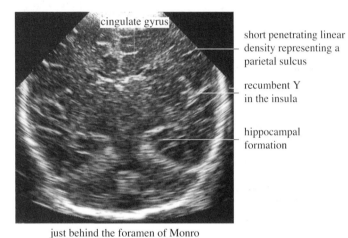

cingulate gyrus

short penetrating linear density representing a parietal sulcus

recumbent Y in the insula

hippocampal formation

just behind the foramen of Monro

Fig. I.1.f.
Frontal sections ———— through the choroid glomus

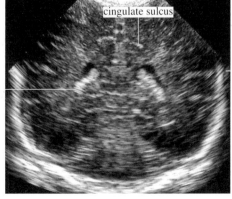

cingulate sulcus

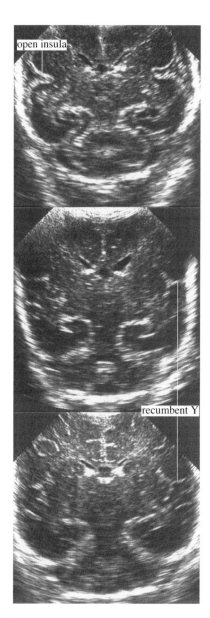
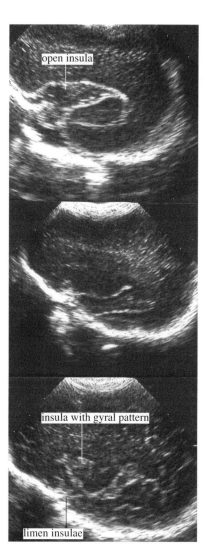

Fig. I.1.g. 7.5 MHz views showing different aspects of maturation of the insula and its opercula: *left*, coronal sections just behind the foramen of Monro; *right*, outward parasagittal sections through the insular cortex. In each case, the *top* images are from an infant at 25 weeks gestation, the *centre* ones at 32 weeks and the *bottom* ones at 40 weeks. Between 26 and 32 weeks the opercula meet and hide the insular cortex: on coronal images this produces an inverted Y, the limbs of which lengthen with increasing gestational age; on parasagittal images the open triangular island of 25 weeks turns into a covered triangular area with complex linear echodensities (short and long gyri) fanning out from the limen insulae.

I.2 LATERAL VENTRICLES

The lateral ventricles are cavities filled with cerebrospinal fluid (CSF), showing as echofree zones. They are found on both sides of the falx and are inferolaterally bordered by the head of the caudate nucleus. Their shape resembles a horseshoe curled round the caudate nucleus, thalamus and cerebral peduncles.

The lateral ventricles each consist of a body (corpus), an atrium and three horns (Figs. I.2.a, I.2.b). On a cross section, the corpus shows as a triangle pointing laterally upwards. On its floor there is vascular tissue resting on thalamic neurons, while medially the fornix borders the ventricular floor. The frontal horn has an elliptical slit-shaped lumen, partly covered by the corpus callosum and situated laterally to the septum pellucidum. The temporal or sphenoidal horn ends in the ventricular atrium. Medially the temporal horn is bordered by the pes hippocampi; its existence can be detected echographically via the plexus that hangs in it. The occipital horn is hardly visible, its dimensions differing from one individual to another. It projects horizontally in the occipital lobe. The choroid plexus of the lateral ventricle is found on the floor of the ventricular corpus, and continues into the roof of the temporal horn. Frontal and occipital horns do not contain plexus.

The foramen of Monro is the connecting passage between third ventricle and frontal horn of the right or left lateral ventricle. Under ordinary circumstances it is not always visible. It can be localized as the place where third ventricle plexus curves into the lateral ventricle in the foramen's upper caudal margin.

In normal children and neonates the lateral ventricles are often asymmetric (*i.e.* the diagonals of the right and left lateral ventricle differ by more than 2 mm in a frontal section at the level of the foramen of Monro). Mild asymmetric dilatations are most noticeable in the corpus and/or occipital horn. The right ventricle most often tends to be larger, a predilection that does not correlate with head position at vertex delivery. Dilatation of the lateral ventricles mostly begins in the occipital horns. Their failing to show up (a frequent phenomenon) constitutes a serious argument against dilatation. In case of clear ventriculomegaly, the concavity that tends to characterize the floor of the frontal horn disappears. Most writers prefer to define lateral ventricle width as a function of cranial width (Fig. I.2.c). This produces indices which, under normal circumstances, tend to remain constant during the first months of life. They are good tools for early recognition of hydrocephalus. In term neonates the following data are found:

- On an axial corporeal section through the lateral ventricles the ratio

$$\frac{[\text{midline to lateral wall of the ventricle}]}{[\text{midline to internal table of the skull}]}$$

varies between 0.25 and 0.35 (0.22–0.33 according to Helmke and Winkler).
- On a frontal section through the head of the caudate nucleus the ratio

$$\frac{[\text{laterolateral diameter between the points of the frontal horns}]}{[\text{distance between the left and right internal table on that section}]}$$

averages 0.32 (95% reliability margin 0.23–0.42).

Slightly higher ratios have been found in preterm (0.32–0.36) than in term infants (0.25–0.30). Term values are achieved around 36 weeks gestation. Such a ratio measured behind the foramen of Monro, at the level of the corpus of the lateral ventricle, tends to be 0.35 at or around term. It has been customary to talk about ventriculomegaly for values between 0.36 and 0.4 and about hydrocephalus for values above 0.4. The ventricular diameter can be followed serially on axial sections by measuring the distance between the falx and the external wall of the body of the opposite ventricle: 97th centile measurements are 10 mm around 26 weeks, 13 mm around 33 weeks and 14 mm around 40 weeks. The diagonal width of the lateral ventricle in a frontal section rarely exceeds 3 mm at the foramen of Monro. One speaks of ballooned frontal horns when this diagonal measure exceeds 6 mm. A final method consists of measuring the surface of the corpus of the lateral ventricle on a cross section behind the foramen of Monro, through the pons and hippocampal structures. In the case of preterm infants with gestational ages of 27–36 weeks, values thus obtained show a broad range: around birth the surface varies between 5 and 15 mm^2, with an average value of about 8 mm^2. Values over 15 mm^2 during the first week of life, and over 20 mm^2 during the first month of life, appear to exceed the normal. Any such value must be considered in conjunction with the child's head circumference.

REFERENCES

Helmke, K., Winkler, P. (1987) 'Sonographisch ermittelte Normwerte des intrakraniellen Ventrikelsystemes im ersten Lebensjahr.' *Monatsschrift für Kinderheilkunde*, **135**, 148–152.
Levene, M.I. (1981) 'Measurement of the growth of the lateral ventricles in preterm infants with real-time ultrasound.' *Archives of Disease in Childhood*, **56**, 900–904.
McArdle, C.B., Richardson, C.J., Nicholas, D.A., Mirfakhraee, M., Hayden, C.K., Amparo, E.G. (1987) 'Developmental features of the neonatal brain: MR imaging. Part II. Ventricular size and extracerebral space.' *Radiology*, **162**, 230–234.
Perry, R.N.W., Bowman, E.D., Murton, L.J., Roy, R.N.D., de Crespigny, L.C.H. (1985) 'Ventricular size in newborn infants.' *Journal of Ultrasound Medicine*, **4**, 475–477.
Poland, R.L., Slovis, T.L., Shankaran, S. (1986) 'Normal values for ventricular size as determined by real time sonographic techniques.' *Pediatric Radiology*, **15**, 12–14.
Saliba, E., Bertrand, P., Gold, F., Vaillant, M.C., Laugier, J. (1990) 'Area of lateral ventricles measured on cranial ultrasonography in preterm infants: reference range.' *Archives of Disease in Childhood*, **65**, 1029–1032.
Shen E-Y., Huang, F-Y. (1989) 'Sonographic finding of ventricular asymmetry in neonatal brain.' *Archives of Disease in Childhood*, **64**, 730–732.

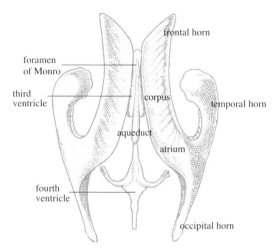

Fig. I.2.a. The ventricular cavities seen from above. (Adapted by permission from Paturet 1964.)

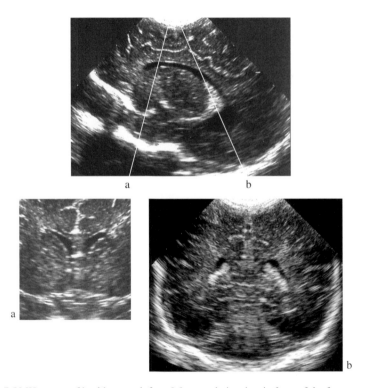

Fig. I.2.b. 7.5 MHz scans of healthy term infant: [a] coronal view just in front of the foramen of Monro and [b] coronal view through choroid glomus. These images demonstrate normal lateral ventricle cavities at term, with an equal width of frontal and parietal size; asymmetry in volume is not uncommon, but is always abnormal if the difference is marked.

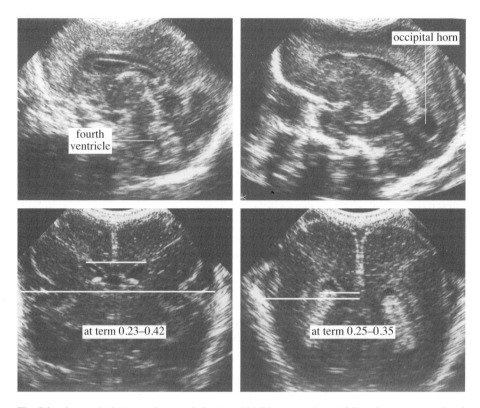

Fig. I.2.c. Parasagittal *(top)* and coronal *(bottom)* 10 MHz scans taken at 25 weeks postconceptional age, showing two examples of indices relating lateral ventricular width to width of the middle cranial fossa. The rather wide variation of these ratios in normal children precludes interindividual use to a certain extent; intraindividual serial use is more important.

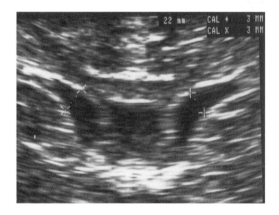

Fig. I.2.d. Coronal detail (at 7.5 MHz) in a term infant. Diagonal ventricular width may be used as a reliable indicator of ventriculo-megaly; values exceeding 5 mm are associated with ballooning of the ventricle and suggest the need for treatment.

10

I.3 THIRD VENTRICLE

The third ventricle is a slit-shaped rectangular cavity filled with CSF. It is situated in the sagittal plane between the thalami and above the bony sella turcica.

On a *sagittal* section the echogram shows a clearly delineated echopoor zone of rounded triangular shape (the aqueductal entry and the epiphyseal recess are too close to show up separately) (Fig. I.3.a). Ventrocranially and slightly laterally, one finds the interventricular foramen (foramen of Monro). Ventrocaudally there is the pointed anterior recess around the chiasma, and dorsocranially there is the pineal recess. In fact, the anterior recess consists of a supra-optic recess and an infundibular recess, rarely distinguishable by ultrasonography. Often one can see the aqueduct appearing in the space between the pineal and anterior recesses. Sometimes one suspects an indentation of the ventricular floor by the mamillary bodies. Superiorly is found echogenic linear choroid plexus. Ventrally the latter bifurcates and, via the interventricular foramina, it courses on as plexus from right and left lateral ventricles. The echopoor interpeduncular cistern is visible under the third ventricle. Behind it one can find the particularly dense bifurcation of the basilar artery and, further dorsally, the echopoor cerebral peduncles. The front wall of the third ventricle, between the interventricular foramina and optic chiasm, is formed by the strongly echogenic lamina terminalis and its commissures.

Sometimes it is hard to recognize the third ventricle on frontal sections because it is narrow and because its lateral walls course parallel to the direction of the sound waves (Fig. I.3.b). On both sides of the third ventricle one finds (sub)thalamic and under the third ventricle hypothalamic nuclei.

The massa intermedia is a cylindrical echogenic structure in the third ventricle, interconnecting the lateral walls. The size of this commissure is highly variable. On frontal and axial sections the width of the third ventricle normally averages 2.8 mm and 3.8 mm respectively for age groups 0–3 and 9–12 months. In the early neonatal period the third ventricle is no wider than 2 mm. When its anatomic boundaries are clearly distinguishable in the sagittal plane, the ventricle has already dilated (Fig. I.3.c).

REFERENCE

Helmke, K., Winkler, P. (1987) 'Sonographisch ermittelte Normwerte des intrakraniellen Ventrikelsystemes im ersten Lebensjahr.' *Monatsschrift für Kinderheilkunde*, **135**, 148–152.

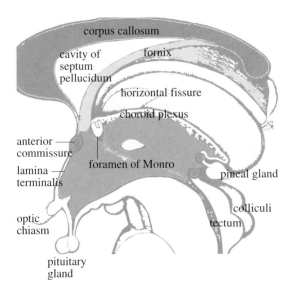

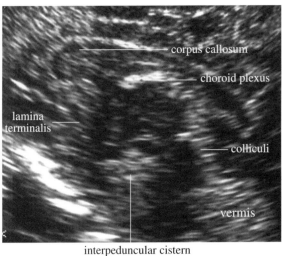

interpeduncular cistern
with basilar artery

Fig. I.3.a. Sagittal section through third ventricle and prosencephalic commissures (diagram adapted by permission from Smith and van der Koy 1985), compared with sagittal 7.5 MHz ultrasound picture of a term infant. The third ventricle contour is not sharp, but its cavity can be recognized because of a decrease in sound reflections from the area.

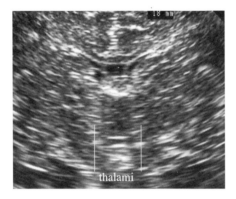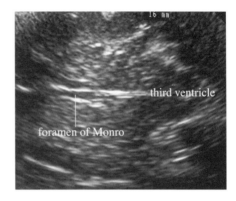

Fig. I.3.b. Coronal *(left)* and axial *(right)* 7.5 MHz scans through the foramen of Monro in a healthy term infant. Under normal conditions the third ventricle is barely recognizable and can only be suspected in coronal views because there is an area of hypodensity between discretely echogenic thalamic substructures; axial imaging permits clear recognition of the third ventricle as both cavity walls generate bright linear echoreflections.

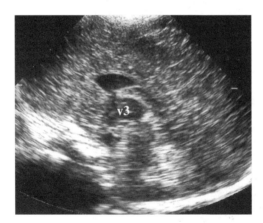

Fig. I.3.c. 7.5 MHz sagittal scan of growth retarded term infant with severe cystic leukomalacia of antenatal onset. The easily recognized third ventricle (v3) contour suggests ventriculomegaly. White matter injury resulted in atrophy of the corpus callosum in this infant.

I.4 CHOROID PLEXUS

The choroid plexus is a highly vascularized organ that produces CSF. Echographically, plexus tissue shows up as a hyperreflective structure with micropulsations. This organ courses from the roof of the third ventricle via the interventricular foramina to corpora and temporal horns of the lateral ventricles (Fig. I.4.a). Its echogenic potential is caused by frequent liquid–solid transitions in the villous crypts and is also due to its extreme vascularity.

The tela choroidea and plexus of the third ventricle constitute one single echogenic sickle-shaped strip. As the plexus courses dorsally in the lateral ventricle, its diameter increases. In the corpus of the lateral ventricle it lies against the lateral fornical wall. On a frontal section plexus in the temporal horns shows as an elliptical density. Near the trigone, dorsal to the posterior nucleus of the thalamus, the plexus forms a local widening: the choroid glomus, situated in the atrium of the lateral ventricle. On a frontal section it tends to be slightly wider towards the base of the cranium and smaller on the calvarial side. The glomus is seen as a laterolateral bulge on posterior parietal coronal sections through the atrium. Changes in width may help to diagnose plexus haemorrhage. Glomus may take different shapes: a projecting finger of choroid tissue or apparent layering (Figs. I.4.b, I.4.c). In the fetus between 12 and 18 weeks gestation, the choroid plexus completely fills up the lateral ventricle.

REFERENCE

Riebel, T., Nasir, R., Weber, K. (1992) 'Choroid plexus cysts: a normal finding on ultrasound.' *Pediatric Radiology*, **22**, 410–412.

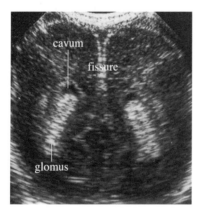 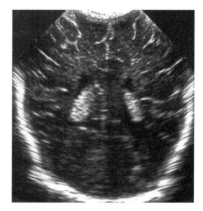

Fig. I.4.a. Coronal views through the choroid glomus: *(left)* 10 MHz scan of an infant of 25 weeks gestation; *(right)* 7.5 MHz scan of a term infant. Note the relative abundancy of choroid plexus tissue at low gestational age.

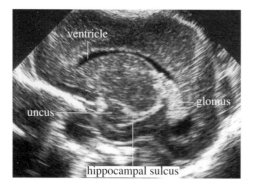

Fig. I.4.b. Parasagittal 7.5 MHz scan of one hemisphere in an infant of 25 weeks gestation. Relatively abundant choroid plexus fills the atrium in the form of a globular structure (glomus); one often perceives lamination in the glomus because of the presence of a hypodense layer between two denser outer parts.

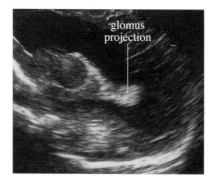

Fig. I.4.c. Infant with delayed development; MR demonstrated virtual absence of white matter and ponto-cerebellar hypoplasia or atrophy; parasagittal 7.5 MHz view. Instead of forming a glomus, choroid plexus projects from the ventricle atrium into the occipital horn, like a finger in an oversized glove.

I.5 PARENCHYMA

In the normal brain a difference in echogenicity can be noticed between cerebral cortex on the one hand and the underlying white matter on the other. The latter is slightly more echogenic, probably because vessels are relatively more numerous. Myelination, which is mainly a postnatal phenomenon, is probably not accompanied by an increase in echogenicity. It is possible to observe in different locations pia mater separated from white matter by cortex, especially on parasagittal 7.5 MHz sections through the cingulate sulcus. The thickness of the cortex does not exceed a few millimetres. A frontal section with a 10 MHz transmitter also offers a good view on the cortico-medullary differentiation. Venous congestion and leukomalacia increase this difference by rendering white matter more echogenic (see chapter on asphyxia). A tangential view of a sulcus or fissure may create the impression of an echogenic focus in the parenchyma. Subtle rotations of the scanhead allow differentiation of this normal variant from a lesion.

Temporal lobe and hippocampus

The mesial part of the temporal lobe (with the hippocampus and inferior horn of the lateral ventricle) can be examined both with parasagittal and frontal sections through the anterior fontanelle (Fig. I.5.a).

A *parasagittal section* through the pes hippocampi and the choroid fissure (Fig. I.5.b): The amygdaloid nucleus, the inferior horn, the pes hippocampi and the hippocampal sulcus produce a typical layered picture. The hippocampus is located above the choroid plexus and below the echogenic hippocampal fissure and the pulvinar. On a section through the limen insulae one can sometimes see the whole echopoor inferior horn underneath plexus, which is echodense, and the hippocampal structures.

A *coronal section through the foramina of Monro* and the hypothalamus (Figs. I.5.b, I.5.c): Generally two echodense lines show up in the poorly echogenic temporal lobe. The upper line, which is a relatively broad tubular echodensity, corresponds to the hippocampal fissure and laterally to the plexus of the temporal horn. The lower, which is a fine echoline, corresponds to the floor of the ventricle and medially and anteriorly to the hippocampal sulcus. The dentate gyrus lies above this sulcus, and below it curls the subiculum. This layered echographic constellation varies according to depth and direction of sulcal section. The reflection from the pes hippocampi and dentate gyrus is low in density and found between the hippocampal fissure and sulcus. The echogenicity of the amygdaloid nucleus is also limited and can be seen above the inferior horn in the temporal uncus, which shows as the curled tip of a Moor slipper. Further towards the posterior fossa, the parahippocampal gyrus, the collateral sulcus and the middle occipitotemporal gyrus can be seen. The echodense suprasellar cistern between both temporal lobes near the foramina of Monro produces a butterfly-like picture as it appears to penetrate into the thalamus. A frontal horn section creates a different picture: the basal cistern is star-shaped. Temporal, collateral and occipitotemporal sulci divide the temporal lobe into five gyri, two of which are situated laterally, one basally and two mesially.

A *coronal section through the thalamus* and the lateral ventricle: Poorly echogenic regions alternate with echodense lines. The fimbria and dentate gyrus are small, echopoor and hard to distinguish. The hippocampal sulcus is seen as a small, echodense line. The parahippocampal gyrus is echopoor. The collateral sulcus shows up as an echodense line in the mesial curve of the temporal lobe.

A *coronal section between the trigona* (Fig. I.5.d): The echodense choroid plexus is easily recognizable. Medially we find the splenium of the corpus callosum, the isthmus of the cingulate gyrus, the parieto-occipital sulcus and the lingual gyrus. The hippocampus cannot be identified on this section.

Calcar avis

The calcar avis is a piece of white matter mesial to the incurved calcarine fissure. The calcarine fissure is formed around the 16th postconceptional week. Between the 32nd and the 40th week it stretches, thus binding off a piece of cortex and white matter, that is pressed against the occipital horn. The calcar avis will be more or less prominent dependent upon the depth of the gyri. An echogram through the posterior fontanelle sometimes shows the calcar avis. Distinction should be made with resorbing haemorrhage in the occipital horn, in that case showing as dense reflections from the lower margin of the occipital horn rather than its lateral wall (Fig. I.5.e).

Frontal lobe

The frontal lobe is posteriorly bordered by the central sulcus and by the lateral fissure along the external part of the hemisphere. Mesially the posterior border is the central sulcus encircled by the paracentral lobule. The frontal lobe extends mesially below the cingulate gyrus. An anterior coronal section displays a number of sulci and gyri against the orbital roof (Fig. I.5.f): the gyrus rectus is situated against the falx, with the olfactory sulcus just beside it (a short linear density rising from below the midline, upwards and laterally away from it, on which rests the olfactory tract). The external orbital sulcus will be found laterally at the base of this lobe. It is difficult to provide a more detailed description of the gyrational pattern in the frontal lobe via transfontanellar echography.

Parietal lobe

The parietal lobe on the lateral hemispherical wall extends from the central sulcus to the indentation of the parieto-occipital sulcus. The intraparietal sulcus starts at the postcentral sulcus, penetrating the parietal lobe behind the lateral sulcus. In between lies the supramarginal gyrus. The angular gyrus is situated between the intraparietal sulcus and the superior temporal sulcus. Some of those anatomical landmarks can be located by means of extremely lateral scans using a 10 MHz transducer (Fig. I.5.g). On the mesial hemisphere wall the parietal lobe consists only of the cuneus, hemmed in between the calcarine and parieto-occipital sulci (Fig. I.1.d).

Occipital lobe

This is echographically the lobe least accessible through the anterior fontanelle. It is usually not possible to recognize the calcarine sulcus, but the experienced sonographer may suspect its presence on a juxtasagittal section (Fig. I.5.e). Apart from that this lobe shows up as a hypoechogenic zone behind the parieto-occipital sulcus.

DiPietro, M.A., Brody, B.A., Teele, R.L. (1985) 'The calcar avis: demonstration with cranial US.' *Radiology*, **156**, 363–364.
Sasaki, M., Nakasato, T., Goto, H., Yanagisawa, T., Suzuki, T., Matsuda, I., Fujiwara, M., Hashimoto, S., Saito, K. (1989) 'Normal sonographic findings of the infant temporal lobe in coronal sections.' *Brain and Development*, **11**, 230–235.

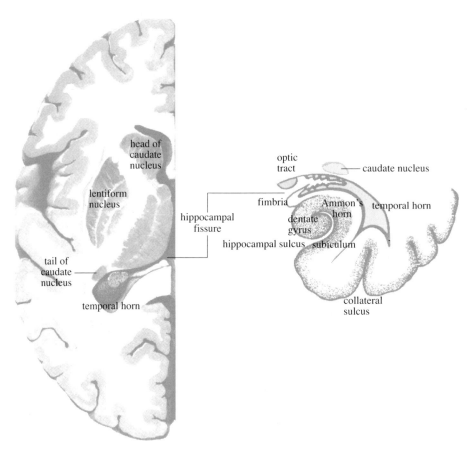

Fig. I.5.a. Structures in an axial section through the right hemisphere (*left*, adapted from Netter 1986) and in a coronal section through the left hippocampal formation *(right)*. (Adapted from Paturet 1964.)

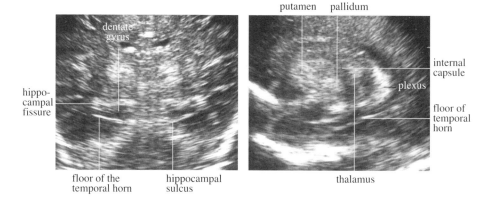

Fig. I.5.b. Term infant with birth asphyxia: *(left)* coronal view behind the foramen of Monro; *(right)* parasagittal view; both 7.5 MHz. Neuronal injury is the cause of thalamic and striatal echogenicity; the hippocampal structures are well delineated in both coronal and parasagittal sections; it is not always easy to distinguish between the layers of hyperdense reflections from plexus, the hippocampal fissure and sulcus, and the floor of the temporal horn of the lateral ventricle.

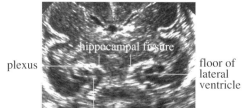

Fig. I.5.c. Coronal 10 MHz section just behind the foramen of Monro in preterm infant of 25 weeks gestation, scanned on day 1. Visualization of the hippocampal formation is better than at term.

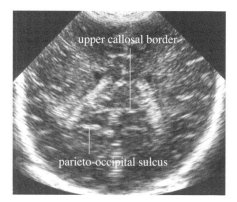

Fig. I.5.d. Coronal 7.5 MHz section through the choroid glomus in a term infant. This section passes through the sulcus of the corpus callosum and the parieto-occipital sulcus; coronal sections do not permit reliable recognition of the calcarine sulcus.

19

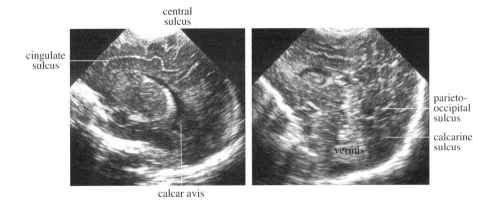

central sulcus

cingulate sulcus

parieto-occipital sulcus

calcarine sulcus

vermis

calcar avis

Fig. I.5.e. Parasagittal *(left)* and sagittal *(right)* 7.5 MHz scans of a term infant. The calcar avis appears as a soft echogenicity in the mesial wall of the occipital horn of the lateral ventricle; the calcarine sulcus is a vague undulating hyperdense line between vermis and parieto-occipital sulcus in the sagittal plane.

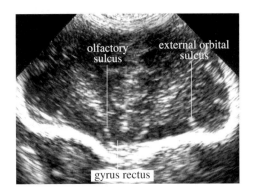

olfactory sulcus

external orbital sulcus

gyrus rectus

Fig. I.5.f. Coronal 7.5 MHz section through the anterior fossa and orbital roof of a term infant. The olfactory and external orbital sulci are easily recognized in an outward anterior coronal view; the gyrus rectus is cut between the interhemispheric fissure and the olfactory sulcus, on top of which rests the olfactory tract.

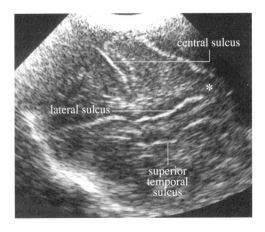

central sulcus

lateral sulcus

superior temporal sulcus

Fig. I.5.g. Preterm infant of 31 weeks gestation, with non-immune hydrops associated with antenatal intestinal infarction; outward parasagittal section lateral to the insula, 10 MHz. Mild dilatation of the arachnoid space permitted good visualization of the convexity's sulci in this infant: the lateral and central sulci are easily recognized; parallel below the former, the superior temporal sulcus is seen; at the right margin of the image the supramarginal gyrus is just visible *(asterisk)*; increasing gestational age reduces the chance of good visualization of these structures.

I.6 MIDLINE STRUCTURES (Fig. I.6.a)

The corpus callosum

A *sagittal* section shows the corpus callosum as a thin, longitudinal, echopoor structure arching from front to back. It is located on the floor of the longitudinal cerebral fissure. The frontal curved part is the genu. The genu courses anteriorly down into the rostrum, which becomes narrower and touches the upper part of the lamina terminalis. Posteriorly the genu continues into the middle part. This part bends towards the back and slightly upwards, to course through in the splenium, which is the thicker and most rounded dorsal part of the corpus callosum. The upper boundary is the pericallosal cistern, also containing the pericallosal arteries. The cingulate gyrus rests on the pericallosal cistern. Under the corpus callosum there are the two leaflets of the septum pellucidum, containing the cavum. In a sagittal section one observes how the laminae of the septum pellucidum touch the concave surface of the middle part, the genu, the rostrum and the fornix. An immediate *parasagittal* section shows the corpus callosum as the roof of the lateral ventricle. Upwards the splenium is in touch with the falx cerebri and the inferior sagittal sinus. Towards the back the splenium touches the border of the tentorium near the great vein of Galen. The vein itself courses in the transverse fissure, a horizontal echodense band under the splenium laterally ending in the choroidal fissures of the temporal horns. In a *frontal* section, the corpus callosum is visible as a thin, narrow echopoor plate. At the front it is slightly curved, concave on the upper side, and it forms the roof of the lateral ventricles. The upward boundary of the corpus callosum is again the pericallosal cistern, underneath the cingulate gyrus.

Cavum of the septum pellucidum and Verga's ventricle

Both cavities are lined by glia and not ependyma. They are situated between the fornix and corpus callosum. The cavum of the septum pellucidum is almost always easily recognizable in the perinatal period, although its diameter rarely exceeds 8 mm (Fig. I.6.b). Around the sixth postnatal month and for the rest of life, it can be identified in one person out of six on average. The walls of the cavum consist of two septal leaflets, which during infancy gradually tend to merge into one single membrane from back to front. There rarely is a well-defined transition area towards Verga's ventricle. Verga's ventricle runs into the occipital side of the cavum of the septum pellucidum, above the choroid plexus and underneath the splenium of the corpus callosum. Laterally this cavum is bordered by the crura of the fornix, which end in the alveus and fimbria of the hippocampus. Both subcallosal cavities must be differentiated from an aneurysm of the great vein of Galen.

A *sagittal* section shows the cavum as an echofree zone with concave rims towards the base of the brain. Under normal circumstances it is sometimes possible to see fenestrations in the partitions of the septum pellucidum on a discretely laterally toppled sagittal section. A *frontal* view nearly always shows a triangular or trapezoid echofree space with its base under the corpus callosum and its apex against the fornix. Pointed and short linear densities in the septal walls are normal reflections from the medial subependymal veins. The cavum of the septum pellucidum is situated above the fringes of choroid plexus in the foramina of Monro. Occipitally directed *coronal* sections show Verga's ventricle as a cavity between the choroid glomera.

21

REFERENCES

Babcock, D.S. (1984) 'The normal, absent, and abnormal corpus callosum: sonographic findings.' *Radiology*, **151**, 449–453.

Farruggia, S., Babcock, D.S. (1981) 'The cavum septi pellucidi: its appearance and incidence with cranial ultrasonography in infancy.' *Radiology*, **139**, 147–150.

Gebarski, S.S., Gebarski, K.S., Bowerman, R.A., Silver, T.M. (1984) 'Agenesis of the corpus callosum: sonographic features.' *Radiology*, **151**, 443–448.

Mott, S.H., Bodensteiner, J.B., Allan, W.C. (1992) 'The cavum septi pellucidi in term and preterm newborn infants.' *Journal of Child Neurology*, **7**, 35–38.

Shaw, C-M., Alvord, E.C. (1969) 'Cava septi pellucidi et Vergae: their normal and pathological states.' *Brain*, **92**, 213–224.

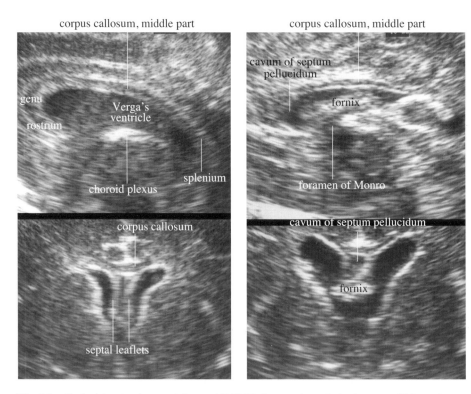

Fig. I.6.a. Sagittal *(top)* and coronal *(bottom)* 7.5 MHz images through the foramen of Monro in two different preterm infants with posthaemorrhagic hydrocephalus. The midline structures are accentuated because of mild ventricular dilatation and ventricle wall echogenicity due to haemorrhagic remnants; fornical reflections can only be seen separately when the ventricles are somewhat dilated; otherwise their reflections are mixed with those from plexus and ventricular walls.

22

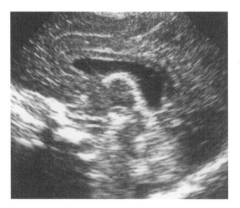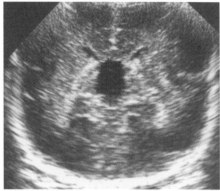

Fig. I.6.b. Sagittal *(left)* and coronal *(right)* 7.5 MHz sections of a ventilated preterm infant (gestational age 29 weeks) without brain injury. The cavum of the septum pellucidum and Verga's ventricle may be relatively large in preterm infants.

I.7 CISTERNS

Cisterns are accumulations of liquid between brain structures and the cranium. Normally they rarely show up on echograms. Their existence can be suspected because the walls, consisting of leptomeninges and blood vessels, are strongly echogenic. An enlarged cistern looks like an irregularly rimmed cavity and generally indicates a proximally located obstruction to the circulation of CSF. The cisterna magna and the prepontine cistern normally show as a cavity. It follows they play an important part when looking for subarachnoid haemorrhage in a sagittal ultrasound section (extensively illustrated by Paneth *et al.* 1994).

• *Basal (suprasellar) cistern*: This comprises the chiasmatic (see below) and interpeduncular cisterns.

• *Cisterna magna* (cerebellomedullary cistern, Fig. I.7.a): This cistern, located under the echogenic vermis above the occipital bone, is of variable size. If large, it will be viewed as an accumulation of liquid in the posterior fossa, around the cerebellum. In this cistern are found the postero-inferior cerebellar artery, cranial nerves IX–XII and the cerebellar tonsils.

• *Pontine cistern* (Fig. I.7.b): This is an echogenic zone ventrally above the pons, in front of the cerebral peduncles, under and behind the anterior recess of the third ventricle. The particularly echodense zone with arterial pulsations in this cistern corresponds with the bifurcation of the basilar artery. It ends in the interpeduncular cistern.

• *Quadrigeminal cistern* (Fig. I.7.c): This is an echogenic line between the plexus of the third ventricle and the vermis. A cyst of the quadrigeminal cistern lies behind this third ventricle. This cistern contains the posterior cerebral and posterior choroidal arteries, the IVth cranial nerve and the great vein of Galen. There is a direct lateral communication with the retrothalamic cistern behind the pulvinar. The thickness of this echogenic zone (normally no more than 3 mm) often increases in case of subarachnoid haemorrhage. Towards the vermis this echogenic line can, under normal circumstances, be covered by an echopoor zone of 1–3 mm.

• *Ambient cistern*: This constitutes the lateral connection between the prepontine and interpeduncular cisterns in front, and the quadrigeminal cistern behind. In this cistern we find the posterior cerebral artery, the superior cerebellar artery, the mesencephalic vein, cranial nerve IV and the optic tract. On a frontal section through the hippocampus the ambient cistern shows as the vertical part of a C, encircling the brainstem on both sides. The upward curve of the C corresponds to the hippocampal fissure and the plexus of the temporal horn, whereas the lower curve corresponds with the tentorium. This echogenic curve is 1–3 mm wide in preterm infants around 26 weeks postconceptional age.

• *Chiasmatic cistern*: This is a pentagonal echodense zone around the optic chiasm. Its angles correspond to the arteries of the circle of Willis: in front we find the anterior cerebral arteries; laterally, the carotid siphon with the origin of the middle cerebral arteries; and at the back, the posterior cerebral arteries. Sideways the cistern ends, together with the middle cerebral artery, in the lateral cistern which fills out the sylvian fossa.

REFERENCE

Paneth, N., Rudelli, R., Kazam, E., Monte, W.(1994) *Brain Damage in the Preterm Infant. Clinics in Developmental Medicine No. 131*. London: Mac Keith Press.

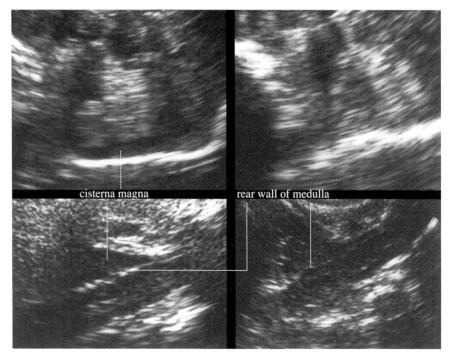

Fig. I.7.a. *(Top)* 7.5 MHz sagittal images zoomed in on the posterior fossa from the anterior fontanelle; *(bottom)* 10 MHz sagittal images through the neck, with the spinal cord to the right of the picture; both subjects were healthy term infants.

Nuchal echography may permit fine visualization of structures within the posterior fossa if the cisterna magna is patent; a small cisternal size makes recognition of the rear brainstem wall difficult.

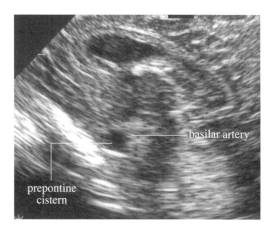

Fig. I.7.b. Term infant: 7.5 MHz sagittal image. The size of the prepontine cistern differs between individuals; in this child it is an easily recognized dark space in front of the dense reflections from the basilar artery.

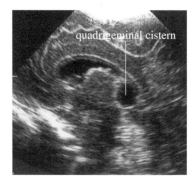

Fig. I.7.c. Term infant: 7.5 MHz sagittal image. Behind the echodense tectal plate and underneath the splenium of the corpus callosum a darker space, variable in size, represents the quadrigeminal cistern; an increase in its volume on serial echograms may indicate arachnoid cyst formation.

I.8 BASAL GANGLIA, THALAMUS AND INTERNAL CAPSULE

The thalamus is a spherical, echopoor zone constituting the lateral border of the third ventricle in a frontal and axial section. In a parasagittal section the thalamus is bordered above and in front by the mildly echogenic caudate nucleus. Cranially, dorsally and caudally the thalamus is encircled by choroid plexus. The thalami are interconnected by the inter-thalamic adhesion. The lentiform nucleus, containing the basal nuclei (pallidum and putamen), is echopoor. The caudate nucleus and putamen constitute the neostriatum, the paleostriatum being the globus pallidus. On a frontal section the lentiform nucleus is medially bordered by thalamus and caudate nucleus, and laterally by the insula. Under the lentiform nucleus courses the lateral sulcus containing the horizontal part of the middle cerebral artery.

A parasagittal section through the caudothalamic groove is the best way of showing the thalamus, the lentiform nucleus, the internal capsule and their mutual relationship (Figs. I.8.a, I.8.b). It shows the thalamus and basal ganglia as an egg-shaped structure bordered by: at the upper front, the frontal horn of the lateral ventricle; at the upper back, the rest of the lateral ventricle; below in front, the rostral corpus callosum; and below at the back, the ambient cistern and choroid fissure.

In the floor of the lateral ventricle, behind and above the gangliothalamic region it is possible to identify the choroid plexus. No plexus is visible below because this parasagittal section bisects the temporal horn. The upper part of the structure splits into two parts at the caudothalamic groove: the front one corresponds to the caudate nucleus, the rear part to the thalamus. The lower margin is split into three parts by the cerebral peduncles: a frontal ganglionic arch, a medial peduncular arch and a posterior thalamic arch. Inside the structure the internal capsule forms an arch of white matter that resembles an inverted Greek ν (nu). The anterior limb of the internal capsule is more echogenic than the caudate nucleus, which is separated from the underlying putamen and pallidum by this capsule. This phenomenon of echogenicity is highly variable: on the one hand it is dependent on vascular texture and on the other on the perpendicular interposition of fibres of the capsule itself and caudoputa-minal connections.

An echographic parasagittal section through the caudothalamic groove shows four bands with different echodensity, bands 1 and 3 being more echogenic than bands 2 and 4 (Fig. I.8.c). Band 2 is the easiest to identify: it is a broad and hypoechogenic band that con-tains the genu and posterior limb of the internal capsule, the cerebral peduncles, and also the medial and lateral nuclei of the globus pallidus. Behind band 2 there is a broad hyper-echogenic band (band 3), consisting of the ventral and lateral nuclei of the thalamus, with the exception of the pulvinar. This third band is softly hyperechogenic with some inter-individual variation. Band 4 is situated behind band 3 and is hypoechogenic. It comprises the pulvinar. Band 1 is least homogenic. It is located in front of and above band 2, is slightly hyperechogenic and consists of the caudate nucleus and parts of the putamen. Band 1 may make interpretation of pathological hyperdensity more difficult. It is crossed by the anterior limb of the internal capsule, which has highly variable density and, in case of congestion, is a strikingly echogenic zone. Just outside and above this zone we often encounter frontal leukomalacia.

Around the gangliothalamic region the orbital gyri of the frontal lobe are perceived to be relatively hypoechogenic. In a frontal section they are separated from it by radiations of the corpus callosum and its corona radiata. The lateral fissure is seen as a hyperechogenic fissure between the frontal and temporal lobes. The ambient cistern and choroid fissure constitute a broad hyperechogenic arch, separating the gangliothalamic region from the temporal lobe. The temporal lobe is hypoechogenic and resembles the tip of a Moor slipper. In fact, it is quite difficult to identify the hypoechogenic internal capsule on a frontal section through the third ventricle, as a thick line situated between the caudate nucleus and the thalamus on the one side, and the lentiform nucleus on the other. It runs from laterally above to medially under. The claustrum is not visible on an echogram. On a dorsally oriented coronal section, it can be seen that the lateral thalamic nuclei are more echogenic than the medial ones.

REFERENCES

Feess-Higgins, A., Larroche, J-C. (1987) *Le Développement du Cerveau Foetal Humain. Atlas Anatomique.* Paris: Masson.
Naidich, T.P., Gusnard, D.A., Yousefzadeh, D.K. (1985) 'Sonography of the internal capsule and basal ganglia in infants: I. Coronal sections.' *American Journal of Neuroradiology*, **6**, 909–917.
— — Yousefzadeh, D.K., Gusnard, D.A., Naidich, J.B. (1986) 'Sonography of the internal capsule and basal ganglia in infants. Part II: Localization of pathologic processes in the sagittal section through the caudo-thalamic groove.' *Radiology*, **161**, 615–621.

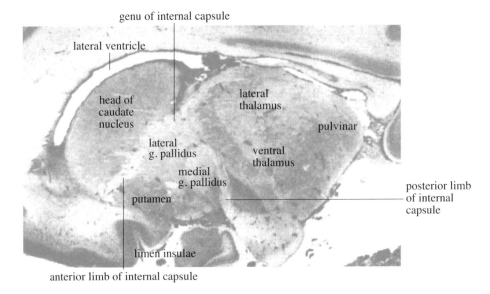

genu of internal capsule

lateral ventricle

head of caudate nucleus

lateral thalamus

pulvinar

lateral g. pallidus

ventral thalamus

medial g. pallidus

putamen

posterior limb of internal capsule

limen insulae

anterior limb of internal capsule

Fig. I.8.a. Drawing reconstructed after a parasagittal scan through the basal ganglia of a term infant. (Adapted by permission from Feess-Higgins and Larroche 1987.)

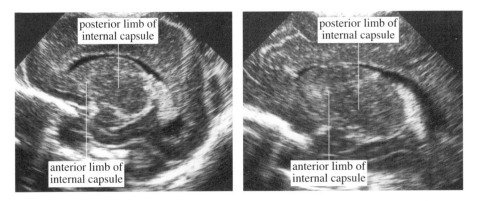

posterior limb of internal capsule

posterior limb of internal capsule

anterior limb of internal capsule

anterior limb of internal capsule

Fig. I.8.b. Parasagittal 7.5 MHz sonograms, *(left)* of an infant of 25 weeks gestation, *(right)* of a term infant. Due to more advanced myelination separate recognition of the basal ganglia is slightly easier at term, because of increased contrast between the echogenic thalamus and the hypoechogenic internal capsule and globus pallidus.

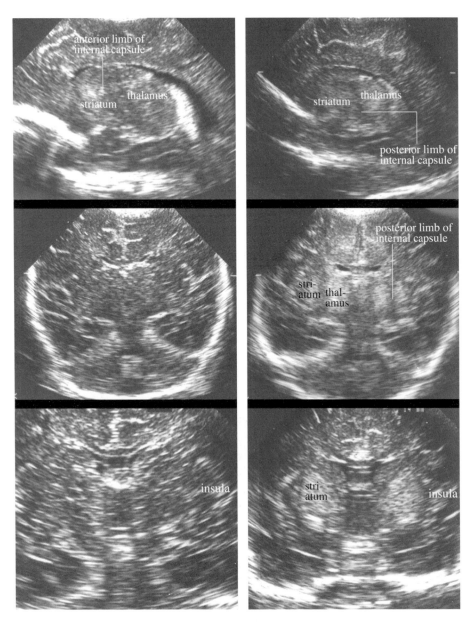

Fig. I.8.c. 7.5 MHz sonograms of *(left)* a healthy term infant, and *(right)* a term infant who suffered from severe birth asphyxia, with subsequent ischaemic necrosis in thalamus and striatum; the top pictures are parasagittal, the others coronal sections just posterior or anterior to the foramen of Monro.

In the normal state one can separate thalamic (mildly echogenic) from striatal nuclei (also mildly echogenic) because of the presence of a hypoechogenic linear structure in between, the posterior limb of the internal capsule; the caudate head is separated from the rest of the striatum by the variably hyperechogenic anterior limb of the internal capsule; delineation of these nuclei and structures is much easier in the presence of neuronal necrosis, as following asphyxia.

I.9 BRAINSTEM

The cerebral peduncles, pons and medulla oblongata (Fig. I.9.a) are situated in line and show as echopoor structures. They can be shown both through the anterior—albeit with a certain loss of visibility on account of the distance—and posterior fontanelles. Pre- and postauricular sections provide more information (Figs. I.9.b–h).

On a parasagittal section the cerebral peduncles show as a craniocaudal echopoor zone under the third ventricle. In front of this zone there is a moderately to highly echodense spherical area that corresponds to the bifurcation of the basilar artery situated in the basal (interpeduncular) cistern. Behind the peduncles one sometimes notices a slightly taller echopoor quadrigeminal cistern. On a coronal dorsally oriented section the peduncles show as an echopoor zone between the parahippocampal gyri. Cranially they bifurcate towards left and right crus cerebri, both bordered by the dense cisterna cruralis. Laterally the brainstem is encircled by the ambient cisterns. Between the peduncles it is possible to see, rostrally, the echofree third ventricle, especially when it is dilated. An axial section through the sphenoidal fontanelle shows the sylvian aqueduct as a pointed dense structure between both peduncles. By a stretch of the imagination, one can identify two structures in the mesencephalon: the substantia nigra, which is slightly echogenic, and the nucleus ruber which shows between the substantia nigra and the aqueduct as a hypoechogenic circle. The frontal midline of the mesencephalon is highly echogenic.

The *pons* is located caudally to the peduncles. A sagittal section through the pons shows two parts: a posterior echopoor zone between the peduncles and the medulla oblongata and a moderately spherical echogenic zone high in front of this echopoor zone. The echogenicity of the latter part is probably due to the transverse fibres of the pons. The clivus is located in front of the pons and between them rises the basilar artery, with visible pulsations. On a frontal section one should first look for the dorsum sellae and then topple the scanhead backwards: the pons is moderately echodense and is to be found between the parahippocampal gyri resting on the clivus. Caudally the pons continues into the echopoor medulla oblongata, which in turn courses through the foramen magnum to the spinal cord. The vertebral arteries are located ventrolaterally to the medulla oblongata. The inferior olives are very faintly echogenic.

The *fourth ventricle*, containing choroid plexus, is nearly always clearly distinguishable. On a preauricular section, 45° to the canthomeatal line (see below), it shows as a triangular, echopoor structure under the cerebral aqueduct (visible as an echodense line). On such sections it is sometimes possible to notice the foramina of Magendie. On a sagittal section through the anterior fontanelle the fourth ventricle shows as a small, triangular echofree zone in front of and half the height of the echodense cerebellar vermis. The front part of the ventricle, the base of this triangle, cannot be separated from the dorsal poorly echogenic part of the pons.

The caudal medullary velum is loaded with choroid plexus and consequently is echogenic. The fourth ventricle cavity can be obliterated by plexus tissue and a differentiation should be made with haemorrhage or tumour. The rostral medullary velum carries the echogenic lingula of the cerebellar vermis. On a frontal section, following the longitudinal axis of the crura cerebri, the fourth ventricle shows as a fine echofree band. It follows a laterolateral

30

course between the partitions of the tentorium cerebelli. Dorsolaterally it is bordered by the echodense cerebellar vermis.

As it is possible to correctly delineate the brainstem circumference on an axial section through the inferior colliculi, it is also possible to make a reliable estimation of the *mesencephalic* surface in that section. It could thus be shown, for example, that the brainstem is smaller in babies affected by trisomy 18, as related to the duration of pregnancy. This does not come as a surprise as their average weight is also lower than the average weight of healthy neonates.

In order to come to an extensive, adequate and systematic view of the brainstem, certain specific sections can be used, starting from the canthomeatal line (CML). For an individual patient the appropriate angle should be sought, with the CML providing the best view of certain structures:

(1) Pre-auricular, parallel to the CML. The echopoor brainstem looks like a butterfly. The cerebral peduncles and the tectal lamina are surrounded by echodense structures corresponding with cisterns and parts of the tentorium. These tentorial rims can be traced proximally to the anterior clinoid process. The two echodense reflections in the posterior part of the brainstem coincide with the walls of the cerebral aqueduct. In the basal cisterns the arteries of the circle of Willis clearly show as short, pulsating lines.

(2) Pre-auricular, 45° to the CML. The lateral and third ventricles are clearly visible. The cerebral aqueduct, the fourth ventricle and the foramina of Magendie are also noticeable on this section.

(3) Retro-auricular, 90° to the CML. On account of the echogenicity of choroid plexus the lateral ventricles can be identified. The brainstem appears as a cruciform structure. The central echodense lines are due to the cerebral aqueduct. The arms of the cross correspond to the cerebellar peduncles. The pons is located under the mesencephalon. The medulla oblongata is partly visible.

(4) Through the posterior fontanelle, 135° to the CML. The brainstem is recognized by the winglike shape of the cerebellar peduncles. Again, the cerebral aqueduct shows as a double linear reflection before the echodense tectal lamina.

REFERENCES

Hashimoto, K., Takeuchi, Y., Takashima, S., Takeshita, K. (1994) 'Morphometric evaluation of neonatal brainstem development by means of the ultrasonographic method.' *Brain and Development*, **16**, 209–212.
Helmke, K., Winkler, P., Kock, C. (1987) 'Sonographic examination of the brain stem area in infants. An echographic and anatomic analysis.' *Pediatric Radiology*, **17**, 1–6.
Yousefzadeh, D.K., Naidich, T.P. (1985) 'US anatomy of the posterior fossa in children: correlation with brain sections.' *Radiology*, **156**, 353–361.

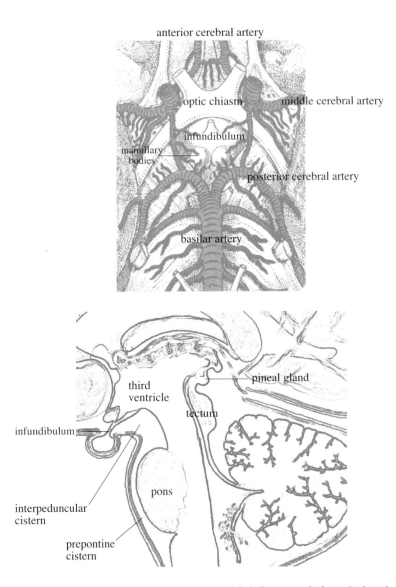

anterior cerebral artery

optic chiasm   middle cerebral artery

infundibulum

mamillary
bodies

posterior cerebral artery

basilar artery

third
ventricle

pineal gland

tectum

infundibulum

interpeduncular
cistern

pons

prepontine
cistern

Fig. I.9.a. Details of the base of the brain with the arterial circle *(top)* and of a sagittal section through brainstem and cerebellar vermis *(bottom)*. (Adapted by permission from Paturet 1964.)

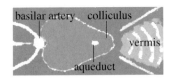

basilar artery   colliculus

vermis

aqueduct

Fig. II.9.b. Axial section through the mesencephalon, showing relationships between the main structures.

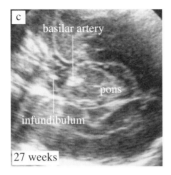

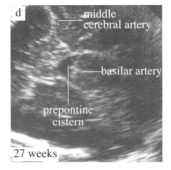

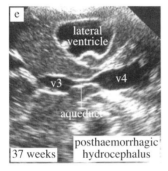

Figs. I.9.c–f. Preauricular axial 7.5 MHz images.

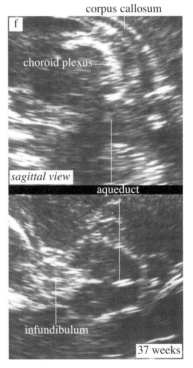

Figs. I.9.g,h. Retroauricular axial 7.5 MHz images.

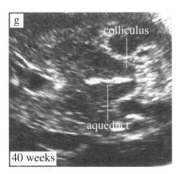

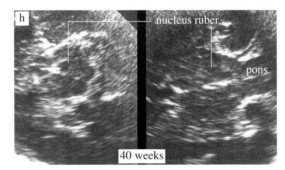

I.10 CEREBELLUM

The cerebellum can be visualized via both the anterior and posterior fontanelles. However, its structures are best seen through the small lateral fontanelles, provided they are sufficiently open (as often occurs in preterm infants or in those with hydrocephalus and intracranial hypertension). Regrettably, the anterior fontanelle offers a lesser image quality due to the relatively large distance to be covered.

The cerebellum consists of two hemispheres connected by the vermis. The cerebellar hemispheres are echopoor to moderately echogenic. The vermis is particularly echodense and shows up like a band on a frontal section and like a sphere on a sagittal section. On a sagittal section it is difficult to clearly separate its different lobules. In the part facing the tentorium, the primary fissure from time to time shows behind the anterior lobe. In the caudal part of the vermis the posterolateral fissure can be seen between tuber and pyramid. In a frontal view the cerebellar tonsils show owing to an increased echogenicity on their back walls, laterally to and behind the vermis: these echogenic zones are the cerebral membranes and blood vessels contrasting with the echopoor cisterna magna and the discretely echogenic substance of the cerebellum (Fig. I.10.a). Paramedially it is also possible to capture reflections of tissue in the hemispheres.

On a sagittal section the ventral part of the vermis takes the shape of an echopoor letter E, consisting of CSF (above: quadrigeminal cistern; in the middle: fourth ventricle; below: cisterna magna) (Fig. I.10.a). Sometimes a triangular echofree zone can be seen between cerebellum and occipital bone: the cerebellomedullary cistern, a prolongation of the cisterna magna (Fig. I.10.b). Cranially the cerebellum is bordered by the echogenic tentorium cerebelli, which clearly shows on a dorsally directed frontal section. Dorsally and caudally the boundary consists of bony cranium. The echodense lines visible in the cerebellar hemispheres correspond to the double cortex layer when two lobules are juxtaposed. Hyperechogenic fissures and hypoechogenic folia consequently alternate on a parasagittal section through the posterior fontanelle or an axial section through the temporal squama (Fig. I.10.c).

A sagittal 7.5 MHz section starting from the neck allows clear visualization of the cisterna magna as an echo-free triangle with its point located on the transition of the occiput towards the neck at the foramen magnum. As a rule this cistern is less than 8 mm wide. In the case of Chiari II malformation it is possible to see a tongue of cerebellar tissue filling the triangle and protruding on through the foramen magnum.

Measurement of the fetal cerebellum may allow the determination of gestational age. The transverse diameter of the cerebellum appears to be a good alternative for the biparietal diameter, in those cases where the latter appears to be unreliable (breech presentation, oligohydramnios, uterine anomalies, etc.). In no direction does the diameter of the fourth ventricle exceed 4 mm in the neonatal period. A relatively reliable and objective method for evaluating the size of the vermis consists of measuring the surface with a cursor in a sagittal section. Term babies show surfaces of 31–62 mm^2 (an average of 42 mm^2); after one month those figures have increased to 42–77 mm^2 (average 57 mm^2).

REFERENCES

Helmke, K., Winkler, P. (1987) 'Sonographisch ermittelte Normwerte des intrakraniellen Ventrikelsystemes im ersten Lebensjahr.' *Monatsschrift für Kinderheilkunde*, **135**, 148–152.
Ichiyama, T., Hayashi, T. (1991) 'Ultrasonic measurements of the posterior cranial fossa structures in neonates and infants.' *European Journal of Pediatrics*, **150**, 719–721.
McLeary, R.D., Kuhns, L.R., Barr, M. (1984) 'Ultrasonography of the fetal cerebellum.' *Radiology*, **151**, 439–442.
Yousefzadeh, D.K., Naidich, T.P. (1985) 'US anatomy of the posterior fossa in children: correlation with brain sections.' *Radiology*, **156**, 353–361.

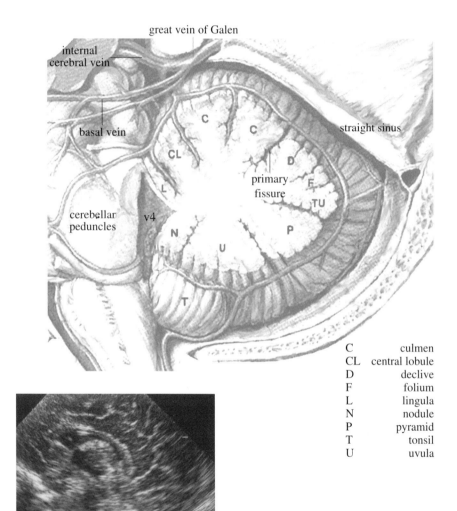

C	culmen
CL	central lobule
D	declive
F	folium
L	lingula
N	nodule
P	pyramid
T	tonsil
U	uvula

Fig. I.10.a. *(Above)* Sagittal view through the adult cerebellar vermis (adapted from Netter 1986); and *(left)* corresponding 7.5 MHz sonogram through the anterior fontanelle of a term infant.

35

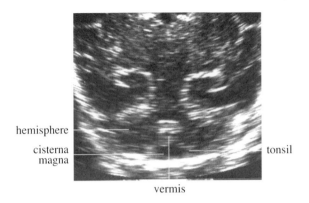

hemisphere

cisterna
magna

tonsil

vermis

Fig. I.10.b. Frontal 5 MHz view of cerebellar structures in a healthy preterm infant of 32 weeks gestation.

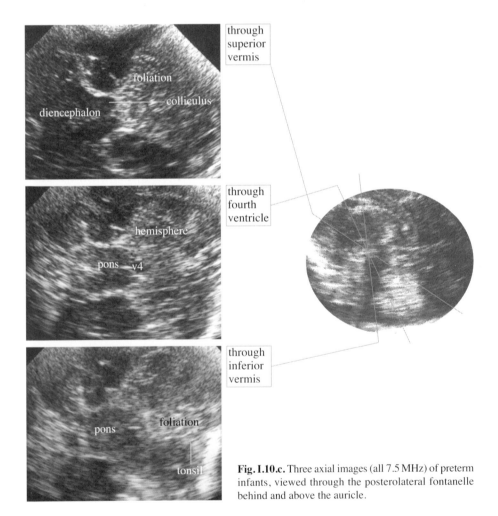

through
superior
vermis

foliation

colliculus

diencephalon

through
fourth
ventricle

hemisphere

pons   v4

through
inferior
vermis

pons   foliation

tonsil

Fig. I.10.c. Three axial images (all 7.5 MHz) of preterm infants, viewed through the posterolateral fontanelle behind and above the auricle.

I.11 GENERAL REFERENCES

Babcock, D.S. Han, B.K. (1981) *Cranial Ultrasonography of Infants*. Baltimore: Williams & Wilkins.
— — — — (1981) 'The accuracy of high resolution, real-time ultrasonography of the head in infancy.' *Radiology*, **139**, 665–676.
Bejar, R., Coen, R.W., Ekpoudia, I., James, H.E., Gluck, L. (1985) 'Real time ultrasound diagnosis of hemorrhagic pathological conditions in the posterior fossa of preterm infants.' *Neurosurgery*, **16**, 281–289.
Couture, A., Veyrac, C., Baud, C. (1994) *Echographie Cérébrale du Foetus au Nouveau-né. Imagerie et Hémodynamique*. Montpellier: Sauramps Médical.
de Vries, L.S., Dubowitz, L.M.S., Dubowitz, V., Pennock, J.M. (1990) *A Colour Atlas of Brain Disorders in the Newborn*. Brighton: Wolfe Medical.
Grant, E.G. (1986) *Neurosonography of the Pre-term Neonate*. Springer-Verlag.
Levene, M.I., Williams, J.L., Fawer, C-L. (1985) *Ultrasound of the Infant Brain. Clinics in Developmental Medicine No. 92*. London: Spastics International Medical Publications.
Maklad, N.F. (1986) 'Ultrasound of the neonatal brain.' *In: Ultrasound in Perinatology. Clinics in Diagnostic Ultrasound Vol. 19*. New York: Churchill Livingstone, pp. 129–156.
Naidich, T.P., Quencer, R.M. (1987) *Ultrasound of the Central Nervous System. Clinical Neurosonography*. Berlin/New York: Springer-Verlag.
— — Yousefzadeh, D.K., Gusnard, D.A. (1986) 'Sonography of the normal neonatal head. Supratentorial structures: state-of-the-art imaging.' *Neuroradiology*, **28**, 408–427.
Netter, F.H. (1986) *The CIBA Collection of Medical Illustrations. Vol. 1. Nervous System. Part I: Anatomy and Physiology*. West Caldwell, NJ: CIBA Pharmaceutical.
O'Rahilly, R., Müller, F. (1994) *The Embryonic Human Brain. An Atlas of Developmental Stages*. New York: Wiley–Liss.
Paneth, N., Rudelli, R., Kazam, E., Monte, W. (1994) *Brain Damage in the Preterm Infant. Clinics in Developmental Medicine No. 131*. London: Mac Keith Press.
Paturet, G. (1964) *Traité d'Anatomie Humaine. Tome IV. Système Nerveux*. Paris: Masson.
Rumack, C.M., Johnson, J.L. (1984) *Perinatal and Infant Brain Imaging: Role of Ultrasound and Computed Tomography*. Chicago: Year Book Medical.
Smith, C.G., van der Kooy, D.J. (1985) *Basic Neuroanatomy. 3rd Edn*. Toronto: Collamore Press.
Yousefzadeh, D.K., Naidich, T.P. (1985) 'US anatomy of the posterior fossa in children: correlation with brain sections.' *Radiology*, **156**, 353–361.

SECTION II
PATHOLOGY: MALFORMATIONS AND HYDROCEPHALUS

II.1 DISORDERS OF NEURULATION

Following induction by the notocord, the neural plate has been transformed into a neural tube 26 days after conception. Should this fail to happen a disorder of neurulation is present. Apart from craniorachischisis, iniencephaly, myeloschisis, cranium bifidum and spina bifida occulta, anencephaly and spina bifida cystica (aperta) are two notable examples of disturbed neurulation. Besides the primary spinal lesion, a number of recurrent central nervous system anomalies have been described with spina bifida cystica (Fig. II.1.a).

The presence of an Arnold–Chiari malformation type II is nearly obligatory: it is a herniation of the inferior vermis (nodule, pyramid and uvula), a caudal piece of fourth ventricle and a part of the tegmentum of the pons through the foramen magnum and behind the medulla oblongata. This wedge sometimes reaches the thoracic spine. It causes the medulla oblongata to bend forwards toward the spinal cord. These changes are now classified as deformative, secondary to the primary malformation, *i.e.* a disturbance in neural tube closure.

The pontine segment is tubular rather than spherical. A caudal shift is more pronounced for structures in the tegmentum than in the base of the brainstem. The posterior fossa is smaller than usual, with a low insertion of the torcula Herophili. The cerebellar hemispheres may embrace the brainstem. An unusually broad tentorial notch may be filled with chronically herniated cerebellar or occipital cerebral tissue. Hydrocephalus almost always develops when an Arnold–Chiari malformation type II is present.

Rarely one will find *heterotopias* of abnormally migrated neuronal tissue in the lateral ventricle (Figs. II.1.h, II.1.i). They can take irregular shapes with unusual liquid levels and are often located in front. A solid longitudinal and mobile club-like band of choroid plexus is often seen (Fig. II.1.h). The mesencephalic tectum extends occipitally as a beak due to fusion of the quadrigeminal bodies. This phenomenon shows best in axial sections (Fig. II.1.b). An echogram may sustain suspicion of Arnold–Chiari malformation following identification of unusually low and eccentric location in the vermis of a small or unrecognizable fourth ventricle, all of this in a sagittal section (Figs. II.1.c, II.1.g). This ventricle may be laterolaterally widened. Obliteration of the cisterna magna must necessarily be present in the case of an Arnold–Chiari malformation and consequently is an important element for antenatal diagnosis. Axial sections of an infant with spina bifida show that the cerebellum leans against the bone and is concave towards the back, producing the so-called 'banana sign'. The herniated tongue of cerebellar tissue itself does not show up on an echogram through the anterior fontanelle. Often the same sagittal section shows a large intermediate mass in the middle of a widened third ventricle (Fig. II.1.g). Generally, the normal gyrational triangle of the insula cannot be traced on an extreme parasagittal section. Instead of this spina bifida is often accompanied by *polygyria*: this non-histological term refers to more numerous and smaller gyri between shallow sulci (Fig. II.1.e). The septum pellucidum may be absent or fenestrated.

Hydrocephalus, often limited to the supratentorial compartment, is caused by narrowing of the aqueduct (hardly ever atresia) and—probably at first—obliteration of the CSF pathways in the malformed posterior fossa (Fig. II.1.d). It is considered secondary to the other anomalies and does not have its onset until the second part of gestation. Ventricular dilatation may be asymmetric. This dilatation is visible prenatally in more than 80% of the cases. Discrepant occipital rather than frontal ventricular dilatation in the early fetal period induces a cranial malformation, often referred to as 'lemon skull'. The frontal horns are rostrally almost pointed. Axial sections are better for evaluating the relationship between the third ventricle and surrounding structures.

Sometimes cystic dilatation of the midline cavities can be seen (*e.g.* the cavity of Verga). Agenesis of the corpus callosum and the olfactory tract may accompany spina bifida. Often the falx is short and fenestrated. Lack of space may cause gyral interdigitation on the midline, between both cerebral hemispheres. The frontal interhemispheric fissure may be wider than under normal circumstances (Fig. II.1.f).

REFERENCES

Babcock, D.S., Han, B.K. (1981)'Cranial sonographic findings in meningomyelocele.' *American Journal of Roentgenology*, **136**, 563–569.

Bliesener, J.A. (1985) 'Die Diagnostik der Arnold–Chiarischen Mißbildung beim Neugeborenen.' *Röntgenblätter*, **38**, 305–311.

de la Cruz, R., Millan, J.M., Miralles, M., Muñoz, M.J. (1989) 'Cranial sonographic evaluation in children with meningomyelocele.' *Child's Nervous System*, **5**, 94–98.

Goldstein, R.B., Podrasky, A.E., Filly, R.A., Callen, P.W. (1989) 'Effacement of the fetal cisterna magna in association with myelomeningocele.' *Radiology*, **172**, 409–413.

Netanyahu, I., Grant, E.G. (1986) 'Prominent choroid plexus in meningomyelocele: sonographic findings.' *American Journal of Neuroradiology*, **7**, 317–321.

Peach, B (1965) 'Arnold–Chiari malformation. Anatomic features of 20 cases.' *Archives of Neurology*, **12**, 613–621.

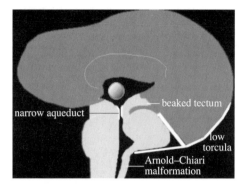

Fig. II.1.a. Some typical findings in spina bifida indicated on a sagittal section of the brain.

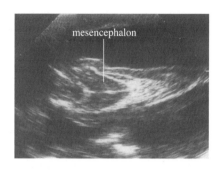

Fig. II.1.b. Axial 7.5 MHz view of the mesencephalon of a term infant with spina bifida cystica. At collicular level the quadrigeminal plate is pointing posteriorly due to collicular fusion and beaking of the tectum.

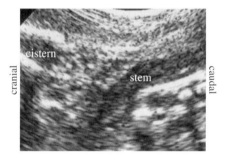

Fig. II.1.c. Sagittal nuchal 10 MHz section through the brainstem at the level of the foramen magnum in a term infant with spina bifida cystica. The area between the cisterna magna and the medulla of the brainstem is filled with nodular echogenic reflections obscuring the foramen: Arnold–Chiari malformation type II.

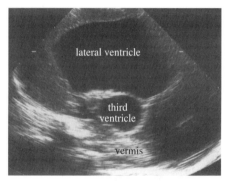

Fig. II.1.d. Sagittal 7.5 MHz view in a newborn infant with lumbar myelomeningocele and macrocephaly. The picture is dominated by massively dilated lateral and third ventricles, whereas the fourth ventricle and cerebellar vermis are barely visible due to aqueductal stenosis. Ballooning of the third ventricle is typical of this condition.

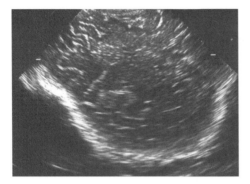

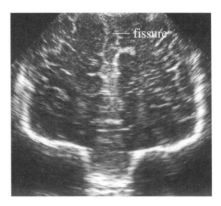

Fig. II.1.e. Lateral parasagittal 7.5 MHz view in an infant with spina bifida cystica. Convolutions are often abnormal in this condition, with typical appearance of polygyria: an abundance of smaller than normal gyri (not to be confused with the histological entity called polymicrogyria). Consequently the normal triangular appearance of the insula is lacking.

Fig. II.1.f. Frontal coronal 7.5 MHz view in a term infant with spina bifida cystica. Dilatation of the frontal interhemispheric fissure is common in this condition.

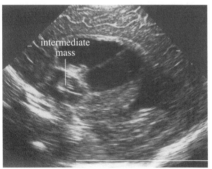

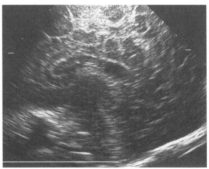

Fig. II.1.g. Sagittal 7.5 MHz views of two term infants with spina bifida cystica and hydrocephalus. The posterior fossa is small, with difficult recognition of normal landmarks, such as the obliterated cisterna magna. The intermediate mass is conspicuous in the left infant, who presented with dilatation of the supratentorial ventricles.

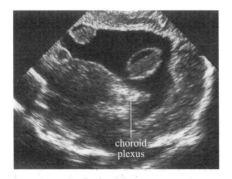

Fig. II.1.h. Term infant with lumbar myelomeningocele and macrocephaly; 7.5 MHz parasagittal view of lateral ventricle and its contents. The ventricle is irregularly dilated and contains two nodules, both with a peculiar fluid–tissue level, suggestive of heterotopic parenchyma. The choroid plexus projects toward the occipital horn.

41

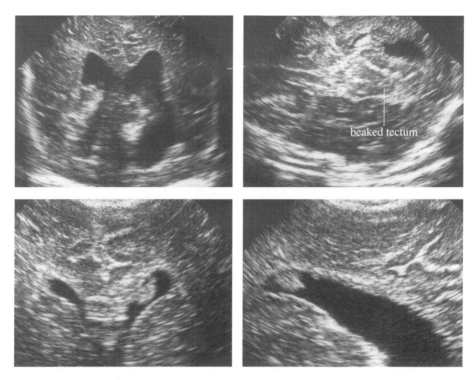

Fig. II.1.i. Term infant with spina bifida cystica; 7.5 MHz images (*left*—coronal; *top right*—axial; *bottom right*—parasagittal). There is ventriculomegaly with dangling plexuses; a heterotopic nodule lies in the left frontal horn; the mesencephalon appears elongated towards the occiput.

II.2 CEPHALOCELE

The nomenclature for this disorder is confusing and rarely correctly used (Fig. II.2.a). If only cerebral membranes are involved in this process of transosseous herniation, we use the term craniomeningocele. Should brain parenchyma with a certain amount of gyri leave the cranium via a bone defect, it is called encephalocele. When part of the ventricle exists in this tissue bridge, the entity is termed encephalocystomeningocele. If in the meningocele a loose piece of neural tissue is present without clear signs of gyration, one talks about a myelomeningocele of the cranium. Craniorachischisis is a disorder whereby a cranial encephalocele is caudally prolonged by a bony defect at the cervical or thoracic level.

The overall incidence is estimated at about 1 in 5–10,000 live births per year. In three quarters of those cases the lesions are located occipitally, and in 15% parietally. Frontal, nasopharyngeal, nasal and orbital forms are rare. Any such cephaloceles may be flat and resemble congenital aplasia of the skin (atretic cephalocele, sometimes with intact calvarium). Associated intracranial changes may include hydrocephalus, microcephaly, agenesis of the corpus callosum, Dandy–Walker malformation and Arnold–Chiari malformation (Fig. II.2.f). As a rule a brain ventricle will be affected by the malformation: the third or lateral ventricle (Figs. II.2.b–d) above the tentorium, the fourth ventricle in the case of an infra-tentorial lesion (Figs. II.2.e,f). A mesenchymal (bone) defect is considered to be the primary cause, whereas in certain cases early hydrocephalus may provoke a cephalocele due to pressure (blow-out). Cephaloceles may be associated with anomalies in other systems.

Contributions by sonography in the evaluation of a cephalocele consist of detecting associated intracranial anomalies and inspecting the contents of the lesion (Fig. II.2.b–f). For the latter purpose scanning of the cephalocele is mandatory.

REFERENCES

Brown, M.S, Sheridan-Pereira, M. (1992) 'Outlook for the child with a cephalocoele.' *Pediatrics*, **90**, 914–919.
Hunter, A.G.W. (1993) 'Brain.' *In:* Stevenson, R.E., Hall, J.G., Goodman, R.M. (Eds.) *Human Malformations and Related Anomalies. Vol. II. Oxford Monographs on Medical Genetics No. 27.* Oxford: Oxford University Press, pp. 114–119.
Jeanty, P., Shah, D., Zaleski, W., Ulm, J., Fleischer, A. (1991) 'Prenatal diagnosis of fetal cephalocele: a sonographic spectrum.' *American Journal of Perinatology*, **8**, 144–149.
Nishimura, H., Okamoto, N. (1976) *Sequential Atlas of Human Congenital Malformations.* Tokyo: Igaku-Shoin.

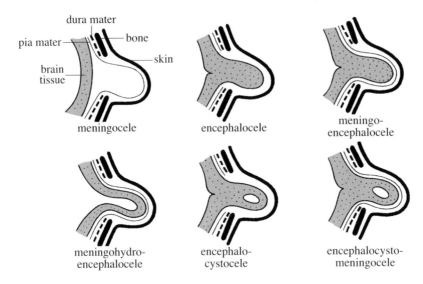

Fig. II.2.a. The constituents of various kinds of cephalocele determine the nomenclature. (Adapted from Nishimura and Okamoto 1976.)

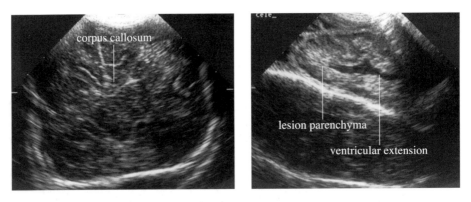

Fig. II.2.b. Term infant with median occipital cephalocele and microcephaly: *(left)* coronal view of the brain through the anterior fontanelle; *(right)* sagittal section through the lesion itself (both 7.5 MHz). Due to displacement of an important brain component, intracranial structures are difficult to recognize; the presence of parenchyma, ventricle and probably meninges permits classification as encephalocysto-meningocele.

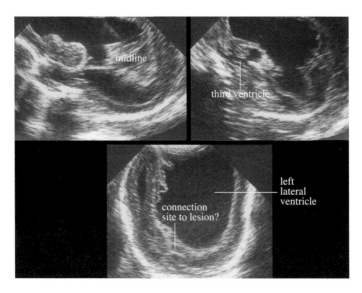

Fig. II.2.c. Preterm infant with median occipital encephalocystomeningocele without other anomalies. All images are 7.5 MHz scans through the anterior fontanelle: *top left*—parasagittal; *top right*—sagittal; *bottom*—coronal view through the occipital area. Dilatation of the left lateral and third ventricles in the presence of a small posterior fossa is suggestive of aqueductal stenosis. The midline is shifted to the right and appears attached to the right choroid glomus; the left hemisphere is the apparent site of brain herniation with massive ventricular dilatation and wrinkling of its telencephalic wall.

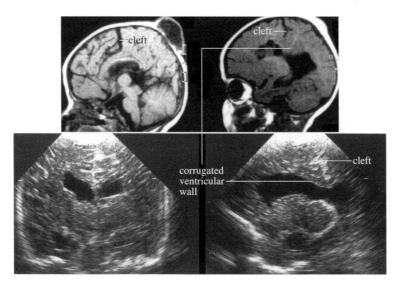

Fig. II.2.d. 3-month-old infant with median parietal meningocele; *top:* sagittal *(left)* and parasagittal *(right)* MR images; *bottom:* coronal *(left)* and parasagittal *(right)* 7.5 MHz sections through the anterior fontanelle. Asymmetric ventricular dilatation with corrugation of their outer margins is diagnostic of neuronal heterotopia associated with this type of cephalocele.

45

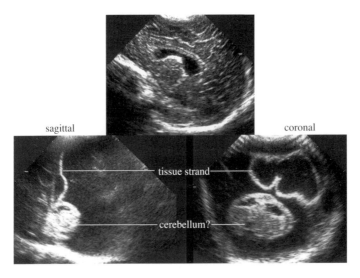

sagittal   coronal

tissue strand

cerebellum?

Fig. II.2.e. Term infant with occipital encephalomeningocele; *(top)* 7.5 MHz sagittal section through the anterior fontanelle; *(bottom)* 7.5 MHz sagittal and coronal sections through the lesion. Normal posterior fossa structures are not recognized in their usual location (vermis and fourth ventricle undetectable). Within the lesion a mass of tissue, probably cerebellar in origin, is seen behind the occipital squama. The likely site of herniation in cases like this is immediately above the foramen magnum.

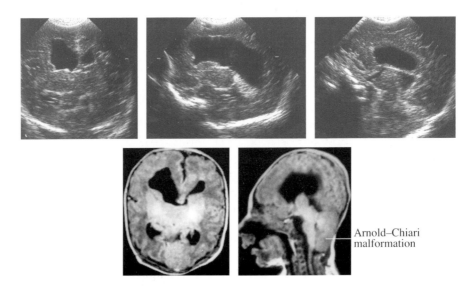

Arnold–Chiari malformation

Fig. II.2.f. Term infant without spina bifida, with a small occipital cephalocele; severe apnoeic episodes persisted after resection of the lesion. *(Top)* 7.5 MHz sections: left coronal, middle parasagittal, right sagittal; *(bottom)* corresponding MR images. The right lateral ventricle is irregularly dilated. A mass of cerebellar tissue fills the space behind the medulla in the foramen magnum: Arnold–Chiari malformation type I with brainstem dysfunction. Structures within the posterior fossa are difficult to define with ultrasound through the anterior fontanelle.

II.3 MEDIAN PROSENCEPHALIC DYSGENESIS
(holoprosencephaly and related anomalies)

A disturbance of the interaction between adjacent mesoderm and the cranial end of the neural groove in the course of the third and fourth postconceptional week may interrupt development of the interhemispherical commissures, so that the prosencephalon will not split into diencephalon and telencephalon. Under normal circumstances the optic chiasm, anterior commissure, corpus callosum, hippocampal commissure and septum pellucidum develop in the lamina terminalis. Together with a dysgenesis of these interhemispheric connections one may, in severe forms, expect fusion of the deep grey nuclei and the existence of a simple telencephalic ventricle (the holosphere) without any indication of hemisphere formation. The telencephalic contributions to the striatum are often lacking and also, quite frequently, any form of pituitary anlage. This sequence of malformations is generally called holoprosencephaly. Its incidence is estimated at 3 per 10,000 live births. Anomalies of the karyotype are commonly causal: trisomy 13 is responsible for around 70% of cases. Holoprosencephaly is often, but not always, accompanied by facial dysmorphism.

Allowing for some simplification, three variants may be distinguished (Fig. II.3.a). Only in the alobar variety, a dorsal median pouch is present: a CSF-filled space located above the cerebellum and the parieto-occipital cerebrum. This pouch is just the dorsal extension of the holosphere. Heterotopic tissue can bulge into this cavity. The tentorium is absent. There is no falx and quite often a sagittal parietal cephalocele is found. Similar median porencephalic cavities have been described in association with hydrocephalus, for instance due to aqueductal stenosis. Isolated absence of the olfactory tract and bulbs should be called *partial arhinencephaly* and does not, as such, belong to the group of the holoprosencephalies. In those places where telencephalic segmentation is absent, the falx and superior sagittal sinus are also absent. The septum pellucidum and its cavity are nearly always absent together with the corpus callosum, but the inverse is not the case. The combination of agenesis of the septum pellucidum with hypothalamic dysfunction and optic nerve hypo- or aplasia is known as septo-optic dysplasia.

Alobar prosencephalies are characterized by a varying amount of residual holospheric mantle and enjoy graphic labels, popular in the world of fetal echography: a pancake (remnants only against the frontal basicranium), a bowl (with a peel of frontal cerebrum) and a ball (complete parenchymal lining of the holosphere without dorsal pouch) (Fig. II.3.b). In the alobar form the ventricular cavity communicates over a horseshoe-like ridge of hippocampal remnants with the dorsal pouch. On the floor of the holosphere plexus lies on the merged diencephalic halves, covering a glial crust lying directly on the thalamus. A rudimentary third ventricle may be present or replaced by ependymal rosettes. A striatal nucleus may be absent or rest in the midline in front of the thalamic mass. The structures in the posterior fossa are, as a rule, normal. From the outside one notices lissencephaly (with a few remnant sulci running from nose to occiput) and cerebellar hypoplasia. The cortex has an architecture particular to holoprosencephalies, a mixture of impaired neuronal production, migration and organization. Depending on the degree of cortical dysplasia, the pyramidal tracts are hypoplastic to absent. Cerebellar dentate and inferior olive nuclei are malformed in most instances. Prenatal sonography provides us with the best descriptions. The *lobar* form of holoprosen-

TABLE II.1
Types of median prosencephalic dysgenesis

	Alobar	*Semilobar*	*Lobar*
Ventricular system	Holosphere with choroid plexus	Posterior segmentation with formation of the third ventricle	Segmentation to the front; quadrangular frontal horns
Corpus callosum	Absent	Absent or rudimentary or normal	Absent, hypoplastic
Septum pellucidum	Absent	Absent	Absent
Striata/thalami	Complete fusion	Partial fusion	Partial fusion
Olfactory tract	Absent	Absent or hypoplastic	Absent or hypoplastic
Hemispheres	Undivided; disturbances of migration	Occipital division	Fusion of frontal gyri

cephaly can show up by the absence of a falx, merger of caudate nuclei, a large massa intermedia, interdigitation of the frontal gyri across the midline (sinuous fissure), or absence of the septum pellucidum and/or corpus callosum (even partial anterior callosal agenesis) (Figs. II.3.c–e).

In order to make a distinction between holoprosencephaly with a dorsal cyst and hydrocephalus with a *midline diencephalic cyst*, it is important to examine the basal nuclei: fusion will support the former, a clear separation by third ventricle the latter (Figs. II.3.f, II.3.g). Other kinds of interhemispheric cavitation may stem from arachnoid or dural cysts, porencephaly or true midline cyst with callosal agenesis.

REFERENCES

Cohen, M.M. (1989) 'Perspectives on holoprosencephaly: Part 1. Epidemiology, genetics, and syndromology.' *Teratology*, **40**, 211–235.

Fitz, C.R. (1983) 'Holoprosencephaly and related entities.' *Neuroradiology*, **25**, 225–238.

Gorlin, R.J., Cohen, M.M., Levin, L.S. (1990) *Syndromes of the Head and Neck. 3rd Edn. Oxford Monographs on Medical Genetics No. 19.* Oxford: Oxford University Press, pp. 573–582.

Griebel, M.L., Williams, J.P., Russell, S.S., Spence, G.T., Glasier, C.M. (1995) 'Clinical and developmental findings in children with giant interhemispheric cysts and dysgenesis of the corpus callosum.' *Pediatric Neurology*, **13**, 119–124.

Hunter, A.G.W. (1993) 'Brain.' *In:* Stevenson, R.E., Hall, J.G., Goodman, R.M. (Eds.) *Human Malformations and Related Anomalies, Vol. II. Oxford Monographs on Medical Genetics No. 27.* Oxford: Oxford University Press, pp 1–19.

Leech, R.W., Shuman, R.M. (1986) 'Holoprosencephaly and related midline cerebral anomalies: a review.' *Journal of Child Neurology*, **1**, 3–18.

Pilu, G., Romero, R., Rizzo, N., Jeanty, P., Bovicelli, L., Hobbins, J.C. (1987) 'Criteria for the prenatal diagnosis of holoprosencephaly.' *American Journal of Perinatology*, **4**, 41–49.

Sener, R.N. (1995) 'Anterior callosal agenesis in mild, lobar holoprosencephaly.' *Pediatric Radiology*, **25**, 385–386.

Yokota, A., Oota, T., Matsukado, Y. (1984) 'Dorsal cyst malformations. Part I: Clinical study and critical review on the definition of holoprosencephaly.' *Child's Brain*, **11**, 320–341.

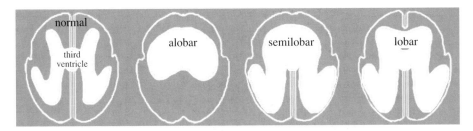

Fig. II.3.a. Schematic representation of gradual increase in hemispheric formation in several variants of holoprosencephaly.

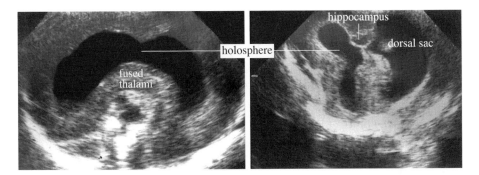

Fig. II.3.b. Preterm infant of 33 weeks gestation with trisomy 13 and cebocephaly: 5 MHz sections (*left*, coronal; *right*, sagittal). Alobar holoprosencephaly of the 'ball type' is characterized by the presence of two CSF pouches; towards the nose one can see the holosphere, in this case lined completely by abnormal white matter and cortical plate; towards the occiput an extracerebral dorsal sac is observed; in between a ridge of hippocampal remnants is seen in the sagittal plane; notice fusion (non-division) of the thalami.

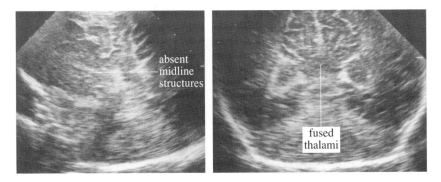

Fig. II.3.c. Term infant with median cleft lip and palate, micropenis, dysthermoregulation and diabetes insipidus: 7.5 MHz sections (*left*, sagittal; *right*, coronal behind the foramina of Monro). In lobar holoprosencephaly one may use fusion of thalami and agenesis of the corpus callosum as sonographic markers.

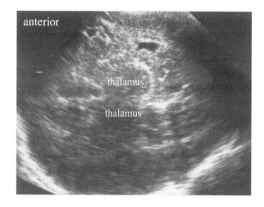

anterior

thalamus

thalamus

Fig. II.3.d. Term infant with cyanotic heart disease due to partial trisomy 13: axial 7.5 MHz view. Non-recognition of the third ventricle in an axial section through the diencephalon is due to thalamic fusion.

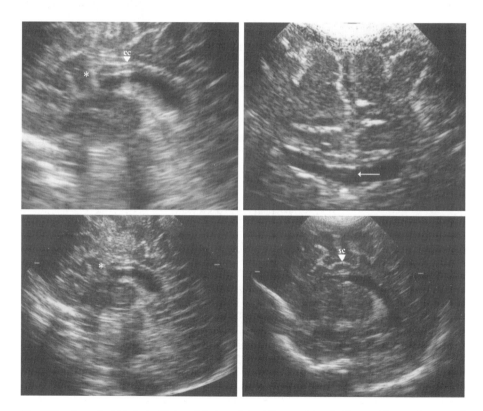

Fig. II.3.e. 4-week-old infant with hypotelorism, flat midface, stridor, feeding problems, seizures and temperature instability: sagittal 7.5 MHz *(left)*, coronal 10 MHz *(top right)* and parasagittal 7.5 MHz *(bottom right)* echograms. The corpus callosum (cc) is invisible at its rostral end *(asterisk)*, whereas the corpus and splenium are present together with the cingulate sulcus (sc) and gyrus. The septal leaflets are absent *(arrow)*. MRI confirmed fusion of the caudate nuclei, suspected due to absence of an orbital interhemispheric fissure. This is a rare variant of lobar holoprosencephaly.

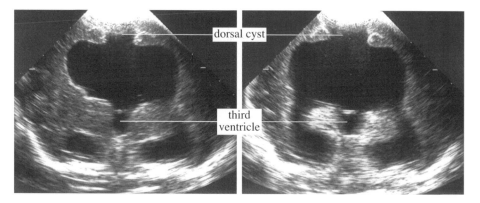

Fig. II.3.f. Macrocephaly diagnosed *in utero*; induction at 33 weeks. 7.5 MHz views: *(top left)* coronal at the foramina of Monro; *(top right)* posterior coronal; and *(opposite)* corresponding MR image. Median prosencephalic dysgenesis is unlikely in this case, because one sees clear evidence of hemispherical development: the falx is present on MRI and the basal ganglia are separated by a dilated third ventricle. Given exclusively supratentorial hydrocephalus, the final diagnosis was aqueductal stenosis with median dorsal cyst and agenesis of the corpus callosum and septum pellucidum.

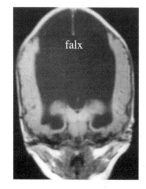

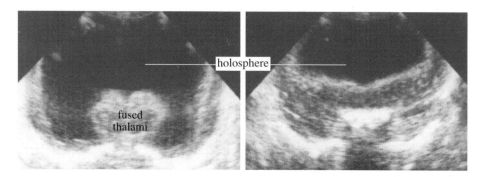

Fig. II.3.g. 30 weeks gestation infant with median cleft lip, who died in the delivery room: 5 MHz coronal sections at the level of the posterior *(left)* and anterior *(right)* cranial fossa indicate alobar holoprosencephaly with median dorsal cyst. The holosphere is lined by parenchyma only at the base and sides ('cup type'); the basal ganglia are fused.

II.4 ANOMALIES OF THE CORPUS CALLOSUM

The major interhemispheric commissure, the corpus callosum, develops in the dorsal part of the lamina terminalis 11 to 12 weeks after conception. The genu of the corpus callosum is present around 13 weeks. The cingulate sulcus and gyrus are visible by the 16th post-conceptional week. The whole corpus callosum (rostrum, corpus and splenium) is complete around the 20th week. MR imaging has demonstrated that the genu and rostrum quickly thicken in early infancy (around 2 to 3 months), whereas the splenium tends to swell usually around 5–8 months. The genu and splenium at the moment of birth of a term infant will be about 4 mm thick and the corpus about 2 mm. The prevalence rate of agenesis of the corpus callosum is estimated at 0.7–2% of the population. The boy:girl ratio is 3:2.

Complete absence of the corpus callosum may be a consequence of a dysgenesis of the midline and is, in such a case, accompanied by one of the types of holoprosencephaly (Fig. II.4.a). It may be associated with disorders of neuronal migration such as lissencephaly or be the result of a degeneration or atrophy of an *ab initio* normally formed structure. Classic exogenous causes are congenital rubella, fetal alcohol syndrome and insulin dependent maternal diabetes. The typical agenesis of the corpus callosum probably results from insufficiently programmed glial degeneration in a part of the lamina terminalis, the so-called 'glial sling', whereby normally forming commissural axons are not guided across the midline. The result is a posterior deviation of the axons along the mesial wall of the lateral ventricle: Probst bundles. The presence of that structure, incurving the mesial wall of the lateral ventricle (concave wall), is characteristic of this type of embryogenesis. For a complete discussion of the syndromology of callosal agenesis the reader is referred to Norman *et al.* (1995).

Agenesis of the corpus callosum can be associated with astroglial festering due to neuroectodermosis. Isolated forms are mostly inherited as autosomally recessive or X-linked, but have been described with autosomal dominant transmission. As there normally is a rostrocaudal progression in the formation of callosal fibres (genu and corpus before the splenium), agenesis, if incomplete, is virtually by exclusion limited to the posterior part. It follows that *partial* agenesis is found after the 12th postconceptional week. In that case the rostrum of the corpus callosum may be much thinner and form an acute angle with the rest. Yet, cases have been described of (apparent) agenesis of the anterior part of this structure, amongst others in alobar holoprosencephaly (Fig. II.3.e). Focal thinning has also been mentioned in the literature. Global hypotrophy is noticed with hydrocephalus or leukomalacia (Fig. I.3.c).

Cranial ultrasound enables one to make this diagnosis (Figs. II.4.b–e). The divergence of separated frontal horns of the lateral ventricle, with calvarially prolonged cavities showing a median concave rim (*bat wings*) are typical phenomena. The complex of lateral and third ventricles shows up on a coronal section as a bull's head. The tips of the frontal horns frequently bend slightly inwards. Discrepant dilatation of the occipital horns is called colpocephaly. *Colpocephaly* is the consequence of the absence of a number of posterior commissural fibres. The third ventricle is usually widened and lifted up between the lateral ventricles (*true midline cyst* with callosal agenesis, to be differentiated from other interhemispheric cavitations discussed with median prosencephalic dysgenesis) (Figs. II.3.f, II.4.i).

52

Also common is a fissure-like elongation of the foramina of Monro. The cingulate sulcus and the pericallosal artery do not show up in a sagittal section in those places where the corpus callosum has not developed. Surrounding gyri radially converge on the area where the corpus callosum is absent. As myelination of the corpus callosum is a postnatal phenomenon, often the volume of the Probst bundles is too small to show on a neonatal ultrasound scan. Partial absence will consequently be best identified by means of the 'bat wings' and of radial gyration (Fig. II.4.h). In more than half of the cases there is no massa intermedia. The presence of the cavity of the septum pellucidum almost certainly excludes agenesis of the corpus callosum.

Dysgenesis of the corpus callosum may be a marker of underlying neurometabolic disease (Figs. II.4.f, II.4.g). It may be presumed that the metabolic disturbance has its pernicious effect after the 18th week, upon completion of the formation of this structure. The corpus is very thin and sunk in between the lateral ventricles and the cingulate sulcus. If the corpus callosum remains rudimentarily present, other indicators of dysgenesis will be changes of the shape of the frontal horns and not colpocephaly or agenesis of the cingulate gyrus.

In the case of a child with erythroblastosis fetalis we observed unusual *hyperechogenicity* of the corpus callosum (Fig. II.4.j). This phenomenon, undiscussed in the literature, appears to be secondary to vascular changes and not malformative. It may sonographically resemble a flat lipoma in that area. Exceptionally one will come across a lesion in the corpus callosum in association with haemorrhage in the germinal matrix with a parenchymal component (see section on matrix bleeding).

A *lipoma* of the corpus callosum shows as an echogenic mass in the middle of the interhemispheric fissure, sometimes with connections into the lateral ventricles, between the hemispheres or in choroid plexus. The mass corresponds to a hypodensity on CT, often with a calcified wall (see section on tumours). Ordinarily the normal corpus callosum has been replaced by this lipoma. This is because its growth is obstructed by the lipoma, which had been formed by the end of the first month of pregnancy due to incomplete closure of the anterior neuropore. The lesion is often found in children suffering from spinal dysraphism.

In a child with oesophageal and duodenal atresia associated with trisomy 21, we noted an unusually *broad* corpus callosum (5mm in genu and corpus) (Fig. II.4.k). We know nothing about the frequency of the phenomenon, nor about its underlying mechanism.

REFERENCES

Atlas, S.W., Shkolnik, A., Naidich, T.P. (1985) 'Sonographic recognition of agenesis of the corpus callosum.' *American Journal of Neuroradiology*, **6**, 369–375.

Auriemma, A., Poggiani, C., Menghini, P., Bellan, C., Colombo, A. (1993) 'Lipoma of the corpus callosum in a neonate: sonographic evaluation.' *Pediatric Radiology*, **23**, 155–156.

Babcock, D.S. (1984) 'The normal, absent and abnormal corpus callosum: sonographic findings.' *Radiology*, **151**, 449–453.

Barkovich, A.J., Kjos, B.O. (1988) 'Normal postnatal development of the corpus callosum as demonstrated by MR imaging.' *American Journal of Neuroradiology*, **9**, 487–491.

— — Norman, D. (1988) 'Anomalies of the corpus callosum: correlation with further anomalies of the brain.' *American Journal of Neuroradiology*, **9**, 493–501.

Bodensteiner, J., Schaefer, G.B., Breeding, L., Cowan, L. (1994) 'Hypoplasia of the corpus callosum: a study of 445 consecutive MRI scans.' *Journal of Child Neurology*, **9**, 47–49.

Fisher, R.M., Cremin, B.J. (1988) 'Lipoma of the corpus callosum: diagnosis by ultrasound and magnetic resonance.' *Pediatric Radiology*, **18**, 409–410.

Gebarski, S.G., Gebarski, K.S., Bowerman, R.A., Silver, T.M. (1984) 'Agenesis of the corpus callosum: sonographic features.' *Radiology*, **151**, 443–448.

Griebel, M.L., Williams, J.P., Russell, S.S., Spence, G.T., Glasier, C.M. (1995) 'Clinical and developmental findings in children with giant interhemispheric cysts and dysgenesis of the corpus callosum.' *Pediatric Neurology*, **13**, 119–124.

Hunter, A.G.W. (1993) 'Brain.' *In:* Stevenson, R.E., Hall, J.G., Goodman, R.M. (Eds.) *Human Malformations and Related Anomalies. Vol. II. Oxford Monographs on Medical Genetics, No. 27.* Oxford: Oxford University Press, pp. 52–60.

Jinkins, J.R., Whittemore, A.R., Bradley, W.G. (1989) 'MR imaging of callosal and corticocallosal dysgenesis.' *American Journal of Neuroradiology*, **10**, 339–344.

Loeser, J.D., Alvord, E.C. (1968) 'Agenesis of the corpus callosum.' *Brain*, **91**, 553–570.

Norman, M.G., McGillivray, B.C., Kalousek, D.K., Hill, A., Poskitt, K.J. (1995) 'Crossing the midline.' *In: Congenital Malformations of the Brain.* Oxford: Oxford University Press, pp. 309–331.

Schaefer, G.B., Shuman, R.M., Wilson, D.A., Saleeb, S., Domek, D.B., Johnson, S.F., Bodensteiner, J.B. (1991) 'Partial agenesis of the anterior corpus callosum: correlation between appearance, imaging, and neuropathology.' *Pediatric Neurology*, **7**, 39–44.

Vade, A., Horowitz, S.W. (1992) 'Agenesis of corpus callosum and intraventricular lipomas.' *Pediatric Neurology*, **8**, 307–309.

Wariyar, U.K., Welch, R.J., Milligan, D.W.A., Perry, R.H. (1990) 'Sonographic and pathological features of callosal hypoplasia in non-ketotic hyperglycinaemia.' *Archives of Disease in Childhood*, **65**, 670–671.

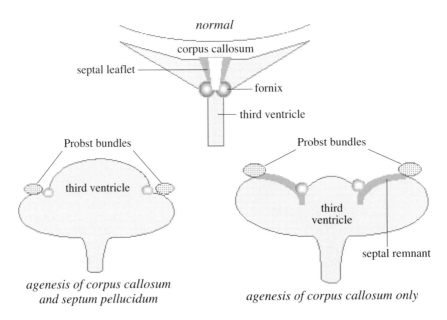

Fig. II.4.a. Pathological findings in agenesis of the corpus callosum. The *upper drawing* shows normal anatomical relationships between the septal leaflets, corpus callosum and fornix; while that at *lower left* shows Probst bundles next to the fornices in the case of agenesis of both corpus callosum and septum pellucidum. (Adapted by permission from Loeser and Alvord 1968.)

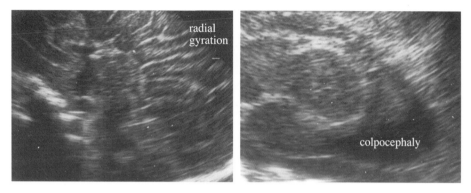

Fig. II.4.b. Term growth retarded infant with cyanotic heart defect associated with fetal alcohol syndrome: 7.5 MHz sections (*left*, sagittal; *right*, parasagittal). In the area where the corpus callosum is absent, gyration is abnormal: instead of forming the cingulate gyrus, gyri display a radial pattern converging on the absent structure. Discrepant dilatation of the occipital horn is termed colpocephaly.

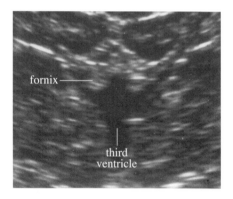

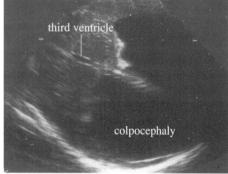

Fig. II.4.c. Term infant with neurofibromatosis: detail of coronal 7.5 MHz section through the foramina of Monro, showing callosal agenesis with preservation of septal remnants; fornical axons are appended at the overlying cerebral cortex.

Fig. II.4.d. Term infant with macrocephaly and hypertelorism: axial 7.5 MHz section. This child and his father had an autosomal dominant type of isolated agenesis of the corpus callosum, associated in the parent with mild mental retardation. Obvious colpocephaly is seen, contrasting with a normal sized third ventricle.

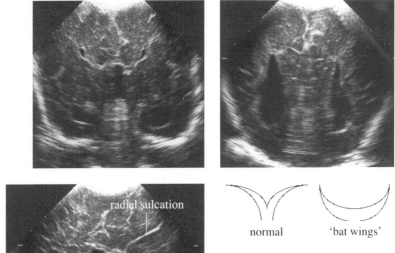

Fig. II.4.e. Preterm infant (28 weeks gestation) with trisomy 8 mosaicism: coronal *(top)* and sagittal *(left)* 7.5 MHz images. The tips of the lateral ventricles point to the vertex in agenesis of corpus callosum (bat wing appearance). Gyral formation is abnormal at this early stage, given the appearance of a radial sulcus instead of the cingulate sulcus.

radial sulcation

normal   'bat wings'

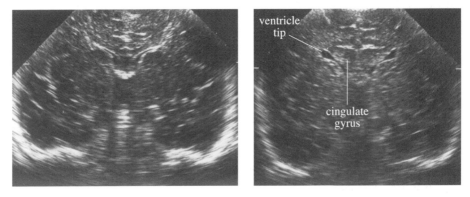

ventricle
tip

cingulate
gyrus

Fig. II.4.f. 7.5 MHz coronal sections at the foramen of Monro in *(left)* normal term infant, and *(right)* newborn infant with non-ketotic hyperglycinaemia. Dysgenesis or hypotrophy of the corpus callosum induces a change in shape of the lateral ventricles, which appear as small slits but with nodular enlargement of the tips; the cingulate gyrus sinks into the cavities due to poor support by callosal fibres.

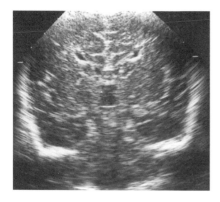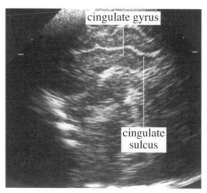

Fig. II.4.g. Coronal *(left)* and sagittal *(right)* views of term infant with Pierre Robin syndrome and non-ketotic hyperglycinaemia. Notice presence of the cingulate gyrus and sulcus and sonographic absence of the corpus callosum.

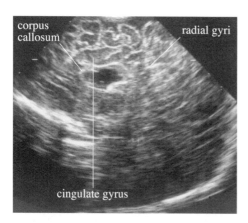

Fig. II.4.h. Term infant with acrocallosal syndrome: sagittal 7.5 MHz view. Partial agenesis of the corpus callosum affects the posterior portion because of normal rostrocaudal development. Note that the cingulate gyrus is replaced by radial gyri at the point of callosal agenesis.

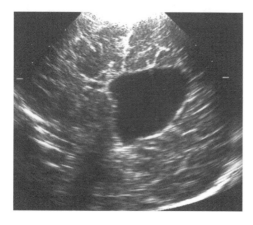

Fig. II.4.i. Term microcephalic infant with seizures at 3 weeks of age: sagittal 7.5 MHz image showing callosal agenesis associated with a posterior midline cyst.

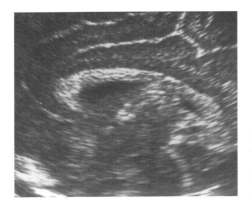

Fig. II.4.j. Term infant with immune hydrops: detail from sagittal 7.5 MHz section, showing unusual echogenicity of the entire callosal structure. The context suggested an acquired pathogenesis, like ischaemia or congestion.

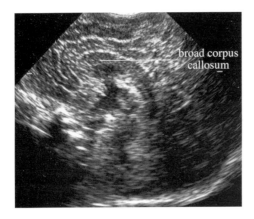

broad corpus callosum

Fig. II.4.k. Term infant with oesophageal and duodenal atresia associated with trisomy 21: 7.5 MHz sagittal section. The middle part of the corpus callosum measured 4 mm in this newborn infant, whereas the upper limit of normal is at or below 3 mm; this observation needs verification and explanation.

II.5 ANOMALIES OF THE SEPTUM PELLUCIDUM

A septum pellucidum cavity can be shown in most neonates and many young infants. It develops early in the second trimester following physiological necrosis in the commissural plate between the anterior commissure, the hippocampal commissure and the growing corpus callosum. The surrounding septal nuclei belong to the limbic system and are a relay site between hippocampus and hypothalamus. On a frontal section the cavity is a triangle with its base against the corpus callosum. Slow disappearance of this cavity, with a glial border, has been well described in the literature. Around the time of birth, the cavity should not be broader or deeper than 10 mm, and in most cases it is less than 6 mm wide. Around the 34th week the normal width may increase to a physiological maximum of 9 mm. Dorsally, behind the top of the fornix column, the prolonging cavity is called the cavity of Verga. In normal newborn infants fenestration of one or both septal laminae can be found (Fig. II.5.f). Linear densities along the cavity are probably caused by septal veins (Fig. II.5.g). Abnormal sizes and shapes have been associated with certain disease profiles. In some very rare cases the whole will constitute a cystic structure pushing against the foramina of Monro or the frontal horns. It is possible for one of the walls to stick to the adjacent caudate nucleus, thereby causing unilateral hydrocephalus. In extremely rare cases a colloidal cyst will develop in the cavity.

We observed *angular widening* of the cavity in term children with a chromosomal anomaly (trisomy 18, dup q15) and — more pronounced — in two children with the neonatal presentation of glutaric aciduria type II. The latter disease is also associated with hypoplasia of the corpus callosum and impairs myelination. Similar dilatation of the cavity, but associated with hypothalamo-pituitary anomalies, has been described as 'pseudo-monoventricle due to a malformation of the septum pellucidum' (Figs. II.5.a–c). The frontal horns are then pushed aside by a rectangular cavity. A widened cavity has also been noted in the syndromes of Sotos and Weaver (both showing exaggerated somatic growth). Some believe a persistently wide cavity to be a minimum grade in the range of midline anomalies described with median dysgenesis of the prosencephalon.

Serious developmental disorders of the lamina terminalis (holoprosencephaly, agenesis of the corpus callosum) will obviously be associated with *absence* of the septum pellucidum cavity (Figs. II.5.a, II.5.d). Absence of the cavity and yet presence of the corpus callosum is well-known in septo-optic dysplasia, where the optic chiasm and the optic nerve are hypoplastic probably due to a disturbance around the sixth week of gestation (Fig. II.5.e). Often colpocephaly is seen without widening of the frontal horns. On a coronal section the lateral ventricles lose their boomerang shape, have a proper lateral wall and show an indentation in the floor at the caudothalamic junction. The fornices are lying loose of the corpus callosum. Another clinical picture combines agenesis of the septum pellucidum, symmetric polymicrogyria and porencephaly.

Prolonged hydrocephalus may cause secondary regression of the cavity (Fig. II.5.h). An example of this was a preterm infant with post-haemorrhagic hydrocephalus and regression of the left, but not of the right, septal leaflet. This was an intermediary stage toward complete disappearance. Finally, blood clot can be found both in the cavity of the septum pellucidum and in the cavity of Verga or the cavum veli interpositi in preterm infants (Fig. II.5.i). One may assume this to be an extension of a haemorrhage in adjacent germinal matrix or choroid plexus. In such instances obliteration of the cavity with cyst formation may occur in the organizing stage.

REFERENCES

Bodensteiner, J.B. (1995) 'The saga of the septum pellucidum: a tale of unfunded clinical investigations.' *Journal of Child Neurology*, **10**, 227–231.
Böhm, N., Uy, J., Kiessling, M., Lehnert, W. (1982) 'Multiple acyl-CoA dehydrogenation deficiency (glutaric aciduria type II), congenital polycystic kidneys, and symmetric warty dysplasia of the cerebral cortex in two newborn brothers. II. Morphology and pathogenesis.' *European Journal of Pediatrics*, **139**, 60–65.
Butt, W., Havill, D., Daneman, A., Pape, K. (1985) 'Hemorrhage and cyst development in the cavum septi pellucidi and cavum Vergae. Report of three cases.' *Pediatric Radiology*, **15**, 368–371.
Garza-Mercado, R. (1981) 'Giant cyst of the septum pellucidum. Case report.' *Journal of Neurosurgery*, **55**, 646–650.
Heibel, M., Heber, R., Bechinger, D., Kornhuber, H.H. (1993) 'Early diagnosis of perinatal cerebral lesions in apparently normal full-term newborns by ultrasound of the brain.' *Neuroradiology*, **35**, 85–91.
Kuban, K.C.K., Littlewood Teele, R., Wallman, J. (1989) 'Septo-optic-dysplasia–schizencephaly. Radiographic and clinical features.' *Pediatric Radiology*, **19**, 145–150.
Poll-Thé, B.T., Aicardi, J. (1985) 'Pseudomonoventricle due to a malformation of the septum pellucidum.' *Neuropediatrics*, **16**, 39–42.
Siejka, S., Strefling, A.M., Urich, H. (1989) 'Absence of septum pellucidum and polymicrogyria: a forme fruste of the porencephalic syndrome.' *Clinical Neuropathology*, **8**, 174–178.

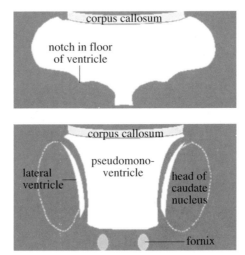

Fig. II.5.a. Two sonographically recognizable anomalies of the septum pellucidum in the neonatal period: *(top)* agenesis with preservation of the corpus callosum; *(bottom)* dilatation of the cavity of the septum pellucidum with compression of the lateral ventricles—frontal pseudomonoventricle. (Redrawn by permission from Poll-Thé and Aicardi 1985.)

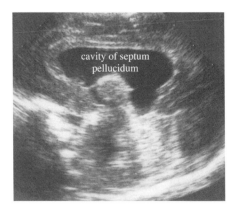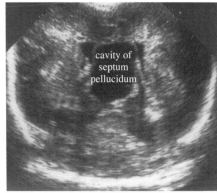

Fig. II.5.b. Newborn infant with glutaric aciduria type II: sagittal *(left)* and coronal *(right)* 7.5 MHz views. Metabolic acidosis in a dysmorphic newborn infant with frontal pseudomonoventricle and cystic kidney disease may well be a constellation unique to this organic aciduria; the cavity of the septum pellucidum is dilated and quadrangular instead of triangular.

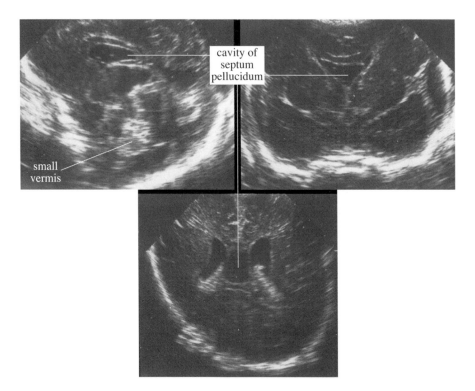

Fig. II.5.c. Two newborn infants with an anomaly of the karyotype: *(top)* 29 week gestation infant with trisomy 18 *(left*, sagittal; and *right*, coronal 7.5 MHz views); *(bottom)* term girl with partial trisomy 15q (coronal 7.5 MHz view). Both children have an enlarged cavity of the septum pellucidum, quadrangular in the latter case. Note the hypoplastic vermis in the child with trisomy 18.

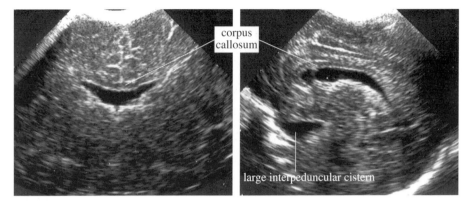

Fig. II.5.d. Preterm infant (34 weeks gestation) with mild mental retardation and a bald patch on the scalp overlying the middle parietal bone. 7.5 MHz views (*left*, coronal; *right*, sagittal) show isolated agenesis of the septum pellucidum, with preservation of the corpus callosum, and an enlarged interpeduncular cistern.

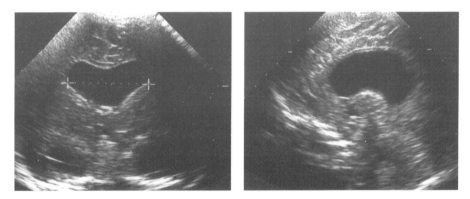

Fig. II.5.e. Term infant with septo-optic dysplasia: 7.5 MHz scans (*left*, coronal; *right*, sagittal). The septal leaflets are absent, whereas a thin corpus callosum is covering an enlarged frontal monoventricle.

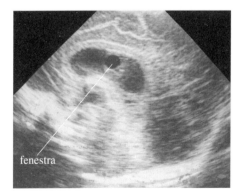

Fig. II.5.f. Preterm infant with congenital toxoplasmosis: sagittal 5 MHz section. Fenestration of one of the septal leaflets is an incidental finding.

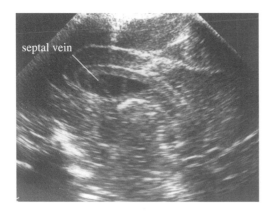

Fig. II.5.g. Healthy preterm infant: sagittal 7.5 MHz section. Septal veins may incidentally draw the attention of the sonographer.

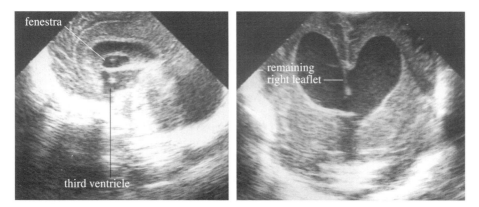

Fig. II.5.h. Preterm infant with posthaemorrhagic hydrocephalus: 5 MHz images (*left*, sagittal; *right*, coronal at the foramina of Monro). Fenestration of the left septal leaflet is an intermediary stage in the evolution to complete regression.

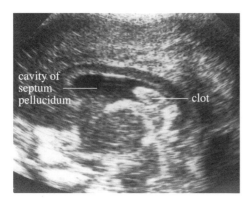

Fig. II.5.i. Preterm infant with subependymal and intraventricular haemorrhage: sagittal 7.5 MHz view. Verga's ventricle is filled with an elliptical clot, possibly indicating extension of bleeding in matrix or plexus, or subarachnoid haemorrhage?

63

II.6 MICROCEPHALY

Insufficient prenatal brain growth (congenital micrencephaly) gives rise to microcephaly at birth. Usually microcephaly can only be determined after the 20th week of gestation. The causes of congenital microcephaly are numerous and diverse. They can be subdivided into two entities:

(1) *Primary microcephaly* due to insufficient cell production and/or insufficient neuronal migration capacity (developed as a rule in the first or second trimester of pregnancy) and/or an excess of 'normal' neuronal death with apoptosis.

(2) *Secondary microcephaly* due to excessive brain cell death following a degenerative process or due to clastic lesions (mostly developed in late second and third trimester).

Ultrasound will reflect the cause. However, the echograms are frequently of poor quality because the fontanelle is too small. Often it is decided to skip sonography and perform an MRI scan straight away. Although precise sonographic descriptions of most syndromes are lacking, some information may be distilled from neuropathological data.

Migration disorders and fetal infections cause typical patterns detailed elsewhere. Antenatal necrosis due to ischaemia will produce some identifiable entity: leukomalacia, porencephaly, hydranencephaly, hydrocephalus *ex vacuo*, germinolysis, densities in the basal grey nuclei. In the cases of microcephalia vera and radial microbrain, two quite distinct histological entities, one expects structurally normal sonograms, with no marked ventricular dilatation and a normal corpus callosum, although the gyrational pattern is simpler than normal and the sulci are less deep. A type of microcephaly with lissencephaly and meningeal vessel proliferation may be recognized through ventriculomegaly and changes of the cortical plate, which contains mainly polymicrogyric zones with calcification and gliosis.

The *atelencephalic* brain consists of a brainstem and a cerebellum with, on top, one small median diencephalic mass without a ventricular cavity. Above the aprosencephalic/atelencephalic brain the cranium is intact, albeit possibly collapsed. These phenomena emerge after closure of the neural tube in the fifth postconceptional week.

A number of *syndromic* microcephalies will be accompanied by an insufficient production of white matter and ventriculomegaly, with agenesis of the corpus callosum, Dandy–Walker malformation and/or intracranial calcification (Fig. II.6.a). In other cases the echogram of the brain is strikingly normal. The echo-anatomy itself may be normal, but dilatation of the arachnoid spaces results in clear delineation of brain contours on coronal sections (Fig. II.6.b). We observed three children in one family with lethal microcephaly whereby the arachnoid spaces were dilated, all ventricles showed moderate dilatation and a small vermis cerebelli floated high in the posterior fossa, above a large cisterna magna (Fig. II.6.c). Other investigations and postmortem examination confirmed atrophy of the olivopontocerebellar region and of the part of the cortex projecting to basal pontine nuclei, without disturbance of neuronal migration. It seems particularly difficult to show atrophy of the brainstem with echographic techniques, but a small vermis with a dilated fourth ventricle against a certain clinical background may be indicative of such olivopontocerebellar atrophy (to be distinguished from the findings in the case of CHARGE association, where brainstem dysplasia is present).

REFERENCES

Harris, C.P., Townsend, J.J., Norman, M.G., White, V.A., Viskochil, D.H., Pysher, T.J., Klatt, E.C. (1994) 'Atelencephalic aprosencephaly.' *Journal of Child Neurology*, **9**, 412–416.

Hunter, A.G.W. (1993) 'Brain.' *In:* Stevenson, R.E., Hall, J.G., Goodman, R.M. (Eds.) *Human Malformations and Related Anomalies. Vol. II. Oxford Monographs on Medical Genetics, No. 27.* Oxford: Oxford University Press, pp 1–19.

Siebert, J.R., Kokich, V.G., Warkany, J., Lemire, R.J. (1987) 'Atelencephalic microcephaly: craniofacial anatomy and morphologic comparisons with holoprosencephaly and anencephaly.' *Teratology*, **36**, 279–285.

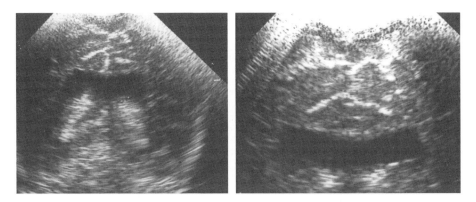

Fig. II.6.a. Term infant with an occipitofrontal circumference of 31 cm: coronal 7.5 MHz sections indicate lobar holoprosencephaly with frontal fusion of supraventricular parenchyma across the midline.

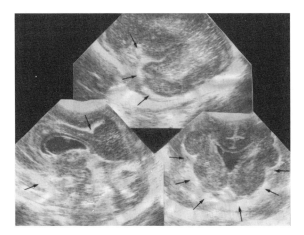

Fig. II.6.b. 28-week-old infant with left diaphragmatic hernia, facial dysmorphism, single umbilical artery and trisomy 20 mosaicism. 7.5 MHz images: *(top)* parasagittal through the insula; *(bottom left)* sagittal; *(bottom right)* coronal. Normal anatomic relations and structures in a small brain, shown at postmortem examination to be affected with verrucous brain dysplasia (warty brain). The leptomeninges are highly echogenic *(arrows)* and there is a clear increase of the bone to brain distance.

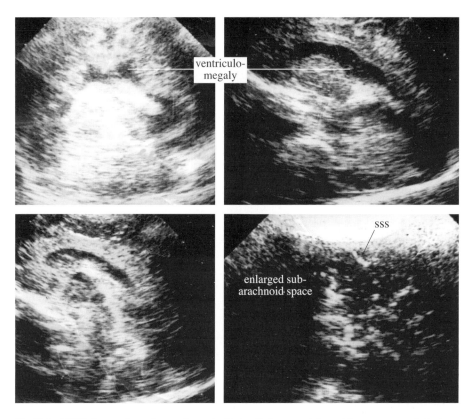

Fig. II.6.c. 5 MHz images through a small anterior fontanelle in a term infant with severe congenital micro-cephaly: *(top left)* coronal; *(top right)* parasagittal; *(bottom left)* sagittal; *(bottom right)* coronal detail (10 MHz). There is dilatation of all ventricles, together with a small vermis (enlarged cisterna magna) and an increase of the sinocortical distance due to enlargement of the subarachnoid space (sss = superior sagittal sinus); the corpus callosum and septum pellucidum are present. The same anomaly was found in two sibs. At postmortem examination there were no anomalies of neuronal migration, although cortical architecture was abnormal and the pyramidal tracts were absent. Meningeal angiomatosis was an additional finding. Brain weight varied around 70 g.

II.7 CEREBRAL HEMIATROPHY

Faced with a striking difference in size between both cerebral hemispheres, a distinction ought to be made between hemimegalencephaly and contralateral hemiatrophy. In both cases the lateral ventricle may be dilated on the affected side. The occipitofrontal circumference does not always tell us enough about the underlying problem, although macrocrania should be associated with megalencephaly and microcrania with hemiatrophy.

In syndromes causing a primary asymmetric disturbance of white matter, for instance on an infective or ischaemic basis, the ventricle will be strongly dilated and dystrophic, or inflammatory calcium deposition may be found together with subcortical cysts.

In the neonatal period cerebral hemiatrophy is particularly rare. We treated a term newborn infant with hypoplasia of the left face, anterior rhinostenosis, left microphthalmia and a remarkable brain anomaly with porencephaly on the left. Starting from a lateral ventricle with corrugated edges, cranial sonography showed a hypodense trajectory leading toward the orbit and ending beneath the left frontal lobe in a cystic terminal. During the first months of life this frontal porencephalic cyst grew and at 18 months surgical removal seemed necessary. CT and MRI confirmed the sonographic suspicions: during the operation it appeared we were dealing with an arachnoid cyst. Around the ventricle and the hypodense trajectory there were nodular masses, probably heterotopia. The ipsilateral hemisphere was globally atrophic. Two comparable observations in the literature lead us to suspect that we were dealing with an early fetal vascular disruption encompassing anomalies of the circle of Willis such as absence of an anterior cerebral artery and/or posterior communicating artery.

Clear cerebral hemispheric asymmetry may also be found in children suffering from septo-optic dysplasia. Focal arterial infarction of the area perfused by the middle cerebral or internal carotid artery may be acquired perinatally. Cerebral hemiatrophy has been reported in a newborn infant with seizures in the hemisphere contralateral to a hemimegalencephalic hemisphere with a lissencephalic appearance.

REFERENCES

Friede, R.L. (1989) *Developmental Neuropathology*. Berlin: Springer-Verlag.
Sarnat, H.B. (1992) *Cerebral Dysgenesis. Embryology and Clinical Expression*. Oxford: Oxford University Press.
Sener, R.N. (1995) 'Hemimegalencephaly associated with contralateral hemispheral volume loss.' *Pediatric Radiology*, **25**, 387–388.
Stewart, R.M., Williams, R.S., Lukl, P., Schoenen, J. (1978) 'Ventral porencephaly: a cerebral defect associated with multiple congenital anomalies.' *Acta Neuropathologica*, **42**, 231–235.
Vosskämper, M., Schachenmayr, W. (1990) 'Cerebral hemiatrophy: a clinicopathological report of two cases with a contribution to pathogenesis and differential diagnosis.' *Clinical Neuropathology*, **9**, 244–250.

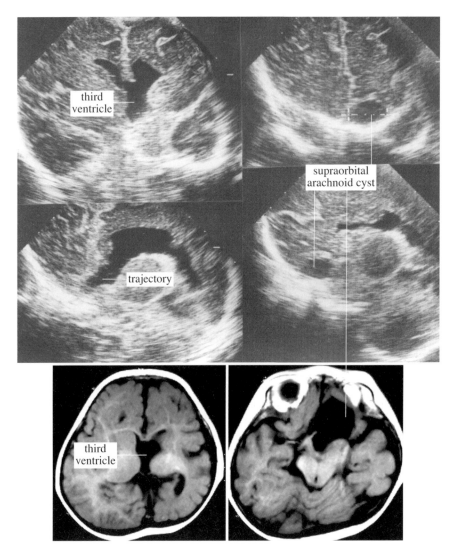

Fig. II.7.a. Term infant with focal right clonic seizures in the neonatal period, with left microphthalmia and left anterior rhinostenosis: 7.5 MHz views (*top*, coronal; *bottom*, parasagittal); and *(below)* two axial MR images (T$_1$-weighted). In association with a dilated left lateral and third ventricle, a tubular hypodense trajectory can be seen projecting underneath the left frontal lobe to reach the orbital roof. Dilatation of the lateral ventricle is irregular, suggesting the presence of heterotopic tissue in the margins of the cleft (ventral porencephaly? ventral schizencephaly?). During neurosurgical intervention at 1.5 years for intractable seizures, the presence of a supraorbital arachnoid cyst was confirmed. The entire left hemisphere was clearly underdeveloped from birth.

II.8 DISORDERS OF NEURONAL MIGRATION

Nearly the entire telencephalic cortex is the result of a stepwise development of the cortical plate due to migration of neuroblasts from the ventricular zone along (mainly radial) glial fibres. Some seemingly erratic non-radial migration is also present. Upon their arrival at the molecular zone (layer I), new neurons displace away from the pial membrane older cells that had already arrived: this pattern is called active inside-out migration. Passive migration, on the other hand, takes place in the diencephalon (thalamus and hypothalamus), spinal cord and brainstem: in this pattern freshly arrived neurons displace the older cells so that these are relocated farthest from their (sub)ventricular origin. The development of the cerebellum is the result of completely different migratory patterns (Figs. II.8.a–c), the anomalies of which cannot yet be studied in life. These phenomena, also called neocortical dysplasias, have been amply described in the literature, in part due to the contribution of MRI to the identification of relatively subtle aberrations. Migration impairment often gives rise to microcephaly. An unusually steep sylvian fossa with primitive gyration around the insula and incomplete opercularization is typical. As pregnancy proceeds, disorders of migration become more subtle. Lissencephaly develops at the beginning of the first or the end of the second trimester, whereas the origin of limited focal cortical dysplasias is in the third trimester (Fig. II.8.d).

It is not easy to identify most of the above entities with brain sonography. Quite often anomalies of the gyrational pattern escape detection even by high frequency scanning. *Lissencephaly* can be divided into four categories. *Type I* is, in turn, subdivided into syndromes with and without dysmorphism. With dysmorphism there is the Miller–Dieker syndrome, a deletion of the short arm of chromosome 17 of varying size (rarely a balanced translocation can be found in one of the parents) (Fig. II.8.e). Without dysmorphic features there is an autosomally recessive form of severe cerebrocerebellar lissencephaly, first described by Barth. Isolated cases without dysmorphism are expected to show microdeletion or focal mutation at the above locus in the genome. This clinical picture is nearly always associated with heterotopia of the inferior olivary nuclei. Complete lissencephaly type I is characterized by absence of gyration underneath the superior sagittal sinus and by a pseudo-liver echopattern of the parenchyma between pia mater and ventricle. This parenchyma consists mainly (80%) of grey matter with neurons in four layers which did not migrate into a proper cortical plate. Only after the 30th gestational week will gyration have developed sufficiently to allow the diagnosis of lissencephaly. The interhemispheric fissure is not flanked by branching sulci. The lateral fissure no longer shows a horizontal Y but has been reduced to a slit, the point of which courses caudally downwards. This is a consequence of the absence of opercularization with a widely patent sylvian fossa that points caudally. Discrepant dilatation of the occipital horns, colpocephaly, is nearly always present. The added neuronal layer, found in the subcortical intermediary zone in lissencephalic brains, cannot be traced echographically. This layer is isointense with the normal cortical plate on T_2-weighted MR images. Sporadically it is possible to identify agenesis of the corpus callosum, periventricular or superficial calcifications and anomalies in the posterior fossa .

The autosomally recessive syndrome of Walker–Walburg (*lissencephaly type II* or *cobblestone lissencephaly*) is characterized by marked generalized ventricular dilatation, usually

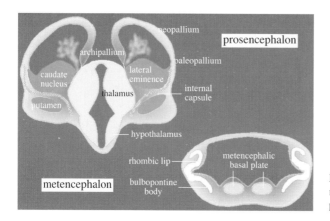

Fig. II.8.a. Sources of neuronal multiplication around the 10th postconceptional week.

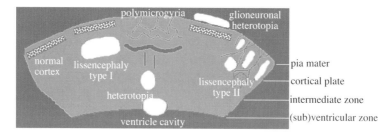

Fig. II.8.b. Typical disorders of neuronal migration (adapted from Barth 1992).

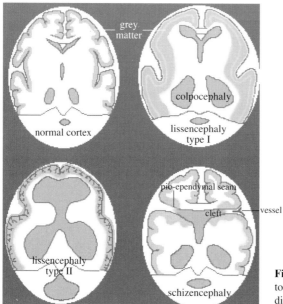

Fig. II.8.c. Relation of telencephalic grey to white matter in classical examples of disturbed neuronal migration.

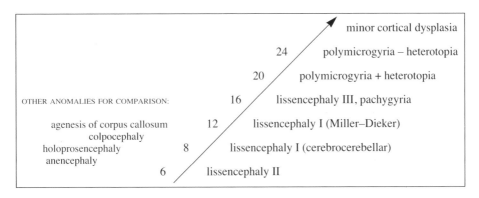

Fig. II.8.d. Chronology (postconceptional weeks) of disorders of telencephalic neuronal migration.

with corpus callosum and falx present as normal (Fig. II.8.f). The third ventricle appears to have a prolongation towards the occiput. Hydrocephalus is of the communicative type due to obliteration of pericerebral CSF spaces. Sometimes one encounters aqueductal stenosis, Dandy–Walker malformation or posterior cephalocele. Deep periventricular heterotopia protrude as nodules into the cavity or cause bizarre malformations of the ventricular lumina. The frontal lobes may partially merge with glial crosslinks, and sometimes the olfactory nerves are absent. Cerebral 'cortex' and white matter are nearly equally thick. A primitive sylvian fissure is the only visible sign of gyration. The cerebellum will be small and dysplastic with hypoplasia of the posterior vermis. *Lissencephaly type III* refers to the agyric brain seen with Neu–Laxova syndrome, which also features agenesis of the corpus callosum and microcephaly. A variant of lissencephaly has been described with microcephaly, polymicrogyria, leptomeningeal vascular proliferation, calcification and gliosis in the cortical plate. Such a constitutional vascular anomaly can also be found in association with fetal hypokinesia (Pena–Shokeir syndrome type I). There exists a *lissencephaly sequence* due to fetal CMV or *Toxoplasma* infection, or resulting from an antenatal brain perfusion disorder.

Partial agyria–pachygyria will show up echographically as ventriculomegaly (Figs. II.8.g, II.8.h). A 10 MHz scan may show very few or no sulci at all under the superior sagittal sinus in the frontotemporal area. The gyri appear to be thicker than normal and scarcer. Against an appropriate background (*e.g.* a chromosomal anomaly), hypoplasia of the cerebellar vermis or coarse parietal gyration may be seen as indicators of dysmigration. Pachygyric zones are mostly found in and on the rim of the areas perfused by the middle cerebral artery: probably this indicates a frequently ischaemic basis. The mildest end of this spectrum is the 'double cortex' or bilateral subcortical band heterotopia syndrome, in which a thin band of white matter separates the (usually normal) sylvian cortical ribbon from a band of subcortical heterotopic neurons.

The dysmigratory pattern of the Zellweger syndrome and related *peroxisomopathies* is well known: subcortical and intracortical heterotopias are found together with a discrepancy in gyral size (smaller around the insula, bigger in the upper parietal and lower temporal areas) (Figs. II.8.k, II.8.l).

Hemimegalencephaly has been found with neurofibromatosis, incontinentia pigmenti, linear naevus sebaceus of Jadassohn (epidermal naevus syndrome), hypomelanosis of Ito and Klippel–Trenaunay–Weber disease. If isolated, hemimegalencephaly is referred to as 'dysplastic' (Fig. II.8.i). In hemimegalencephalic brains it is possible to see a shift of the midline (fissure and pulsating anterior cerebral artery) towards the healthy side, provided the head is placed symmetrically. The ventricle in the megalencephalic hemisphere is dilated and irregular. Ipsilateral cortical gyri are wide and unbranched, with an ill-developed insula and shallow sulci. White matter on the hemimegalencephalic side may already be hyperdense in the neonatal period. In cerebral hemiatrophy one expects ventricular dilatation on the side of the smaller telencephalic half. Hemispheral atrophy has been described contralateral to hemimegalencephaly.

Schizencephaly is an often symmetric lesion developed in embryonic or early fetal life. Most often a parietal fissure throws a bridge between the leptomeninges and the dilated lateral ventricle. This cleft can be wide open or reduced to a slit. It is possible to identify arachnoid vessels in its edges, which is impossible with a clastic porencephalic cyst. The fissure is bordered by neuronal heterotopia which show echographically as crude nodules causing the slit to undulate. The adjacent cortex is polymicrogyric. It is not impossible to identify the finer slit on an echogram. One will concentrate on ventriculomegaly with a colpocephalic character and confirm the diagnosis with MRI.

Heterotopic neuron masses are, echographically speaking, not separable from the encircling parenchyma. Their existence may be suspected due to the presence of round bulges in a ventricular cavity (see section on phakomatoses) (Figs. II.8.h, I.8.m). Unilateral periventricular heterotopias are often non-contiguous, contrary to bilateral symmetric contiguous forms. If the neuron masses are periventricularly located, they may resemble the nodules of a phakomatosis. Heterotopias in the deep grey nuclei have been described in the case of trisomy 18. Quite often cerebellar heterotopias are associated, either of the granular type, of spool-cell type near the dentate nucleus, or else of neuronal type in the cerebellar white matter lateral to the dentate nucleus.

Heterotopic location of neurons in the leptomeninges or *ectopia* is quite frequent in, among others, fetal alcohol syndrome, lissencephaly type II and tuberous sclerosis. Ischaemia in the third trimester or postnatally in preterm infants may disturb the pial barrier and provoke any such ectopion. Mostly we are dealing with small, stalked nodules or planes, and sometimes with plaques of extracerebral cells giving the brain a lissencephalic aspect. In a rare case they will be macroscopically identifiable as an extracerebral tumour. A rare variant of anomalous migration is known as verrucous dysplasia (brain warts). Nodules will be found in the cerebral cortex with a diameter of 2–3 mm, surrounded by a rim and with a pit on top. They contain disorganized neurons from layers II and III. Those small warts are connected to white matter with a strip of myelin and an irrigating artery. No signs of inflammation or gliosis can be documented. The surrounding cortex may be normal or polymicrogyric. The warts are mainly found around the insula in parietal and frontal cortex but sometimes are also orbitofrontally located. The brain as such is often small and may lack a corpus callosum (Fig. II.6.b). Identical subcortical nodules can be seen in cerebrum, cerebellum, brainstem and retina. Locally, meningeal vascularization is often excessive (pseudo-angiomatous). Comparable verrucous dysplasia is observed with glutaric aciduria type II (Fig. II.8.j).

REFERENCES

Aicardi, J. (1991) 'The agyria–pachygyria complex: a spectrum of cortical malformations.' *Brain and Development*, **13**, 1–8.

Barth, P.G. (1989) 'Neocorticale dysplasieën.' *Tijdschrift voor Kindergeneeskunde*, **57**, 197–202.

— — (1992) 'Migrational disorders of the brain.' *Current Opinion in Neurology and Neurosurgery*, **5**, 339–343.

Bird, C.R., Gilles, F.H. (1987) 'Type I schizencephaly: CT and neuropathologic findings.' *American Journal of Neuroradiology*, **8**, 451–454.

Chamberlain, M.C., Press, G.A., Bejar, R.F. (1990) 'Neonatal schizencephaly: comparison of brain imaging.' *Pediatric Neurology*, **6**, 382–387.

Cioffi, V., Bossi, M.C., Ballarati, E., Solbiati, L. (1991) 'Lissencephaly in two brothers detected by US. A "pseudo-liver" pattern.' *Pediatric Radiology*, **21**, 512–514.

DiPietro, M.A., Brody, B.A., Kuban, K., Cole, F.S. (1984) 'Schizencephal: rare cerebral malformation demonstrated by sonography.' *American Journal of Neuroradiology*, **5**, 196–198.

Dobyns, W.B., Truwit, C.L. (1995) 'Lissencephaly and other malformations of cortical development: 1995 update.' *Neuropediatrics*, **26**, 132–147.

— — Pagon, R.A., Armstrong, D., Curry, C.J.R., Greenberg, F., Grix, A., Holmes, L.B., Laxova, R., Michels, V.V., *et al.* (1989) 'Diagnostic criteria for Walker–Warburg syndrome.' *American Journal of Medical Genetics*, **32**, 195–210.

Fariello, G., Malena, S., Lucigrai, G., Tomà, P. (1993) 'Hemimegalencephaly: early sonographic pattern.' *Pediatric Radiology*, **23**, 151–152.

King, M., Stephenson, J.B.P., Ziervogel, M., Doyle, D., Galbraith, S. (1985) 'Hemimegalencephaly —a case for hemispherectomy?' *Neuropediatrics*, **16**, 46–55.

Motte, J., Gomes, H., Morville, P., Cymbalista, M. (1987) 'Sonographic diagnosis of lissencephaly.' *Pediatric Radiology*, **17**, 362–364.

Nakai, A., Shigematsu, Y., Nishida, K., Kikawa, Y., Konishi, Y. (1996) 'MRI findings of Zellweger syndrome.' *Pediatric Neurology*, **13**, 346–348.

Pellicer, A., Cabanas, F., Perez-Higueras, A., Garcia-Alix, A., Quero, J. (1995) 'Neural migration disorders studied by cerebral ultrasound and colour Doppler flow imaging.' *Archives of Disease in Childhood*, **73**, 55–61.

Ramirez, R.E. (1984) 'Sonographic recognition of lissencephaly (agyria.)' *American Journal of Neuroradiology*, **5**, 830–831.

Sarnat, H.B. (1987) 'Disturbances of late neuronal migrations in the perinatal period.' *American Journal of Diseases of Children*, **141**, 969–980.

— — (1992) *Cerebral Dysgenesis: Embryology and Clinical Expression.* Oxford: Oxford University Press.

Schuierer, G., Kurlemann, G., Lengerke, H-J. (1993) 'Neuroimaging in lissencephalies.' *Child's Nervous System*, **9**, 391–393.

Sener, R.N. (1995) 'Hemimegalencephaly associated with contralateral hemispheral volume loss.' *Pediatric Radiology*, **25**, 387–388.

Titelbaum, D.S., Hayward, J.C., Zimmerman, R.A. (1989) 'Pachygyriclike changes: topographic appearance at MR imaging and CT and correlation with neurologic status.' *Radiology*, **173**, 663–667.

Trounce, J.Q., Fagan, D.G., Young, I.D., Levene, M.I. (1986) 'Disorders of neuronal migration: sonographic features.' *Developmental Medicine and Child Neurology*, **28**, 467–471.

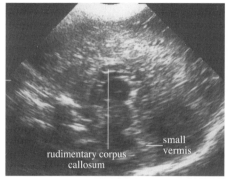

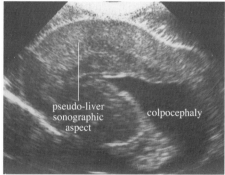

small
vermis

rudimentary corpus
callosum

pseudo-liver
sonographic
aspect

colpocephaly

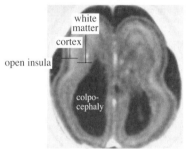

white
matter

cortex

open insula

colpo-
cephaly

Fig. II.8.e. 7.5 MHz sections: *(top left)* sagittal; *(top right)* parasagittal; and *(left)* axial T_1-weighted MR image of a preterm (31 weeks) infant with Miller–Dieker syndrome and unilateral renal agenesis. Colpocephaly, absence of gyration and an open insula are features typical of lissencephaly type I. The corpus callosum is only rudimentary, as is the cerebellar vermis. The pseudo-liver pattern of echoreflections in the telencephalic parenchyma is caused by subcortical heterotopic neurons. An anomaly of the karyotype was documented in this case.

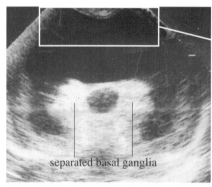

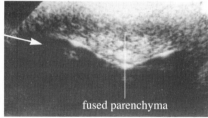

fused parenchyma

separated basal ganglia

Fig. II.8.f. Term infant with apnoea and hypotonia; bilateral retinal dysplasia and elevated muscle enzymes were subsequently found. *(Top left)* coronal section (7.5 MHz); *(top right)* coronal detail (10 MHz); *(left)* sagittal section (7.5 MHz). There is supratentorial hydrocephalus, with clear separation of the basal ganglia and apparent fusion of the sub-fontanellar parenchyma. (The falx cannot be seen with ultrasound.) The third ventricle is prolonged toward the occipital bone. The vermis and posterior fossa are small. These findings are typical of lissencephaly type II, as seen in Walker–Warburg syndrome.

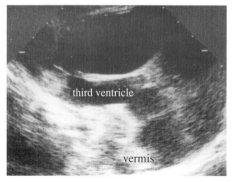

third ventricle

vermis

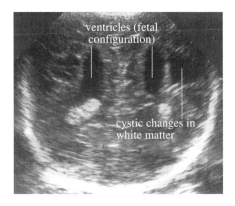

Fig. II.8.g. Term infant of a diabetic mother, with antenatally suspected ventriculomegaly: 5 MHz coronal view. The lateral ventricles have a peculiar angular shape (fetal configuration), with an upstanding dilated part and a horizontal part filled with plexus. Multiple large and small cysts are seen in periventricular white matter. MRI documented pachygyria in both middle cerebral artery fields, suggesting possible early fetal hypoperfusion damage.

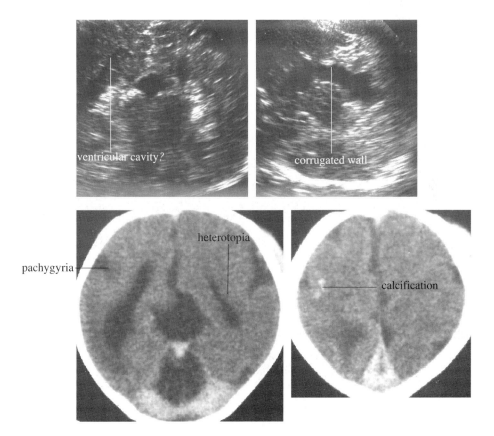

Fig. II.8.h. Term infant with microcephaly, neonatal seizures, facial dysmorphism and a very small anterior fontanelle; the karyotype was normal. *(Top)* 5 MHz coronal *(left)* and parasagittal *(right)* views. The right lateral ventricular lumen is invisible, probably due to heterotopic neuronal masses; the left ventricle's superior wall is corrugated for the same reason. *(Bottom)* CT documented pachygyria and parietal calcifications on the right.

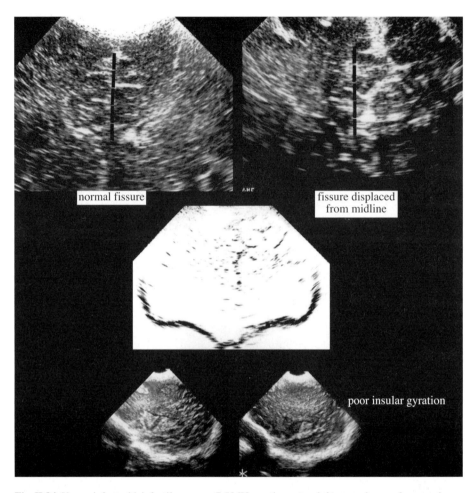

Fig. II.8.i. Young infant with infantile spasms. 7.5 MHz sections: *(top left)* coronal scan of a normal control infant; *(top right)* coronal view in this patient; *(middle)* inverted coronal image; *(bottom)* scans of affected side through the insula (*left*, control; *right*, patient). The interhemispheric fissure is displaced to the left, best seen via the linear density of the anterior cerebral artery on the inverted image. Left insular gyration is hardly present compared with the contralateral side. There was limited left ventriculomegaly; CT confirmed the diagnosis of hemimegalencephaly.

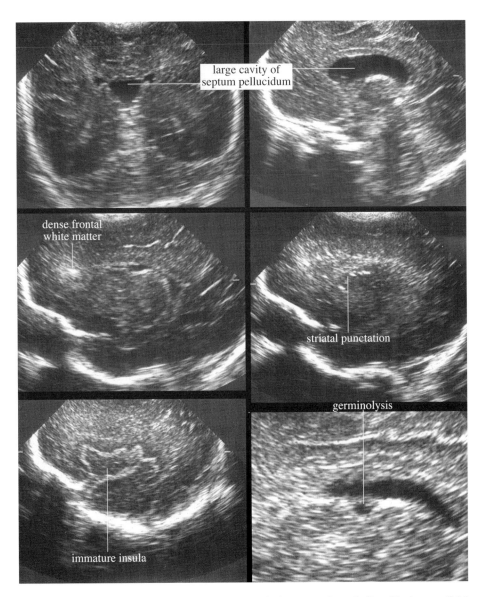

Fig. II.8.j. Term growth retarded infant with dysmorphic features and metabolic acidosis; superficial renal cysts were seen with ultrasound. All 7.5 MHz pictures (*top left*, coronal; *top right*, sagittal; others parasagittal). In this clinical context cerebral sonography can suggest a diagnosis of glutaric aciduria type II: the cavity of the septum pellucidum is enlarged; there are increased reflections from white matter, suggestive of metabolic white matter disease; striatal vessels are echogenic, seen best on parasagittal sections where their cut surfaces show up as a row of bright spots; there is cystic germinolysis in the caudothalamic groove; the insula is poorly gyrated for a term infant, and the short and long gyri are not discernible. Histologically, the brain of this child showed verrucous dysplasia, an unusual type of neuronal dysmigration.

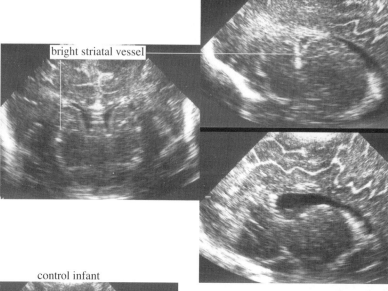

bright striatal vessel

control infant

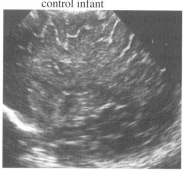

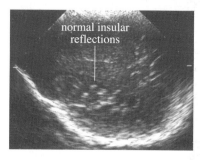

normal insular reflections

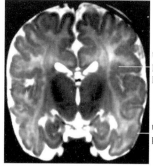

thick cortical plate with polymicrogyria

temporal pachygyria

Fig. II.8.k. Term infant, presenting with severe hypotonia and seizures; the clinical picture was comparable with classical Zellweger syndrome, but biochemical tests suggested an isolated peroxisomal enzyme defect, most likely of bifunctional protein. 7.5 MHz sections: *(top left)* coronal; *(top right)* both parasagittal; *(middle)* outer parasagittal sections through the insula of a normal infant *(left)* and of the patient *(right)*. A striatal artery is very echogenic on the right. The profile of the insular gyri does not differ sonographically from the normal. Broad gyration in the temporal area contrasts with polymicrogyria of the insular cortex seen on the coronal T_2-weighted MR image *(bottom)* but not visible with ultrasound.

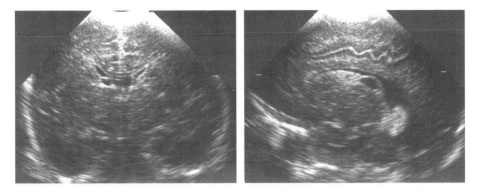

Fig. II.8.l. Term infant with intrapartum asphyxia and hypotonia, subsequently shown to have Zellweger syndrome: 7.5 MHz sections (*left*, coronal; *right*, parasagittal). There is callosal dysgenesis, recognizable by the presence of the cingulate gyrus together with a very thin callosal structure. A subependymal cyst is seen in the right caudothalamic groove.

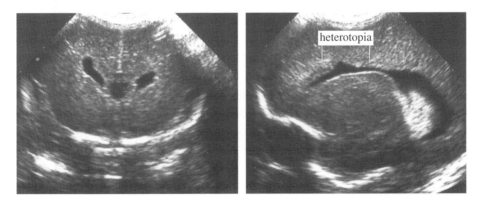

Fig. II.8.m. 28 weeks gestation growth retarded preterm infant: 7.5 MHz sections (*left*, coronal; *right*, parasagittal). The corrugations of the upper lateral ventricle wall were shown at postmortem examination to correlate with periventricular heterotopia.

II.9 POSTERIOR FOSSA ANOMALIES

After the 16th intrauterine week the fourth ventricle is completely covered by vermis. Growth of the vermis is particularly rapid during the third trimester of pregnancy. The greatest absolute depth for the cisterna magna (distance of bone to lower ridge of the vermis) occurs between the 20th and 28th weeks of pregnancy: normal depth is then at a maximum of 10 mm. The upper limit of normal in the term infant is 8 mm. Congenital malformations of the cerebellum are often interwoven with anomalies of the brainstem or diencephalon. They emerge between the 7th and 10th gestational week and, apart from rhombencephalic structures, the adjacent brain membranes are often affected as well. Only manifest cerebellar anomalies can be detected sonographically. Different authors have proposed different subdivisions of congenital cerebellar disorders, an example of which is illustrated in Figure II.9.a.

Hypoplasia or even *aplasia of the cerebellar vermis* is present in the syndromes of Joubert and of Dekaban, in tectocerebellar dysraphism, in rhombencephalosynapsis, in association with holoprosencephaly and with Arnold–Chiari or Dandy–Walker malformation. Three elements obligatory in *Dandy–Walker malformation* are: (1) vermis hypoplasia (especially inferior part) or absence, (2) large posterior fossa with elevated torcula and sinuses; and (3) retrocerebellar cyst starting at the roof of the fourth ventricle and lined with ependyma on a layer of glial tissue with, at the outside, a second layer of meningeal tissue. The occipital squama is thinner than normal above this dilated posterior fossa. Supratentorial hydrocephalus occurs in about 50% of the perinatally recognized cases of Dandy–Walker malformation. This represents about 3% of all instances of congenital hydrocephalus.

A Dandy–Walker malformation can be identified sonographically through the presence of a cyst, communicating with the fourth ventricle and widening the posterior fossa (Figs. II.9.b, II.9.f). The torcula has almost always been moved upwards. The vermis has disappeared caudally. Often vermal remnants have been rotated dorsally and cranially. The broadened fourth ventricle pushes the cerebellar hemispheres aside ('splaying'). Plexus tissue rests against the lateral and dorsal walls of this cyst. In certain manifest cases remnants of cerebellar hemisphere may be found only underneath the tentorium. As this residual cerebellum may be large, a section immediately adjacent to the sagittal plane may suggest the existence of a fourth ventricle: the 'pseudo fourth ventricle'. Correct frontal sonography will show that the ventricle is opened widely toward the retrocerebellar space. Less grotesque forms of the same spectrum are sometimes called Dandy–Walker variant: the fourth ventricle is dilated and communicates with the arachnoid spaces under a partially atrophic inferior vermis (Fig. II.9.g). In this case the posterior fossa is, as a rule, no larger than normal. Independent of the duration of pregnancy the fetal cisterna magna is rarely wider than 10 mm, as measured in an axial section. A 'mega cisterna magna' may be accompanied by hydrocephalus but is by definition not accompanied by any cerebellar anomaly and the fourth ventricle is not enlarged. To refer to that condition the terms 'mega cisterna magna' and 'arachnoid cyst of the posterior fossa' are often used in conjunction.

Global cerebellar hypoplasia or atrophy can be suspected in the presence of a large fourth ventricle and broad pericerebellar cisterns with deep grooves between the foliae, while the normal macrostructure of the cerebellum remains unchanged. Often the internal granular layer is particularly affected. A subgroup of global cerebellar hypoplasias is associated with atrophy of the base of the pons and quite often the inferior olive: ponto-cerebellar atrophies or hypoplasias. At least four variants can be distinguished.

The *Arnold–Chiari malformation type II* is highly associated with spina bifida cystica (Figs. II.1.c, II.2.f). Apart from herniation of the cerebellar tonsils through the foramen magnum (Arnold–Chiari malformation type I), one will also find herniation of vermis and fourth ventricle together with a bend in the cervicomedullary junction. Quite often this anomaly is associated with hydrocephalus and low cervical syringomyelia. Its character-istics have been discussed in the section on neurulation disorders.

Antenatal *arachnoid cysts of the posterior fossa* are not always located in the midline (Figs. II.9.c, II.9.d). They do not lead to dilatation of the fourth ventricle or hypoplasia of the vermis. These cysts may or may not communicate with the surrounding normal arach-noid spaces. Often hydrocephalus is brought about by compression of the structures in the posterior fossa. In a child with hydrocephalus, compression of brainstem and cerebellum by the cyst may make differentiation from the Dandy–Walker malformation particularly difficult. Association with other congenital anomalies is not exceptional.

Rhombencephalosynapsis is a particularly rare phenomenon causing the cerebellar hemispheres to merge, thus giving rise to one single microcerebellar mass behind and on the brainstem. The dentate nuclei have merged on the midline into a horseshoe-shaped nucleus, whereas the central cerebellar nuclei are absent. Thalami, inferior colliculi and cerebral peduncles can be fused as well. Aqueductal stenosis often occurs.

Unilateral hemispheric hypoplasia can be detected in neonates with Moebius syndrome, but it can also be asymptomatic. The ipsilateral inferior cerebellar peduncles and the contra-lateral inferior olivary nucleus are then atrophied.

Vermal hypoplasia can be suggested by dilatation of the fourth ventricle and widened cisterna magna and pericerebellar cisterns. The most serious malformation of the posterior fossa, only found in association with the clinical syndrome of Joubert (characteristic episodes of tachypnoea), is *tectocerebellar dysraphism*. In that case the tectum has been occipitally prolonged into a tissue band which may spill out through the occipital bone (Fig. II.9.e). Due to the absence of the vermis, the fourth ventricle may show on a sagittal section as a hypodense longitudinal structure with, above and below, pieces of cerebellar hemisphere ('hot-dog' picture). Differentiation from Dandy–Walker variant may prove to be difficult on an echogram if there is no occipital encephalocele.

REFERENCES

Adamsbaum, C., Moreau, V., Bulteau, C., Burstyn, J., Lair Milan, F., Kalifa, G. (1994) 'Vermian agenesis without posterior fossa cyst.' *Pediatric Radiology*, **24**, 543–546.
Barkovich, A.J., Kjos, B.O.. (1989) 'Normal postnatal development of the corpus callosum as demonstrated by MR imaging.' *American Journal of Neuroradiology*, **9**, 487–491.
Barth, P. G. (1993) 'Pontocerebellar hypoplasias. An overview of a group of inherited neurodegenerative dis-orders with fetal onset.' *Brain and Development*, **15**, 411–422.
Bawle, E.V., Kupsky, W.J., D'Amato, C.J., Becker, C.J., Hicks, S. (1995) 'Familial infantile olivopontocerebel-lar atrophy.' *Pediatric Neurology*, **13**, 14–18.

Bordarier, C., Aicardi, J. (1990) 'Dandy–Walker syndrome and agenesis of the cerebellar vermis: diagnostic problems and genetic counselling.' *Developmental Medicine and Child Neurology*, **32**, 285–294.

Comstock, C.H., Boal, D.B. (1985) 'Enlarged fetal cisterna magna: appearance and significance.' *Obstetrics and Gynecology*, **66**, 25S–28S.

Charney, E.B., Rorke, L.B., Sutton, L.N., Schut, L. (1987) 'Management of Chiari II complications in infants with myelomeningocoele.' *Journal of Pediatrics*, **111**, 364–371.

Friede, R.L. (1989) *Developmental Neuropathology. Dysplasias of Cerebellum*. Berlin: Springer-Verlag.

Golden, J.A., Rorke, L.B., Bruce, D.A. (1987) 'Dandy–Walker syndrome and associated anomalies.' *Pediatric Neuroscience*, **13**, 38–44.

Goodwin, L., Quisling, R.G. (1983) 'The neonatal cisterna magna: ultrasonic evaluation.' *Radiology*, **149**, 691–695.

Hourihane, J.O'B., Bennett, C.P., Chaudhuri, R., Robb, S.A., Martin, N.D.T. (1993) 'A sibship with a neuronal migration defect, cerebellar hypoplasia and congenital lymphedema.' *Neuropediatrics*, **24**, 43–46.

Hunter, A.G.W. (1993) 'Brain.' *In:* Stevenson, R.E., Hall, J.G., Goodman, R.M. (Eds.) *Human Malformations and Related Anomalies. Vol. II. Oxford Monographs on Medical Genetics, No. 27*. Oxford: Oxford University Press, pp. 82–96.

King, M.D., Dudgeon, J., Stephenson, J.B.P. (1984) 'Joubert's sydrome with retinal dysplasia: neonatal tachypnoea as the clue to a genetic brain–eye malformation.' *Archives of Disease in Childhood*, **59**, 709–718.

Mahony, B.S., Callen, P.W., Filly, R.A., Hoddick, W.K. (1984) 'The fetal cisterna magna.' *Radiology*, **153**, 773–776.

Nakamura, Y., Hashimoto, T., Sasaguri, Y., Yamana, K., Tanaka, S., Morodomi, T., Murakami, T., Maehara, F., Nakashima, T., Fukuda, S., Nakashima, H. (1986) 'Brain anomalies found in 18 trisomy: CT scanning, morphologic and morphometric study.' *Clinical Neuropathology*, **5**, 47–52.

Nyberg, D.A., Cyr, D.R., Mack, L.A., Fitzsimmons, J., Hickok, D., Mahony, B.S. (1988) 'The Dandy–Walker malformation: prenatal sonographic diagnosis and its clinical significance.' *Journal of Ultrasound Medicine*, **7**, 65–71.

Paidas, M.J., Cohen, A. (1994) 'Disorders of the central nervous system.' *Seminars in Perinatology*, **18**, 266–282.

Raybaud, C. (1982) 'Les malformations cystiques de la fosse postérieure. Anomalies associées du développement du toit du 4ème ventricule et des structures méningées adjacentes.' *Journal de Neuroradiologie*, **9**, 103–133.

Saraiva, J.M., Baraitser, M. (1992) 'Joubert syndrome: a review.' *American Journal of Medical Genetics*, **43**, 726–731.

Taylor, G.A., Sanders, R.C. (1983) 'Dandy–Walker syndrome: recognition by sonography.' *American Journal of Neuroradiology*, **4**, 1203–1206.

Welch, K., Lorenzo, A.V. (1991) 'Pathology of hydrocephalus.' *In:* Bannister, CM, Tew, B. (Eds.) *Current Concepts in Spina Bifida and Hydrocephalus. Clinics in Developmental Medicine No. 122*. London: Mac Keith Press, pp. 55–82.

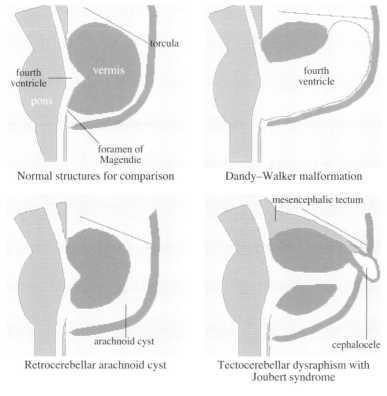

Normal structures for comparison

Dandy–Walker malformation

Retrocerebellar arachnoid cyst

Tectocerebellar dysraphism with
Joubert syndrome

Fig. II.9.a. Sonographically recognizable congenital anomalies in the posterior fossa.

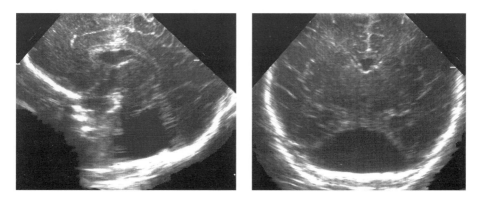

Fig. II.9.b. Term newborn infant with episodic apnoea, interrupted by tachypnoeic episodes: 7.5 MHz sections *(left*, sagittal; *right*, coronal). The supratentorial structures were completely normal in this child; MRI confirmed total absence of the cerebellum, although the question of some infratentorial remnants remained open. The child died because of hypoventilation; postmortem examination was refused. Some of the features of Dandy–Walker malformation were present, but cerebellar absence militates against such a classification.

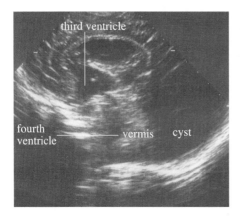
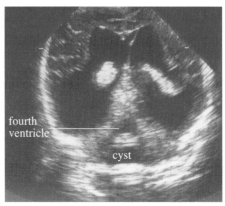

Fig. II.9.c. Term infant with congenital hydrocephalus: 5 MHz sections (*left*, sagittal; *right*, coronal posterior). All ventricles show dilatation (communicating hydrocephalus). A large cystic structure (posterior fossa arachnoid cyst) is present behind the normal cerebellar vermis.

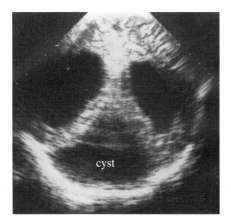
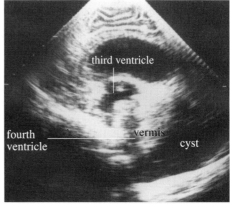

Fig. II.9.d. Term infant with congenital hydrocephalus: 5 MHz sections (*left*, coronal posterior; *right*, sagittal). All ventricles show dilatation (communicating hydrocephalus). A large cystic structure (posterior fossa arachnoid cyst) is present behind the normal but clearly compressed cerebellar vermis.

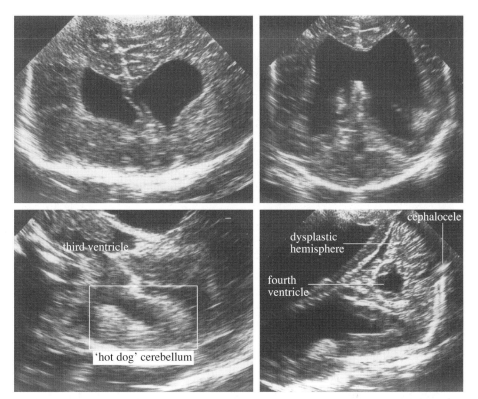

Fig. II.9.e. Term newborn girl with nystagmoid eye movements, episodic tachypnoea interrupted by apnoeic periods, occipital cephalocele, microcystic kidney disease and absence of visual evoked potentials. 7.5 MHz sections: *top*, coronal (*left*, anterior; *right*, posterior to the foramen of Monro); *bottom left*, sagittal; *bottom right*, axial. One anomaly associated with the clinical Joubert syndrome is tectocerebellar dysraphism; the cerebellum is small and dysplastic, with severe vermal atrophy; the fourth ventricle is prolonged, together with tectal tissue remnants, into an occipital meningo-hydro-encephalocele; in sagittal view the cut hemispheric mesial portions create the impression that the fourth ventricle is a sausage-shaped hypodensity with parenchymal roof and floor ('hot-dog' cerebellum). Supratentorial hydrocephalus is associated.

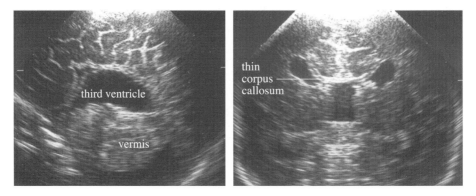

Fig. II.9.f. Term infant with tetralogy of Fallot and talipes. 7.5 MHz sections: *left*, sagittal; *right*, coronal. The corpus callosum is present but severely dysplastic and with abnormal surrounding gyral architecture (normal cingulate gyrus not recognized). There is moderate dilatation of lateral and third ventricles. The posterior fossa is enlarged due to the presence of a cystic structure that pushes the cerebellum up and to the front. It is not possible sonographically to prove Dandy–Walker malformation, but the cluster of changes is suggestive of it.

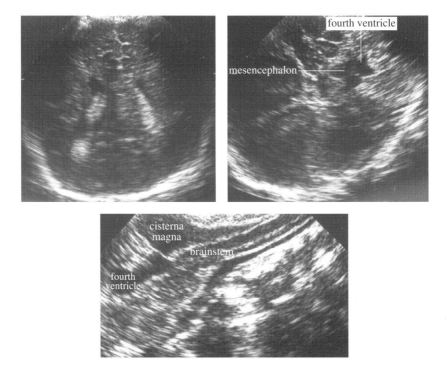

Fig. II.9.g. Term infant with CHARGE association, oesophageal atresia, right cleft hand and bifurcation of the distal end of the right femur: 7.5 MHz sections (*top*, right axial; *bottom*, nuchal sagittal). The fourth ventricle is enlarged, its surface approaching that of the mesencephalon. A wide communication is seen between the fourth ventricle and the cisterna magna.

II.10 INTRACRANIAL FLUID COLLECTIONS

The various types of hydrocephalus (the collection of excessive CSF in normal brain structures such as ventricles and subarachnoid space) are discussed in subsequent sections. Cyst formation in the parenchyma can of course be found after destruction caused by haemorrhage or ischaemia and will be discussed in the appropriate sections. In the midline one should consider a varix of the great vein of Galen, median cavities against the background of holoprosencephaly or anomalies of the corpus callosum and septum pellucidum, a basocranial arachnoid cyst or a cystic tumour (*e.g.* craniopharyngioma).

Quadrigeminal cyst

A sagittal section through the anterior fontanelle quite often shows an echopoor zone behind and above the superior colliculi, under the splenium of the corpus callosum. Follow-up of some of these 'cysts' allowed us to observe that they did not grow but remained visible for months. We were probably dealing with a dilatation of the quadrigeminal cistern (Fig. II.10.a).

Arachnoid cyst

Two thirds of these lesions are supratentorially located, especially in the temporal fossa and along the sylvian fissure. Location above the sella turcica, in the cerebellopontine angle, on the vermis and in the quadrigeminal cistern are less common. In a rare instance the cyst may be located between and in front of the cerebral peduncles, over the cerebral convexity or interhemispherically (Figs. II.10.d, II.10e). Usually we deal with one single cyst, located on the left. In the posterior cranial fossa they are mostly located in the sagittal plane and exert pressure on the aqueduct (if located behind the colliculi) or interfere with CSF circulation around the cerebellum, generally provoking hydrocephalus. It is difficult to make a distinction between an arachnoid cyst and a very big cisterna magna because, in that particular location, the cysts generally adapt in shape to the surrounding structures. Histological examination is the only exact way of confirming a diagnosis of arachnoid cyst formation.

After perinatal subarachnoid haematoma a cyst may fill the temporal lobe, difficult to distinguish *in vivo* from an arachnoid cyst. A cyst may develop in the cisterna magna after intraventricular haemorrhage (Fig. II.10.c). Exceptionally there is association with cerebral hemiatrophy (see related section). Even for antenatal onset cysts it is believed they are the result of a secondary injury to primitive leptomeninges, causing a split that gradually fills with arachnoid fluid. Mature cysts may have lost communication with the arachnoid space.

Ependymal cyst

Ependymal cysts are particularly rare. The intraventricular form or colloid cyst is best known. Those cysts are bordered by ependyma on a neuroglial basis. They may also occur in the frontral lobe or between the hemispheres (Fig. II.10.b). They do not communicate with ventricular cavities. Dependent upon their size and location they may cause neonatal signs such as apnoea on account of pressure exerted, for instance, from within the ambient cistern. Association with other brain anomalies may accelerate clinical presentation.

Neurenteric cyst

These are mostly found in the posterior fossa, exerting pressure on the brainstem. We are dealing with remnants of the neurenteric channel temporarily existing in the embryo.

REFERENCES

Barth, P.G., Uylings, H.B.M., Stam, F.C. (1984) 'Interhemispheral neuroepithelial (glio-ependymal) cysts, associated with agenesis of the corpus callosum and neocortical maldevelopment.' *Child's Brain*, **11**, 312–319.

Meizner, I., Barki, Y., Tadmor, R., Katz, M. (1988) '*In utero* ultrasonic detection of fetal arachnoid cyst.' *Journal of Clinical Ultrasound*, **16**, 506–509.

Naidich, T.P., McLone, D.G., Radowski, M.A. (1986) 'Intracranial arachnoid cysts.' *Pediatric Neuroscience*, **12**, 112–122.

Norman, M.G., Ludwin, S.K. (1991) 'Congenital malformations of the nervous system.' *In:* Davis, R.L., Roberts, D.M. (Eds.) *Textbook of Neuropathology. 2nd Edn*. Baltimore: Williams & Wilkins, pp. 207–280.

Norman, M.G., McGillivray, B.C., Kalousek, D.K., Hill, A., Poskitt, K.J. (1995) 'Abnormalities of the skull, meninges, choroid plexus and blood vessels.' *In: Congenital Malformations of the Brain*. Oxford: Oxford: Oxford University Press, pp. 368–370.

Rahman, N., Adam, K.A.R. (1986) 'Congenital polycystic disease of the brain: report of an unusual case.' *Developmental Medicine and Child Neurology*, **28**, 72–76.

Rengachary, S.S., Watanabe, I. (1981) 'Ultrastructure and pathogenesis of intracranial arachnoid cysts.' *Journal of Neuropathology and Experimental Neurology*, **40**, 61–83.

Zalatnai, A. (1987) 'Neurenteric cyst of medulla oblongata—a curiosity.' *Neuropediatrics*, **18**, 40–41.

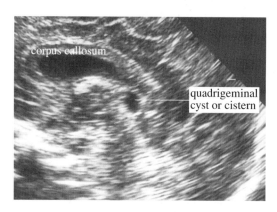

Fig. II.10.a. Routine ultrasound examination (7.5 MHz sagittal section) before discharge of preterm infant with respiratory distress syndrome. Note cystic aspect of the quadrigeminal cistern underneath the splenium of the corpus callosum. At age 1 year a CT scan confirmed the (asymptomatic) presence of a cyst, 1 cm in diameter. A larger tectal plate cyst has been found in unexplained death in infancy (Norman and Ludwin 1991).

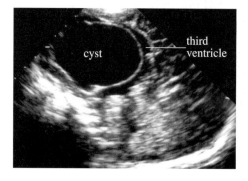

Fig. II.10.b. Term newborn infant with macrocephaly: sagittal 7.5 MHz section. A large median interhemispheric cyst is compressing the third ventricle and foramina of Monro with resultant dilatation of the lateral ventricles (not shown here). Other cysts were seen with sonography and MRI. The probable diagnosis is glio-ependymal cysts.

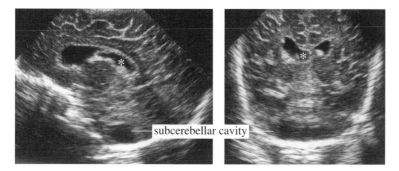

Fig. II.10.c. Preterm infant (26 weeks gestation) with hydrocephalus following bleeding in the right caudothalamic groove matrix: 7.5 MHz sections in the third postnatal month (*left*, sagittal; *right*, coronal). The right lateral ventricle crosses the midline to invade the cavity of Verga (*asterisks*). Underneath the vermis, organizing posterior fossa clot induced a cavity, probably an arachnoid cyst.

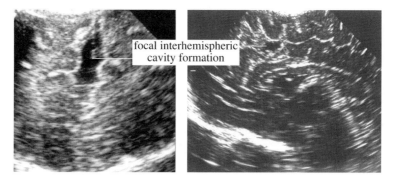

Fig. II.10.d. 7.5 MHz sections of two ventilated term infants (*left*, coronal in front of the foramen of Monro; *right*, sagittal). Both children were incidentally found to have a focal dilatation of the arachnoid space in between the frontal hemispheres. These cavitations were not preceded by parenchymal injury in the area. The significance of this finding is unknown.

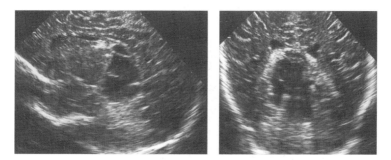

Fig. II.10.e. Term infant with antenatally recognized interhemispheric cyst: 7.5 MHz sections (*left*, parasagittal; *right*, coronal) at 3 months of age. During endoscopy the cavity was shown to be an interhemispheric arachnoid cyst.

Symmetric ventricular dilatation

Hydrocephalus can take three forms: (1) internal and symmetric, with dilatation of at least both lateral ventricles; (2) internal but asymmetric, following focal narrowing or valve mechanism at one of the foramina or a part of a ventricle; (3) external, through excessive accumulation of CSF in the subarachnoid space. The causes are hypersecretion of CSF, obstruction to its circulation, decreased resorption, or loss of parenchyma ('*ex vacuo*'). Any type of early fetal hydrocephalus leads to polygyria: lack of space encourages the formation of abundant but small gyri, with histologically normal cortex.

This section is concerned with symmetric ventriculomegaly of the neonate (Fig. II.10.f). We may exceptionally be confronted with isolated hereditary hydrocephalus: (1) X-linked with or without aqueductal stenosis or cerebellar agenesis; (2) autosomal recessive; (3) sibling of a child with neural tube defect; (4) due to ciliary dyskinesia; (5) due to agenesis of arachnoid villi; (6) familial colpocephaly; (7) familial porencephaly; (8) familial vasculopathy with extreme hydrocephalus. The annual incidence rate of hereditary congenital hydrocephalus is estimated at about 0.5 per 1000 liveborn infants. Overall incidence rates, independent of cause, vary around 3 per 1000.

Aqueductal stenosis (Figs. II.10.g, II.10.i) exists in autosomal and X-linked recessive forms. The distinction between malformative and acquired stenosis is less straightforward than formerly believed. Early clastic or infective lesions do not cause gliosis, and forking has on the other hand been noticed with malformative types (dysplasia of the aqueduct in holoprosencephaly and lissencephaly type II). An association exists between stenosis of the aqueduct near the superior colliculi and pressure on the tectum through the pineal recess of the third ventricle and the temporal horns of the lateral ventricles. Minimal stenosis is sometimes seen with neurofibromatosis: a membrane partially occludes the aqueduct as it enters the fourth ventricle.

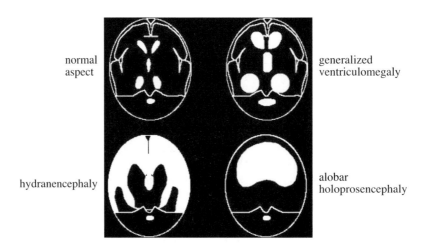

Fig. II.10.f. Types of symmetric ventriculomegaly. The white areas represent CSF collections.

Colpocephaly refers to ventriculomegaly of the occipital horns without clear frontal dilatation. This may be due to a developmental disturbance (in fetal months 1–4) or destruction of occipital periventricular white matter. Colpocephaly may be found in association with lissencephaly and pachygyria, with porencephaly, with agenesis of the corpus callosum and with heterotopia. Due to its non-specific character it is advisable not to consider colpocephaly a disease proper, but rather part of an overlying cerebral anomaly.

It is not difficult to differentiate between obstructive hydrocephalus and encephaloclastic sequelae with hydrocephalus *ex vacuo*: (1) in the latter situation we are dealing with microcephalic children, with normal fontanelle tension; (2) occipital as well as frontal ventricular segments are affected compared with prominent occipital dilatation in obstructive hydrocephalus; (3) with brain atrophy one finds dilated subarachnoid spaces and a dilated interhemispheric fissure (also seen with disordered neurulation); (4) changes in the velocity of cerebral arterial flow may be seen only with obstructive hydrocephalus (high resistance in diastole) (Fig. II.10.k).

REFERENCES

Garg, B.P. (1982) 'Colpocephaly. An error of morphogenesis?' *Archives of Neurology*, **39**, 243–246.
Noorani, P.A., Bodensteiner, J.B., Barnes, P.D. (1988) 'Colpocephaly: frequency and associated findings.' *Journal of Child Neurology*, **3**, 100–104.
Pober, B.R., Greene, M.F., Holmes, L.B. (1986) 'Complexities of intraventricular abnormalities.' *Journal of Pediatrics*, **108**, 545–551.
Raimondi, A.J. (1994) 'A unifying theory for the definition and classification of hydrocephalus.' *Child's Nervous System*, **10**, 2–12.
Welch, K., Lorenzo, A.V. (1991) 'Pathology of hydrocephalus.' *In:* Bannister, CM, Tew, B. (Eds) *Current Concepts in Spina Bifida and Hydrocephalus. Clinics in Developmental Medicine No. 122.* London: Mac Keith Press, pp. 55–82.

TABLE II.2
Brain changes in disorders with symmetric ventricular dilatation

Disorder	Telencephalic tissue	Falx	Median cavity	Choroid plexus	Thalami
Hydrocephalus	Present	Present	If septum pellucidum absent	Prominent	Separated
Hydranencephaly	Regional absence	May be absent	Massive	Normal	Separated, atrophic
Alobar holoprosencephaly	Absent posteriorly	Absent	Holosphere	Lying on basal grey matter	Fused
Callosal agenesis	Present	Present	Elevated third ventricle	Prominent	Separated
Lissencephaly type II	Present	Present	Third ventricle	Unremarkable	Separated

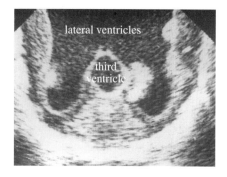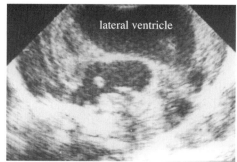

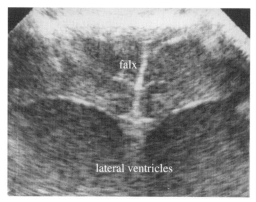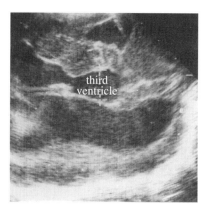

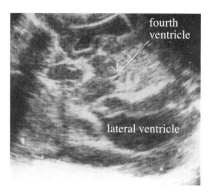

Fig. II.10.g. Stillborn 36 week gestation infant with cloverleaf skull and camptomelic dwarfism: 7.5 MHz sections (*top left*, coronal; *top right*, sagittal; *centre left*, coronal detail (10 MHz); *centre right*, axial; *bottom*, axial). In this child hydrocephalus affected the supratentorial ventricles only. The fourth ventricle is visible but its size is not in accord with obvious dilatation of lateral and third ventricles. The falx is recognizable and the hemispheres are separated. The third ventricle is extended to the rear. These findings suggested aqueductal stenosis, which was confirmed at postmortem examination.

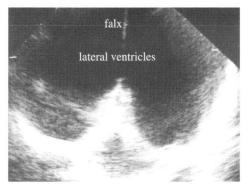

falx

lateral ventricles

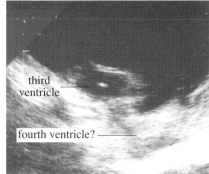

third ventricle

fourth ventricle?

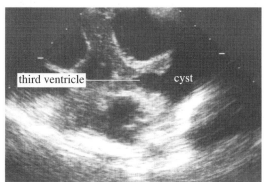

third ventricle   cyst

Fig. II.10.h. Term infant of consanguineous parents, with hexadactyly, retinal dysplasia and macrocephaly; muscular dystrophy was clinically unlikely, and the anterior eye chambers were not dysplastic. 5 MHz images (*top left*, coronal; *top right*, sagittal; *left*, axial). Note dilatation of third and lateral ventricles, with small fourth ventricle in a small posterior fossa. On axial section the aqueduct is seen to open into a cystic structure apparently communicating with a lateral ventricle. The falx is clearly visible.

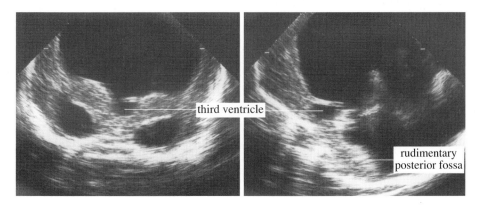

third ventricle

rudimentary posterior fossa

Fig. II.10.i. Monozygotic twin pregnancy, complicated by fetofetal transfusion. The donor twin suffered from cystic periventricular leukomalacia. This child, the recipient, presented with oesophageal atresia and macrocephaly. 7.5 MHz sections (*top*, coronal; *bottom*, sagittal). Dilatation of the supratentorial ventricles, with rudimentary posterior fossa and invisible fourth ventricle suggest aqueductal atresia.

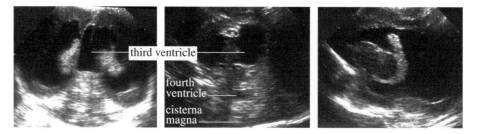

Fig. II.10.j. Term infant of consanguineous parents, with clinical diagnosis of oro-facio-digital syndrome: 5 MHz images (*top*, coronal; *middle*, sagittal; *bottom*, parasagittal). All ventricles are dilated, including the fourth. The cisterna magna is clearly visible and large. A dorsal expansion of the third ventricle obscures the midline image. The corpus callosum and cingulate gyrus are not visible. The choroid plexus points upward from the atrium into the body of the lateral ventricle.

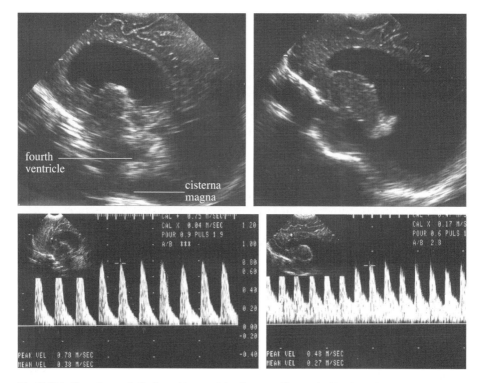

Fig. II.10.k. Growth retarded infant with unexplained postnatally acquired hydrocephalus. *(Top)* 7.5 MHz images (*left*, sagittal; *right*, parasagittal). *(Bottom)* Doppler flow velocities in the anterior cerebral artery before (*left*) and after (*right*) the first lumbar puncture, which yielded 20 mL clear fluid. All ventricles, including the fourth, are dilated; the cisterna magna is enlarged. Conservative treatment with furosemide, acetazolamide and serial lumbar punctures was started. Following initial succes, a ventriculo-atrial shunt was nevertheless needed in early infancy. An increase of diastolic flow velocities is clearly seen following release of the pressure with lumbar puncture. It is impossible to exclude a retrocerebellar arachnoid cyst as the cause of hydrocephalus in this child.

Unilateral hydrocephalus

An asymmetric configuration of the occipital horns is quite common, with one in two newborn infants having a slightly more dilated left horn. The term 'unilateral hydrocephalus' refers to the rare situation whereby a newborn infant shows obvious asymmetric ventricular dilatation.

An obstructive tumoral lesion around the foramen of Monro has to be excluded in the first place. Inflammation within the ventricles may be another mechanism whereby fetal mumps was reported as a cause. We have seen a case of unilateral hydrocephalus with congenital toxoplasmosis (Fig. II.10.l). In spina bifida hypertrophic choroid plexus may exert an occlusive effect. Real malformation of a foramen may exist, quite often in relation with other congenital anomalies. Finally, the foramen of Monro may be obstructed following regression of a major subependymal matrix bleed (Fig. II.10.o).

Exceptionally, unilateral hydrocephalus will regress or stabilize without the need for surgical drainage. In some cases a porencephalic cyst, for instance after an infarct in the area of the middle cerebral artery, blows up under pressure and requires surgical treatment. This is called *expansive unilateral porencephaly* ('*porencéphalie soufflante*') (Fig. II.10.m).

The echographic aspects will depend on the underlying cause. Secondary phenomena are displacement of the midline and possibly asymmetric insertion of the septum pellucidum under the contralateral cingulate gyrus. We came across a strange presentation of asymmetric hydrocephalus (Fig. II.10.n). In the left caudothalamic groove and in the left choroid glomus of an asymptomatic term newborn infant, a hypoechogenic to isodense hourglass-shaped tumour was found. The ipsilateral periventricular white matter had been invaded by echodense strings from the ventricular cavity. Common causes of fetal infection and a disorder of haemostasis were excluded. CT scanning and MR angiography suggested that vascular anomalies were highly improbable. During ventriculoscopy the mass on the left plexus was ablated: the material thus obtained appeared to be old blood and connective tissue. The mother had had a generalized epileptic seizure around the 12th gestational week, and we diagnosed fetal plexus bleeding with hygromatous organization in the form of a tumour. Follow-up excluded a genuine tumour.

REFERENCES

Anderson, N., Malpas, T., Davison, M. (1993) 'Prenatal diagnosis of unilateral hydrocephalus.' *Pediatric Radiology*, **23**, 69–70.
Baumann, B., Danon, L., Weitz, R., Blumensohn, R., Schonfeld, T., Nitzan, M. (1982) 'Unilateral hydrocephalus due to obstruction of the foramen of Monro : another complication of intrauterine mumps infection?' *European Journal of Pediatrics*, **139**, 158–159.
Gaston, B.M., Jones, B.E. (1989) 'Perinatal unilateral hydrocephalus. Atresia of the foramen of Monro.' *Pediatric Radiology*, **19**, 328–329.
Heibel, M., Heber, R., Bechinger, D., Kornhuber, H.H. (1993) 'Early diagnosis of perinatal cerebral lesions in apparently normal full-term newborns by ultrasound of the brain.' *Neuroradiology*, **35**, 85–91.
Pfeiffer, G., Friede, R.L. (1984) 'Unilateral hydrocephalus from early developmental occlusion of one foramen of Monro.' *Acta Neuropathologica*, **64**, 75–77.
Sherer, D.M., Allen, T.A., Ghezzi, F., Epstein, L.G. (1995) 'Prenatal diagnosis of moderate unilateral hydrocephalus subsequently not requiring neonatal decompression.' *American Journal of Perinatology*, **12**, 50–52.
Tardieu, M., Evrard, P., Lyon, G. (1981) 'Progressive expanding congenital porencephalies: a treatable cause of progressive encephalopathy.' *Pediatrics*, **68**, 198–202.

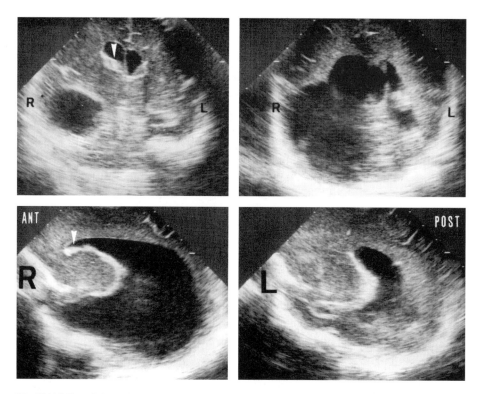

Fig. II.10.l. Term infant with congenital toxoplasmosis: 7.5 MHz views (*upper*, coronal; *lower*, parasagittal). Hydrocephalus is clearly asymmetric; calcific deposits are best seen near the right caudothalamic groove (*arrowheads*), presumably pointing to an intense inflammatory focus.

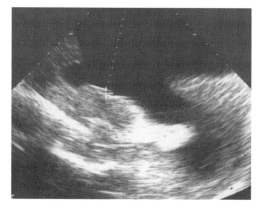

Fig. II.10.m. Term infant with ventriculomegaly, diagnosed prenatally: parasagittal 7.5 MHz section showing unilateral expansive porencephaly, the cause of which remained elusive. Conversion of maternal rubella titres occurred late in the second trimester, but neither the virus nor specific antibodies were found in the newborn infant.

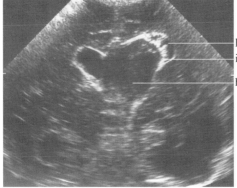

lateral ventricle
irregular dense margin

hygroma

Fig. II.10.n. Ventriculomegaly in a term infant, diagnosed prenatally. The mother had a low-grade astrocytoma, and had two fits during her pregnancy, the first at 12 weeks. Coronal 7.5 MHz scan performed in the early neonatal period shows a hypodense mass filling the foramina of Monro, occluding all but a small part of the left ventricle. The margins of the mass are feathered and hyperechogenic. Following ventriculoscopic surgery, this tissue was found to be an old hygromatous haemorrhagic remnant, resting in choroid plexus.

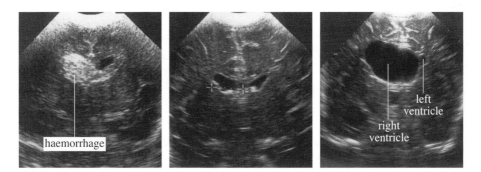

haemorrhage

left ventricle

right ventricle

Fig. II.10.o. Preterm infant (27 weeks gestation), scanned in the first week of life, and at 3 and 6 months (all 7.5 MHz coronal images). A large right germinal matrix haemorrhage lodged near the caudothalamic groove apparently disappears with mild ventriculomegaly at 3 months. However, at 6 months cystic dilatation has affected the occluded right lateral ventricle, shifting the midline and displacing the normal contralateral ventricle.

External hydrocephalus
This term refers to the existence of widened pericerebral and/or pericerebellar arachnoid spaces. It implies that the fissures and sulci are too prominent. The cisterns at the base of the cranium and around the brainstem are more pronounced than normal. In the normal preterm infant there is more extracerebral fluid, especially parieto-occipitally. In the perinatal period, the greatest width in regions other than insular and parieto-occipital is shown to be 4 mm. External hydrocephalus is best interpreted together with the occipitofrontal circumference. In association with normo- or macrocephaly, widened arachnoid spaces may indicate a distal block to the CSF circulation or a decreased resorption of CSF in the cranial sinuses.

In the neonatal period external hydrocephalus is uncommon, but its identification is important on account of its association with serious disorders. In our experience these have included: neonatal presentation of myotonic dystrophy; transient neonatal diabetes insipidus; fetofetal transfusion; arthrogryposis following global fetal brain ischaemia; superior vena cava syndrome due to venous thrombosis; non-immune hydrops associated with antenatal bowel necrosis; Kniest disease (Fig. II.10.u); and lysosomal storage disease. Manifest widening of the extracerebral CSF spaces may also be found with congenital microcephaly.

In infancy progressive widening of the subarachnoid spaces with transient macrocrania is regularly observed, especially in children seen as outpatients after neonatal intensive care. Preterm infants discharged from the neonatal unit may show widened arachnoid spaces. This will only forecast cerebral atrophy if it is accompanied by (cystic) leukomalacia and/or ventriculomegaly. The subarachnoid CSF collection is hypodense (<15 HU) on CT and shows by definition a normal protein content. Infantile macrocephaly is initially best investigated with ultrasound. On routine cranial scans (7.5 MHz) the sulci and gyri under the fontanelles are easily identifiable (Figs. II.10.q–t). The interhemispheric fissure has widened, allowing for immediate identification of the falx.

External hydrocephalus quite often goes hand in hand with a moderate degree of ventriculomegaly, provided the ventricles communicate with the arachnoid spaces and CSF circulation is impeded. One will, in such a case, also find a slightly widened third and fourth ventricle. Those findings do not automatically occur in the case of external hydrocephalus following cerebral atrophy. Widening of the arachnoid spaces can be echographically quantified by measuring the distance between the lateral wall of the superior sagittal sinus and the closest gyral margin (sino-cortical width, SCW) (Fig. II.10.p). Perpendicular 10 MHz sonography at the anterior fontanelle must be carried out, using plenty of gel and applying the scanhead gently. Meningeal hydrops, oedematous dilatation of the leptomeninges, manifests echographically as a deposit of some millimetres on the gyri under the sagittal sinus (Fig. II.10.u). In practice, it is impossible to differentiate between this and subarachnoid fluid accumulation. If dilatation of the arachnoid spaces is the consequence of leukomalacia and/or cortical necrosis and atrophy, one should expect deep and wide sulci which, on account of the absence of a certain amount of white matter, may reach as far as the lateral ventricle.

In chronic subdural haematoma or hygroma, echography (10 MHz) may show a membrane in the spaces around the gyri. The interhemispheric fissure may or may not be widened.

The sulci are not deepened by a pure subdural collection. As a rule there is no ventriculomegaly due to mass-effect of the haematoma. However, any such subdural process may induce subarachnoid CSF accumulation with mild ventriculomegaly. Left and right of the falx, echodensity may differ because there may be fresh(er) bleeding on one side.

REFERENCES

De Vries, L.S., Smet, M., Ceulemans, B., Marchal, G., Wilms, G., de Roo, M., Plets, C., Casaer, P. (1990) 'The role of high resolution ultrasound and MRI in the investigation of infants with macrocephaly.' *Neuropediatrics*, **21**, 72–75.

Gooskens, R.H.J.M., Willemse, J., Bijlsma, J.B., Hanlo, P.W. (1988) 'Megalencephaly: definition and classification.' *Brain and Development*, **10**, 1–7.

Govaert, P., Pauwels, W., Vanhaesebrouck, P., De Praeter, C., Afschrift, M. (1989) 'Ultrasound measurement of the subarachnoid space in infants.' *European Journal of Pediatrics*, **148**, 412–413.

Jaspan, T., Narborough, G., Punt, J.A.G., Lowe, J. (1992) 'Cerebral contusional tears as a marker of child abuse—detection by cranial sonography.' *Pediatric Radiology*, **22**, 237–245.

Lui, K., Boag, G., Daneman, A., Costello, S., Kirpalani, H., Whyte, H. (1990) 'Widened subarachnoid space in pre-discharge cranial ultrasound : evidence of cerebral atrophy in immature infants?' *Developmental Medicine and Child Neurology*, **32**, 882–887.

McArdle, C.B., Richardson, C.J., Nicholas, D.A., Mirfakhraee, M., Hayden, C.K., Amparo, E.C. (1987) 'Developmental features of the neonatal brain: MR imaging. Part II. Ventricular size and extracerebral space.' *Radiology*, **162**, 230–234.

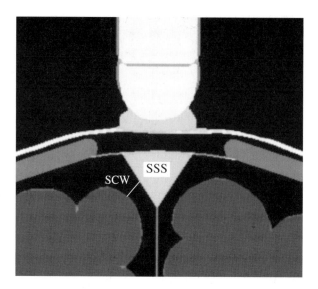

Fig. II.10.p. An approach to measurement of the subarachnoid space in infancy. As shown in the diagram *(above)*, the shortest distance between the lateral wall of the superior sagittal sinus (SSS) and the adjacent cerebral cortex is measured in a coronal plane through the anterior fontanelle, using 10 MHz scanning, plenty of transmission gel and gentle application of the scanhead. The measure is referred to as the sino-cortical width (SCW).

In the graph *(below)*, SCW values are plotted against postconceptional age for a sample of infants from our own neonatal unit (Govaert *et al.* 1989): the *circles* represent patients with external hydrocephalus of known cause and the squares show normal infants without central nervous system anomalies. The broken lines indicate the useful upper limits of normal for SCW.

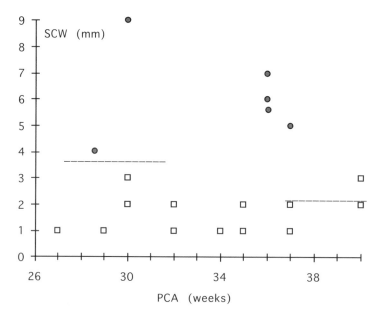

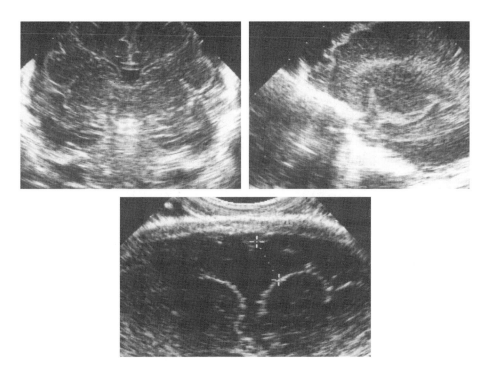

Fig. II.10.q. Infant born preterm with macrocephaly and transient postnatal polyuria, the mother's pregnancy having been complicated by hydramnios: *top*, 7.5 MHz sections (*left*, coronal; *right*, parasagittal); and *bottom*, coronal 10 MHz section. The entire brain, including its parietal surface down to the insula, is displaced from the bone by an extracerebral hypodense fluid collection. The sino-cortical width on day one was measured at 9 mm, subsequently dropping to normal size in the first week of life. The presumed cause was unexplained fetal and transient neonatal diabetes insipidus. Development of this child was entirely normal at 3 years of age.

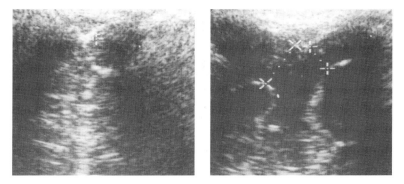

Fig. II.10.r. Monozygotic twins born preterm (29 weeks): coronal 10 MHz sections of the area under the anterior fontanelle at age 6 months. *(Left)* This twin, who showed only mild respiratory distress in the neonatal period, has a normal sino-cortical width, whereas that of his co-twin *(right)*, who required mechanical ventilation for severe respiratory distress syndrome, is clearly increased. As neonatal sonography was not performed, an intracranial haemorrhage may have occurred but gone undiagnosed.

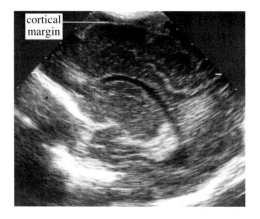

cortical margin

Fig. II.10.s. Floppy newborn infant (36 weeks gestation, pregnancy complicated by hydramnios): 7.5 MHz parasagittal section. Enlargement of the arachnoid spaces and mild ventricular dilatation is not uncommon in the neonatal presentation of myotonic dystrophy. The cortex is easily visible under the anterior fontanelle.

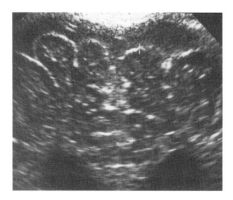
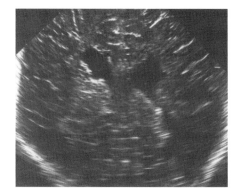

Fig. II.10.t. Preterm infant (25 weeks gestation) with chronic lung disease and catheter-related superior vena cava thrombosis, who developed oedema of the head and neck at 4 months of age: 10 MHz *(left)* and 7.5 MHz *(right)* coronal images. The subarachnoid as well as ventricular spaces were dilated, presumably due to long-standing intracranial venous hypertension as a consequence of jugular vein and superior vena cava thrombosis.

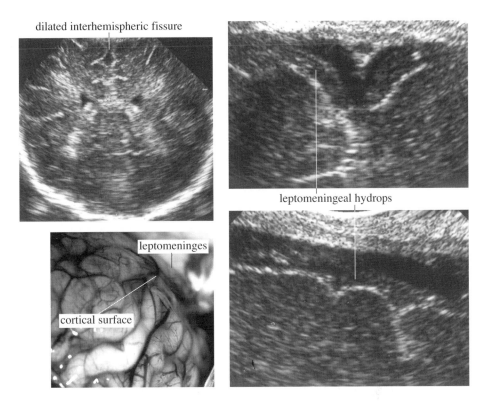

Fig. II.10.u. Term infant with Kniest disease (a type of metatropic dwarfism with associated anomalies): 7.5 MHz coronal *(top left)* and 10 MHz coronal *(top right)* and 10 MHz parasagittal *(bottom right)* sections on the first day of life. The sino-cortical width is increased and the interhemispheric fissure dilated. The arachnoid layer is clearly visible and separate from the cortex, with soft echogenicities in between. At postmortem examination *(bottom left)* this was confirmed to be meningeal hydrops.

II.11 VASCULAR ANOMALIES

Anomalies of brain vessels may cause brain damage with calcification or cystic necrosis in white matter. The family history may be helpful. In some cases accompanied by intracranial haemorrhage, the clinical and sonographic presentation suggests a vascular anomaly at the outset. For references on syndromic vascular anomalies, see Norman *et al.* (1995). It is important to exclude asphyxia, trauma, systemic infection, coagulation anomaly and thrombotic disorders.

In the absence of haemorrhage some of these anomalies may show up sonographically as an unexplained density. We observed an histologically confirmed venous *angioma* in the right occipital lobe of a baby with trisomy 18. It showed as a round opacity with lentiform central clearing, an unusual appearance indicative of vascular anomaly (Fig. II.11.a). Likewise, cavernous haemangiomata and arteriovenous malformations should be very echogenic, due to the presence of haemosiderin and calcium in the former and blood in enlarged, tortuous and thick vessels in the latter (Fig. II.11.h).

Aneurysm of the great vein of Galen is an echopoor sausage-like structure, located in the midline of the quadrigeminal cistern (Figs. II.11.c–g). The varix, in its neonatal presentation, is irrigated by various branches from the anterior and posterior cerebral arteries. In hypertrophied feeding arteries a high systolic and diastolic flow velocity can be measured. During cranial sonography the picture dances up and down because of increased brain pulsatility. In the varix itself flow is turbulent. Colour Doppler sonography further clarifies these findings. Irregular reflections may be visible in the walls of the mass. The varix prolongates occipitally in a dilated straight sinus and torcula, which explains its tennis racket like appearance on a fetal echogram. Increased echodensity in the varix is due to thrombosis, either spontaneous or following treatment. A 'steal-effect' (with hypoperfusion of the arterial domains that are unaffected by the anomaly) and venous congestion may—in the fetus or with postnatal progression—act in concert to give rise to leukomalacia with calcification and cortical necrosis. Dilatation of a number of collateral veins, such as in the back of the falx, has also been reported. These may become very wide.

It may be impossible to identify an *arteriovenous fistula* sonographically, although there may be indirect indications of an intracranial shunt. Clinically, an obviously bulging forehead, pulsatile fontanelle and a cranial bruit may be evident. Sonography shows dilated sinuses with, for instance, enlarged anchor veins draining to the superior sagittal sinus. In those arterialized veins increased velocity will be noted (Fig. II.11.c). Venous hypertension may provoke external hydrocephalus and also discrete communicating ventriculomegaly. MRI, MR angiography, phase contrast MR and/or direct angiography should offer a solution to those problematic cases.

REFERENCES

Baenziger, O., Martin, E., Willi, U., Fanconi, S., Real, F., Boltshauser, E. (1993) 'Prenatal brain atrophy due to a giant vein of Galen malformation.' *Neuroradiology*, **35**, 105–106.

Govaert, P. (1993) 'Differential diagnosis: vascular anomalies.' *In: Cranial Haemorrhage in the Term Newborn Infant. Clinics in Developmental Medicine No. 129.* London: Mac Keith Press, pp. 162–175.

Needell, G.S., Brewer, W.H., Kodroff, M.B., Fernandez, R.E. (1983) 'Midline cerebral arterio-venous anomalies: ultrasound diagnosis.' *Pediatric Radiology*, **13**, 72–76.

Norman, M.G., McGillivray, B.C., Kalousek, D.K., Hill, A., Poskitt, K.J. (1995) 'Abnormalities of the skull, meninges, choroid plexus and blood vessels.' *In: Congenital Malformations of the Brain.* Oxford: Oxford University Press, pp. 368–370.

Saliba, E., Santini, J.J., Pottier, J.M., Chergui, A., Billard, C., Laugier, J. (1987) 'Diagnostic et surveillance de l'anévrysme de l'ampoule de Galien (AAG) du nourrisson par les ultrasons.' *Neurochirurgie,* **33,** 291–295.

Strauss, S., Weinraub, Z., Goldberg, M. (1991) 'Prenatal diagnosis of vein of Galen arteriovenous malformation by duplex sonography.' *Journal of Perinatal Medicine,* **19,** 227–230.

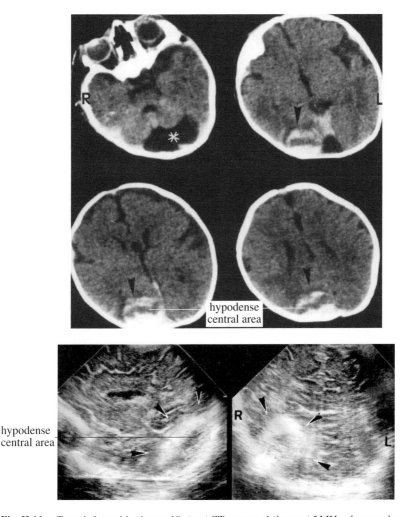

Fig. II.11.a. Term infant with trisomy 18: *(top)* CT scans and *(bottom)* 5 MHz ultrasound sections *(left,* parasagittal through the right hemisphere; *right,* coronal posterior). The corpus callosum is absent. A cystic lesion *(asterisk)* is present behind the cerebellum but extends behind the straight sinus and above the tentorium. A dense (on CT and ultrasound) circular mass *(arrowheads)* lies above and within the right occipital lobe. A peculiar central 'sausage' of hypodensity is difficult to explain. At postmortem examination the falx was absent. The echodense area corresponded histologically with a venous angioma.

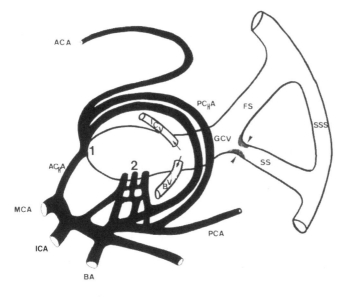

Fig. II.11.b. The complex of feeding arteries and arterial plexuses ends in two collectors, one in front and one in the floor of the varix. Stenosis of regular outflow veins and sinuses may in part explain collateral venous channels of enormous size. (PC_HA = posterior choroidal artery; ACA = anterior cerebral artery; AC_HA = anterior choroidal artery; MCA = middle cerebral artery; ICA = internal carotid artery; BA = basilar artery; PCA = posterior cerebral artery; GCV = great cerebral vein, BV = basal vein; ICV = internal cerebral vein; SS = straight sinus; FS = falx sinus; SSS = superior sagittal sinus.)

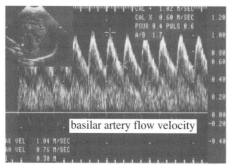

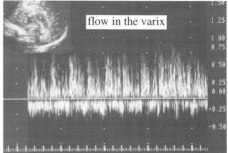

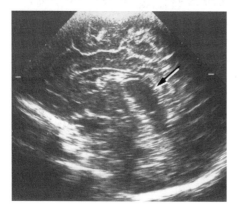

Fig. II.11.c. Term infant with a cranial bruit and generalized oedema due to cardiac failure: Doppler findings in the basilar artery and in the varix; sagittal 7.5 MHz section. There is an elliptoid hypodense very pulsatile structure *(arrow)* behind the splenium of the corpus callosum and resting on the mesencephalic tectum. Within this varix, typical of a vein of Galen aneurysm, turbulent flow is captured, whereas feeding arteries such as the basilar artery display high systolic (even >1 m/s) and diastolic flow velocities; the entire brain pulsates during sonography. At 2 years of age this child had two embolization sessions and is awaiting a final third one.

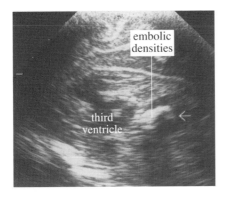

Fig. II.11.d. Term infant with vein of Galen aneurysm: 5 MHz sagittal view. Following transarterial embolization echodense material is seen in the varix.

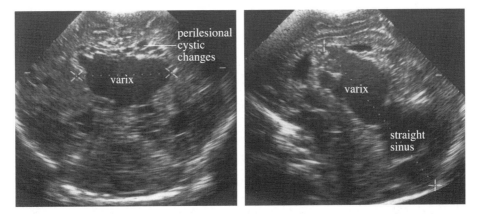

Fig. II.11.e. Term infant with cardiac failure: 7.5 MHz sections (*left*, coronal; *right*, sagittal). This huge vein of Galen aneurysm was associated with perilesional cystic changes, probably venous collaterals. The varix extends into an enormous straight sinus.

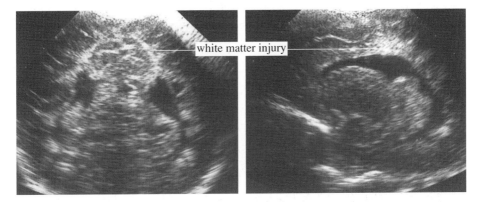

Fig. II.11.f. Preterm infant (36 weeks gestation) with cardiac failure: 7.5 MHz sections (*left*, coronal; *right*, parasagittal) showing periventricular cystic leukomalacia due to vein of Galen aneurysm.

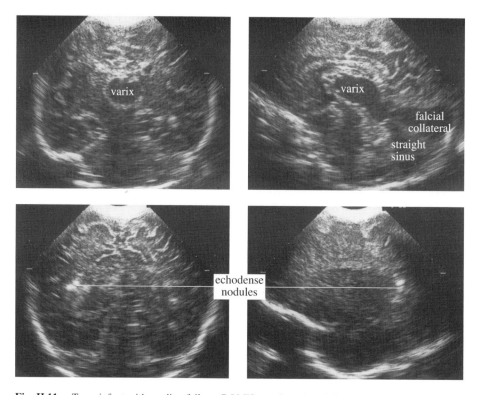

Fig. II.11.g. Term infant with cardiac failure: 7.5 MHz sections (*top left*, coronal; *top right*, sagittal; *bottom left*, coronal; *bottom right*, parasagittal) showing vein of Galen aneurysm. In the back of the falx a very dilated venous collateral can be seen. Such collaterals are the consequence of venous obstruction along the usual drainage system of straight and sagittal sinuses. Nodular echodense lesions in the right occipital area were confirmed as ischaemic changes at postmortem examination.

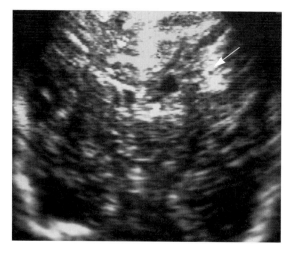

Fig. II.11.h. Term infant with seizures: 5 MHz coronal section showing left periventricular parietal hyperechogenic focus *(arrow)* corresponding with an arteriovenous malformation.

SECTION III
PATHOLOGY: ANTENATAL BRAIN
DAMAGE

III.1 FETAL INTRACRANIAL HAEMORRHAGE

For various reasons haemorrhage may occur in the central nervous system before birth. The three most commonly occurring mechanisms are haemorrhagic diathesis, fetal trauma and ischaemic accident.

The diagnosis of an antenatal intraventricular haemorrhage may be upheld by specific anamnestic data (Fig. III.1.e), revealed by an abnormal fetal brain ultrasound or MR examination, by finding acute heart-rate changes *in utero* or by means of an early brain sonogram after birth. The non-recent and posthaemorrhagic character of a fetal lesion may also show during ventriculoscopic neurosurgery or at postmortem examination.

An extensive necrotic or haemorrhagic lesion that is strikingly echogenic within the first hour after birth is almost certainly not postnatal in origin (Fig. III.1.a). The non-recent character of a ventricular haemorrhage can be echographically defined by some simple observations. After a few days a clot in a ventricle begins to undergo lysis, sometimes giving rise to cavitation (Figs. III.1.b–d). The coagulum starts to retract leaving irregular intraluminal structures with a dense ridge and a hypodense centre. Toward the end of the first week, following a sterile reaction to extravascular blood, the ependyma becomes denser and granular in some spots, a phenomenon that will persist for weeks. Widening of the ventricle without bulky clot is an additional subacute or chronic element. Associated lesions in white matter, if cystic, can of course be indicative of the subacute character of the intrauterine event (Figs. III.1.f, III.1.g). Exceptionally, haemorrhage in choroid plexus or germinal matrix may evolve into a growing hygromatous mass with a capsule analogous to that of a chronic subdural haematoma. In that case a rounded lesion will show up with a fine dense border and discrete intralesional echoreflections. Axial ultrasound may show clot in the widened fourth ventricle. Typical for alloimmune thrombocytopenia is the development of superficial haemorrhage in the parenchyma, usually of the temporal lobe (Fig. III.1.h). This is a subpial haemorrhage that, on growing towards the surface, will start to look like a subarachnoid haematoma. Posthaemorrhagic hydrocephalus may occur if such a haemorrhage extends into the deeper tissues and reaches the ventricle. It is sometimes impossible to make a clear distinction between haemorrhagic conversion of an ischaemic zone and primary haemorrhage, for instance after direct fetal cranial trauma (Fig. III.1.i). As a rule ischaemic echodensities persist for several (≥ 2) weeks, whereas any haemorrhagic area should be cleared of most echogenic foci in two to three weeks.

REFERENCES

Chambers, S.E., Johnstone, F.D., Laing, I.A. (1988) 'Ultrasound *in-utero* diagnosis of choroid plexus haemorrhage.' *British Journal of Obstetrics and Gynaecology*, **95**, 1317–1320.

Candito, M., Richelme, C., Parvy, P., Dageville, C., Appert, A., Bekri, S., Rabier, D., Chambon, P., Mariani, R., Kamoun, P. (1995) 'Abnormal α-aminoadipic acid excretion in a newborn with a defect in platelet aggregation and antenatal cerebral haemorrhage.' *Journal of Inherited Metabolic Disorders*, **18**, 56–60.

Dean, L.M., McLeary, M., Taylor, G.A. (1995) 'Cerebral hemorrhage in alloimmune thrombocytopenia.' *Pediatric Radiology*, **25**, 444–445.

Eken, P., de Vries, L.S., van der Graaf, Y., Meiners, L.C., van Nieuwenhuizen, O. (1995) 'Haemorrhagic–ischaemic lesions of the neonatal brain: correlation between cerebral visual impairment, neurodevelopmental outcome and MRI in infancy.' *Developmental Medicine and Child Neurology*, **37**, 41–55.

Fogarty, K., Cohen, H.L., Haller, J.O. (1989) 'Sonography of fetal intracranial hemorrhage: unusual causes and a review of the literature.' *Journal of Clinical Ultrasound*, **17**, 366–370.

Govaert, P., Bridger, J., Wigglesworth, J. (1995) 'Nature of the brain lesion in fetal allo-immune thrombocytopenia.' *Developmental Medicine and Child Neurology*, **37**, 485–495.

Jackson, J.C., Blumhagen, J.D. (1983) 'Congenital hydrocephalus due to prenatal intracranial hemorrhage.' *Pediatrics*, **72**, 344–346.

Kim, M-S., Elyaderani, M.K. (1982) 'Sonographic diagnosis of cerebroventricular hemorrhage *in utero*.' *Radiology*, **142**, 479–480.

Lustig-Gillman, I., Young, B.K., Silverman, F., Raghavendra, B.N., Wan, L., Reitz, M.E., Aleksic, S., Greco, M.A., Snyder, J.R. (1983) 'Fetal intraventricular hemorrhage: sonographic diagnosis and clinical implications.' *Journal of Clinical Ultrasound*, **11**, 277–280.

Matsui, K., Ohsaki, E., Goto, A., Koresawa, M., Kigasawa, H., Shibata, Y. (1995) 'Perinatal intracranial hemorrhage due to severe neonatal alloimmune thrombocytopenic purpura (NAITP) associated with anti-Yukb (HPA-4a) antibodies.' *Brain and Development*, **17**, 352–355.

McGahan, J.P., Haesslein, H.C., Meyers, M., Ford, K.B. (1984) 'Sonographic recognition of *in utero* intraventricular hemorrhage.' *American Journal of Roentgenology*, **142**, 171–173.

Rypens, F., Avni, E.F., Dussaussois, L., David, P., Vermeylen, D., Van Bogaert, P., Matos, C. (1994) 'Hyperechoic thickened ependyma: sonographic demonstration and significance in neonates.' *Pediatric Radiology*, **24**, 550–553.

Scher, M.S., Belfar, H., Martin, J., Painter, M.J. (1991) 'Destructive brain lesions of presumed fetal onset: antepartum causes of cerebral palsy.' *Pediatrics*, **88**, 898–906.

Stirling, H.F., Hendry, M., Brown, J.K. (1989) 'Prenatal intracranial haemorrhage.' *Developmental Medicine and Child Neurology*, **31**, 807–811.

Tampakoudis, P., Bili, H., Lazaridis, E., Anastasiadou, E., Andreou, A., Mantalenakis, S. (1995) 'Prenatal diagnosis of intracranial hemorrhage secondary to maternal idiopathic thrombocytopenic purpura: a case report.' *American Journal of Perinatology*, **12**, 268–270.

Whitelaw, A., Haines, M.E., Bolsover, W., Harris, E. (1984) 'Factor V deficiency and antenatal intraventricular haemorrhage.' *Archives of Disease in Childhood*, **59**, 997–999.

Zorzi, C., Angonese, I., Nardelli, G.B., Cantarutti, F. (1988) 'Spontaneous intraventricular haemorrhage *in utero*.' *European Journal of Pediatrics*, **148**, 83–85.

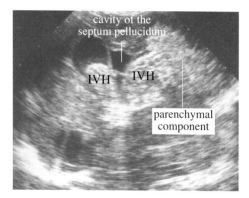

Fig. III.1.a. Preterm infant (28 weeks gestation) with signs of intracranial hypertension from birth: 5 MHz sonogram within the first hour of life shows bilateral grade III intraventricular haemorrhage (IVH) with acute ventriculomegaly and extensive parenchymal involvement on the left. This aspect, together with the history of antenatal maternal salicylate use, suggests a recent ante- or intrapartum onset of haemorrhage.

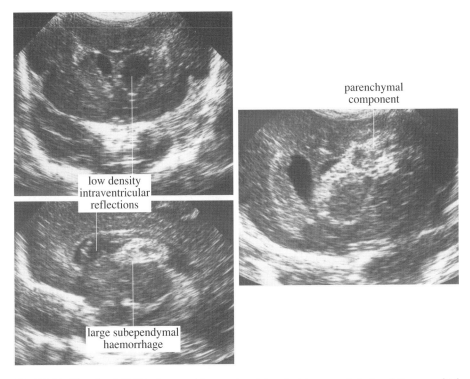

parenchymal
component

low density
intraventricular
reflections

large subependymal
haemorrhage

Fig. III.1.b. First day 7.5 MHz ultrasound images (*top left* and *right*, coronal; *bottom left*, parasagittal through the left hemisphere) of a growth retarded infant whose mother had had pre-eclampsia; during labour the fetal heart rate recordings showed a loss of variability and there was reverse diastolic flow in the umbilical artery. The echographic appearance suggests a large left subependymal haemorrhage with central hypointensity. Reflections from within the ventricle are not very dense. Parenchymal involvement is best seen on a coronal section. The extent of bleeding has caused a midline shift. Progression from subependymal to intraventricular haemorrhage with parenchymal component is unusual in the first hours of life, and given a suitable historical context, is suggestive of antenatal bleeding.

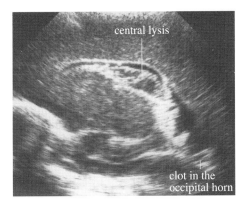

central lysis

clot in the
occipital horn

Fig. III.1.c. Preterm infant (29 weeks gestation): first day 7.5 MHz parasagittal section. Five days before delivery an episode of antepartum haemorrhage had been associated with transient fetal tachycardia (>180 bpm); during labour the fetal cardiotocogram was entirely normal. There was no birth asphyxia and the child did not develop respiratory distress. There is clot in or on top of the left plexus, adjacent to the matrix in the caudo-thalamic groove. Organization within the clot resulted in central hypodensity, a feature not achieved in a couple of hours. There is clot in the occipital horn.

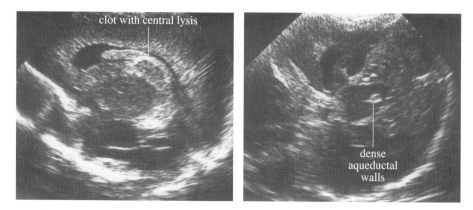

Fig. III.1.d. First day sonograms (*left*, parasagittal; *right*, axial) of a preterm infant without respiratory distress or asphyxia, born after prelabour rupture of the membranes. There is ventriculomegaly with clot sitting on the thalamus; within the clot, changes in echogenicity suggest the non-acute character of this event. The aqueductal wall is hyperechogenic with haemorrhagic changes.

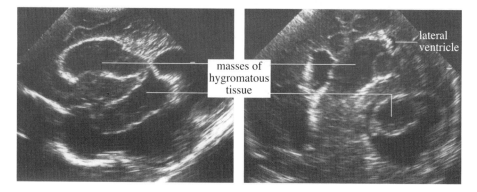

Fig. III.1.e. Parasagittal *(left)* and coronal *(right)* 7.5 MHz scans of a term infant diagnosed antenatally as having ventriculomegaly. Her mother had presented at 12 weeks gestation with seizures due to an astrocytoma. Tumour-like iso- to hypodense changes are seen within the left lateral ventricle, on or in the choroid plexus. The ipsilateral frontal and parietal ventricular cavity is displaced and compressed. The outer surface of the lesion is echodense and irregular. Tissue removed from within these masses during ventriculoscopic surgery contained only siderophages and glial cells. The final diagnosis was hygromatous change of choroid plexus following early fetal haemorrhage, with stenosis of the left foramen of Monro resulting in predominantly ipsilateral hydrocephalus.

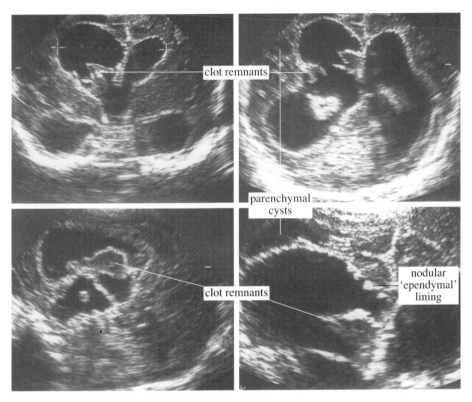

Fig. III.1.f. First day scans from a term girl with ventriculomegaly diagnosed *in utero*: 7.5 MHz sections (all coronal, except *lower left*, sagittal). There is generalized ventriculomegaly except for the fourth ventricle, suggesting aqueductal stenosis. The haemorrhagic nature of this event is indicated by the dense and nodular ependymal lining and the irregular clot remnants scattered throughout the ventricular system. There are cystic changes within the right parietal parenchyma. There was no clue to the aetiology of this third trimester event.

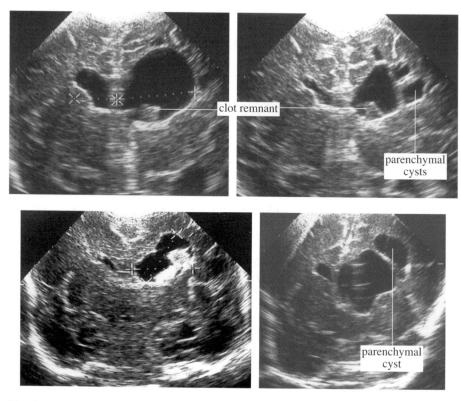

Fig. III.1.g. Two different infants with prenatally established intraventricular haemorrhage with parenchymal infarction, connatal ventriculomegaly and subsequent occlusion of the foramen of Monro.

(Top) First day 7.5 MHz coronal scans [before *(left)* and after *(right)* shunting for hydrocephalus] of a term infant, whose mother had had abdominal pain at 30 weeks gestation.

(Bottom) Preterm infant (33 weeks gestation) with transient hydrops due to supraventricular tachycardia around the 28th week of gestation: 7.5 MHz coronal sections on day 1 *(left)* and at term age *(right)* before shunting for unilateral hydrocephalus.

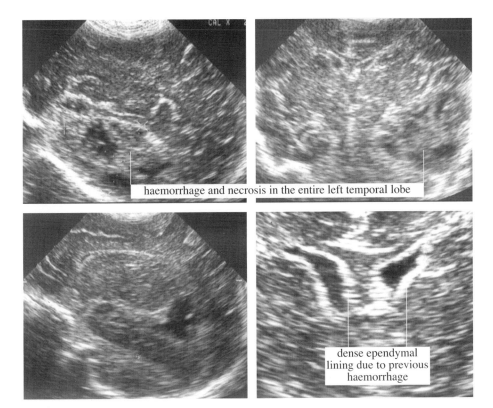

haemorrhage and necrosis in the entire left temporal lobe

dense ependymal
lining due to previous
haemorrhage

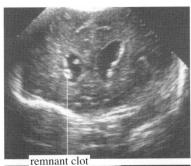

remnant clot

ventricle–cavity
aperture

Fig. III.1.h. First day sonograms (all 7.5 MHz) of two otherwise healthy term infants with petechiae and severe thrombocytopenia (platelets <20.0 × 10⁹/L). In both infants HPA1 (former PlA1) platelet antigen was the target of alloimmunization *in utero*, with ensuing severe haemorrhagic tendency and spontaneous intracranial bleeding long before delivery.

(Above) This infant has a characteristic parenchymal haemorrhage in the left temporal lobe. From evidence not shown here this is thought likely to be a subarachnoid haematoma which started as a small subpial bleed and subsequently grew to involve the entire left temporal lobe. It is not yet understood why bleeding is often restricted to the left. Compare the parasagittal scan through the left temporal lobe *(upper left)* with that of the healthy right side *(lower left)*. Coronal sections focus on the temporal region *(upper right)* and the ventricles at the foramen of Monro *(lower right)*. Some blood has entered the ventricular system as can be deduced from the dense ependymal lining. Development at 2 years was within the normal range.

(Left) This infant presented with occipital porencephaly, hydrocephalus and remnant frontal clots *(top, coronal; bottom, parasagittal sections)*. Mild mental retardation and severe visual sequelae were evident later.

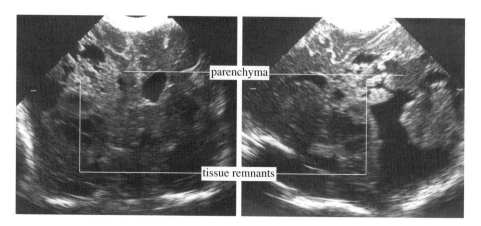

Fig. III.1.i. Preterm infant (36 weeks gestation) whose mother had been physically abused (kicked on the abdomen) four weeks prior to delivery: 7.5 MHz day 1 sonograms (*left*, coronal; *right*, parasagittal). Haemorrhagic and necrotic tissue remnants fill the entire area supplied by the right middle cerebral artery, with extension to the occiput. Destruction of cortical and periventricular parenchyma suggests that intraventricular haemorrhage with parenchymal involvement is not the likely primary mechanism; one would rather suspect the combined occurrence of arterial infarction and direct trauma. (Reproduced by permission from Eken *et al.* 1995.)

III.2 ESTABLISHED WIDESPREAD HYPOXIC–ISCHAEMIC BRAIN DAMAGE PRESENT AT BIRTH

A fetus may, even after intrauterine asphyxia in severity equivalent to prolonged postnatal bradycardia or asystole, survive the acute episode and then, during pregnancy or at birth, show signs of an established brain lesion. The criterion for inclusion into this disease category is the combined presence of necrosis and gliosis in diencephalon, striatum, cerebellum and brainstem. In a number of cases necrosis in deep grey matter is associated with leukomalacia or haemorrhage into germinal matrix. Other causes of prenatal brain damage must be excluded: primary haemorrhage with secondary ischaemia, fetal infection, any genetically determined condition or embryonic anomaly. Important markers of global forebrain ischaemia, be it *in* or *ex utero* in the perinatal period, are neuronal necrosis, gliosis and atrophy of thalamic nuclei. Any episode in pregnancy jeopardizing oxygenation and/or perfusion of the fetus is a potential cause. The absence of growth retardation in over three quarters of cases does not suggest a role for an underlying permanent maternal or placental problem. The clinical presentation can be summarized as follows: polyhydramnios (about 1 in 2), signs of fetal distress (about 1 in 2, typically with decreased or even absent heart beat variation but a normal scalp pH), pulmonary hypoplasia (in over a quarter of cases), a low to normal occipitofrontal circumference, fixed limb contractures due to neurogenic muscle atrophy (about 1 case in 3 is initially diagnosed as an 'arthrogrypoid syndrome'), hypertonia and tendon hyperreflexia from birth, early convulsions, cranial nerve palsies (facial diplegia, swallowing or sucking problems, ophthalmoplegia, tongue fasciculations, stridor), signs of hypothalamic dysfunction (temperature instability), and abdominal fasciculations. The mortality rate associated with diffuse antenatal brain ischaemia is high.

Sonographic observations of this phenomenon are particularly scarce. In one personal observation echogenicity of white brain matter appeared to be normal (Fig. III.2.b). Both lateral ventricles, especially in their occipital part, and also the third, were moderately dilated. On a sagittal section the third ventricle, normally not visible, could be easily seen. The region of thalamus and caudate nucleus appeared atrophic, with a zone of cystic germinolysis in the right caudothalamic groove. Both thalami were moderately hyperdense. There was no focal calcification anterior to the fourth ventricle as sometimes seen in Moebius syndrome. Ischaemic zones in the dorsal part of the brainstem and the thalamus showed up on MR images. Under the anterior fontanelle the arachnoid space was 6–7 mm wide, pointing to discrete global brain shrinkage. The combination of the clinical picture and these subtle sonographic changes allows for a tentative diagnosis of this often misjudged clinical picture. In the case of hypoxic–ischaemic insult in the last few weeks before delivery, the ultrasonographic substrate may be even less striking. One can be confronted with apparent birth asphyxia without a stage of brain swelling and without characteristic flow velocity changes in the cerebral arteries. Recent haemorrhages may still be hyperechogenic in such an instance (Fig. III.2.e). This clinical picture is not limited to the term infant (Figs. III.2.b–d). Even in a preterm baby of 26 weeks gestation, symmetrically increased echodensity laterally in both thalami can suggest preceding global *in utero* brain ischaemia. Ischaemic matrix injury may be recognized in the hyperechogenic, pre-cystic stage (Fig. III.2.d).

REFERENCES

Brazy, J.E., Kinney, H.C., Oakes, W.J. (1987) 'Central nervous system structural lesions causing apnea at birth.' *Journal of Pediatrics*, **111**, 163–175.

DiMario, F.J., Clancy, R. (1989) 'Symmetrical thalamic degeneration with calcifications of infancy.' *American Journal of Diseases of Children*, **143**, 1056–1060.

Eicke, M., Briner, J., Willi, U., Uehlinger, J., Boltshauser, E. (1992) 'Symmetrical thalamic lesions in infants.' *Archives of Disease in Childhood*, **67**, 15–19.

Natsume, J., Watanabe, K., Kuno, K., Hayakawa, F., Hashizume, Y. (1995) 'Clinical, neurophysiologic, and neuropathological features of an infant with brain damage of total asphyxia type (Myers).' *Pediatric Neurology*, **13**, 61–64.

Wigglesworth, J.S., Bridger, J.E. (1994) 'Neuropathological clues to the timing of early brain lesions.' *In:* Lou, H.C., Greisen, G., Larsen, J.F. (Eds.) *Brain Lesions in the Newborn. Hypoxic and Haemodynamic Pathogenesis. Alfred Benzon Symposium No. 37.* Munksgaard. pp. 165–177.

Wilson,E.R., Mirra, S.S., Schwartz, J.F. (1982) 'Congenital diencephalic and brain stem damage: neuropathologic study of three cases.' *Acta Neuropathologica*, **57**, 70–74.

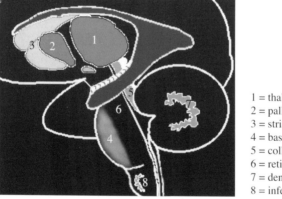

1 = thalamus
2 = pallidum
3 = striatum
4 = base of the pons
5 = colliculi
6 = reticular formation
7 = dentate nucleus
8 = inferior olive

Fig. III.2.a. Deep grey matter structures vulnerable to global forebrain ischaemia in the perinatal period.

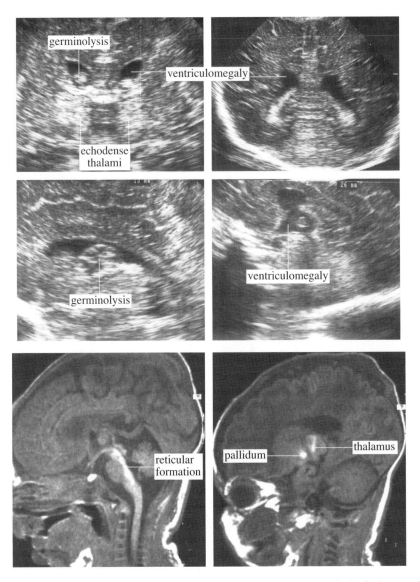

Fig. III.2.b. This infant was the second of twins. Polyhydramnios was present in the fetal sac, and at term there was loss of beat-to-beat variation on CTG. After birth, immobile facies and flexed limb deformities were evident. Sucking and swallowing reflexes and spontaneous eye movements were absent, and apnoeic episodes occurred. The ultrasonograms *(top)* are first day, 7.5 MHz images *(upper*, coronal; *lower*, (para)sagittal). Also shown *(bottom)* are two representative slices of the corresponding (T$_1$-weighted) MRI scans performed on day 5. There is mild dilatation of all ventricles, and other pictures (not shown here) also revealed brain shrinkage. Increased echogenicity of the thalami was shown at postmortem examination to be due to iron-containing neurons. Cystic germinolysis is apparent, especially in the right caudothalamic groove. Necropsy also demonstrated neuronal loss (in the cerebellar cortex and anterior horns of the spinal cord) and iron accumulation in necrotic cells of the brainstem's reticular formation.

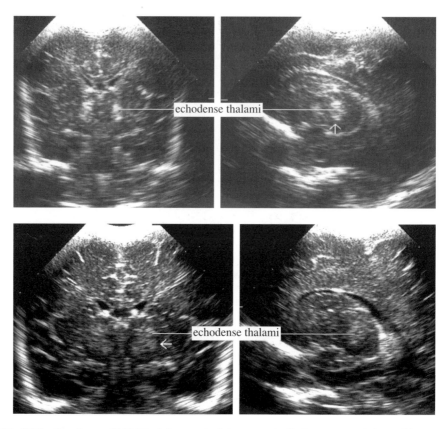

Fig. III.2.c. Day 1 scans (7.5 MHz; *left*, coronal; *right*, parasagittal) of two preterm infants with neurological abnormalities evident at birth.

(Top) This 26 weeks gestation baby presented with facial diplegia and flexed knee deformities and died shortly after birth. Calcification of the thalami and superior colliculi was confirmed at postmortem examination.

(Bottom) Pregnancy in this case was complicated by polyhydramnios and diminished fetal movements. At birth (in the 33rd week of gestation), facial diplegia was evident, there was lack of spontaneous movement, and swallowing and sucking reflexes were absent.

In these two babies ischaemia of the forebrain may have occurred early in the third trimester: these cases show the importance of recognizing thalamic injury as a marker for this entity.

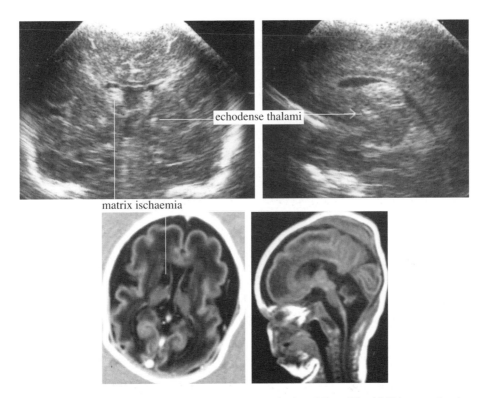

Fig. III.2.d. 7.5 MHz sections (*left*, coronal; *right*, parasagittal) and T$_1$-weighted MR images of an infant born at 33 weeks gestation following a pregnancy complicated by polyhydramnios; this baby had atonia, fixed limb flexion contractures, facial diplegia and abdominal muscle fasciculation, and was unable to breathe spontaneously. Both caudothalamic matrix areas are hyperechogenic but hypointense on MRI, suggesting infarction and not haemorrhage. There are focal echogenicities in the thalamus. The brainstem is slender, and the vermis is clearly atrophied. At postmortem examination, gliosis and neuronal loss was confirmed in cerebrum, cerebellum, brainstem and spinal cord.

121

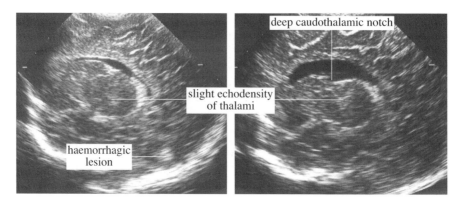

Fig. III.2.e. 7.5 MHz parasagittal views (*left*, day 1; *right*, day 9) of term infant. One week prior to delivery the mother, a farmer's wife, had been injured on the thigh by a bull. From the onset of labour there was diminished fetal heart beat to beat variability and the liquor showed stale meconium staining. Following birth Apgar scores were low, and persistent pulmonary hypertension was diagnosed. Both scans show mild increase of thalamic echogenicity, in the lateral nuclei just behind the posterior limb of the internal capsule. A nodular haemorrhagic and/or ischaemic lesion in the transitional area from temporal to occipital lobe (confirmed by MRI) is seen on the day 1 scan but not on day 9. Dilatation of the lateral ventricle in the second week is suggestive of atrophy of the basal ganglia, also confirmed by the sharp angle between the caudate nucleus and thalamus, where germinal matrix has disappeared. Note the absence of slit ventricles on day 1, suggesting that there has not been true birth asphyxia, the low Apgar scores reflecting established neurological disease.

III.3 HYDRANENCEPHALY

Hydranencephaly is the prototype of an *encephaloclastic* lesion, *i.e.* an anomaly due to a disruption of normally developed structures. Its incidence varies, according to different authors, between 1:5,000 and 1:10,000 live births. Hydranencephaly most commonly occurs *in utero*, usually in the second trimester. Although in some autopsied cases major cerebral arteries were found to be occluded, the primary cause seems to be hypoperfusion rather than actual vascular thrombosis, embolic obstruction or vasculitis. Secondary to infarction, these arteries involute and occlude at a later stage.

Systemic maternal hypoxia with secondary fetal asphyxia and brain hypoperfusion may be the consequence of, *inter alia*, gas intoxication (CO, butane), cocaine abuse, shock after an accident, fetal irradiation or allergic reaction.

Infarction in the region of both middle and posterior cerebral arteries is known to occur following *in utero* demise of a monozygotic co-twin.

Infectious agents associated with hydranencephaly include *Toxoplasma gondii*, cyto-megalovirus (CMV), herpes simplex virus (HSV), varicella-zoster virus (VZV), rubella virus, *Listeria monocytogenes* and *Treponema pallidum*.

Exceptional cases of familial hydranencephaly have been reported.

Extensive global brain necrosis occurring during birth or in the neonatal period may give rise to postnatally acquired hydranencephaly, *e.g.* following bilateral grade IV ventricular haemorrhage (see p. 165 for definitions of IVH grades) and extensive multicystic white matter disease. Unilateral hydranencephaly may occur with unilateral total infarction in the area of the internal carotid artery.

Supratentorial hydranencephaly is the final stage of an infarction in the region of both middle cerebral arteries in the course of the second trimester. In cases with occipital telencephalic remnants only, we are dealing with the consequences of bilateral necrosis of areas supplied by the internal carotid artery (Fig. III.3.a). It follows that cortical layers are no longer present in the affected zones, which constitutes an important differential characteristic. By definition the hippocampus and basal parts of the temporal lobes, occipital lobes and orbitofrontal cortex are maintained if we are dealing with select hypoperfusion of the middle cerebral artery. Due to the resulting echographic appearance this is referred to as a 'basket brain' because the residual structures medially constitute a kind of handle around absent tissue (Fig. III.3.b). The adjacent residual cerebral cortex may undergo polymicrogyric changes. Cerebellum and brainstem structures beneath the oculomotor nucleus are macroscopically normal, but may undergo histologic change (such as atrophy of the pyramidal tracts). The thalamus is present, but may secondarily atrophy in those parts that project onto absent cortex (transsynaptic degeneration). Striatal remnants may be found. Optic nerves and tracts atrophy secondarily. The falx can be absent but does not have to be. Empty spaces caused by necrosis are bordered toward the surface by a gliomeningeal membrane without ependyma and with neuronal encrustation. For as yet unclear reasons, this phenomenon is nearly always associated with hydrocephalus.

In the differential diagnosis one should consider atelencephaly–aprosencephaly (see microcephaly, section II.6).

Isolated *vertebro-basilar hydranencephaly* is a curiosity.

In the absence of hydrocephalus, hemispheric necrosis may present as a 'fetal brain disruption sequence' with collapse of the cranium and a protruding occipital squama giving the appearance of a mast on a sailboat. The scalp covers the cranium in big folds. Such babies always have an open aqueduct. Their occipitofrontal circumference is at least six standard deviations below the mean for age, and at term their brains weigh no more than 100 g.

REFERENCES

Alexander, I.E., Tauro, G.P., Bankier, A. (1995) 'Fetal brain disruption sequence in sisters.' *European Journal of Pediatrics*, **154**, 654–657.

Bordarier, C., Robain, O. (1988) 'Familial occurrence of prenatal encephaloclastic damage: anatomoclinical report of 2 cases.' *Neuropediatrics*, **20**, 103–106.

Crome, L. (1972) 'Hydrencephaly.' *Developmental Medicine and Child Neurology*, **14**, 224–226. *(Annotation.)*

Dublin, A.B., French, B.N. (1980) 'Diagnostic imaging evaluation of hydranencephaly and pictorially similar entities, with emphasis on computed tomography.' *Radiology*, **137**, 81–91.

Fowler, M., Dow, R., White, T.A., Greer, C.H. (1972) 'Congenital hydrocephalus–hydrencephaly in five siblings, with autopsy studies: a new disease.' *Developmental Medicine and Child Neurology*, **14**, 173–188.

Govaert, P., Vanhaesebrouck, P., De Praeter, C., Leroy, J. (1989) 'Hydranencéphalie et prise d'oestrogènes pendant la grossesse.' *Archives Françaises de Pédiatrie*, **46**, 235. *(Letter.)*

Halsey, J.H., Allen, N., Chamberlin, H.R. (1971) 'The morphogenesis of hydranencephaly.' *Journal of the Neurological Sciences*, **12**, 187–217.

Hughes, H.E., Miskin, M. (1986) 'Congenital microcephaly due to vascular disruption: *in utero* documentation.' *Pediatrics*, **78**, 85–87.

Hunter, A.G.W. (1993) 'Brain.' *In:* Stevenson, R.E., Hall, J.G., Goodman, R.M. (Eds) *Human Malformations and Related Anomalies. Vol. II. Oxford Monographs on Medical Genetics, No. 27.* Oxford: Oxford University Press, pp. 1–19.

Lyon, G., Robain, O. (1967) 'Etude comparative des encéphalopathies circulatoires prénatales et para-natales (hydranencéphalies, porencéphalies et encéphalomalacies kystiques de la substance blanche).' *Acta Neuropathologica*, **9**, 79–98.

Moore, C.A., Weaver, D.D., Bull, M.J. (1990) 'Fetal brain disruption sequence.' *Journal of Pediatrics*, **116**, 383–386.

Naidich, T.P., Chakera, T.M.H. (1984) 'Multicystic encephalomalacia: CT appearance and pathological correlation.' *Journal of Computer Assisted Tomography*, **8**, 631–636.

Plantaz, D., Joannard, A., Pasquier, B., Bost, M., Beaudoing, A. (1987) 'Hydranencéphalie et toxoplasmose congénitale. A propos de quatre observations.' *Pédiatrie*, **42**, 161–165.

Roessmann, U., Parks, P.J. (1978) 'Hydranencephaly in vertebral-basilar territory.' *Acta Neuropathologica*, **44**, 141–143.

Russell, L.J., Weaver, D.D., Bull, M.J., Weinbaum, M. (1984) 'In utero brain destruction resulting in collapse of the fetal skull, microcephaly, scalp rugae, and neurologic impairment: the fetal brain disruption sequence.' *American Journal of Medical Genetics*, **17**, 509–521.

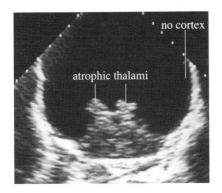

no cortex

atrophic thalami

Fig. III.3.a. Term infant with macrocephaly: 5 MHz coronal section illustrating classic supratentorial hydranencephaly. Note complete absence of cortical plate and white matter in the entire hemispheric wall (except for some occipitotemporal remnants not shown here). The thalami are present but atrophic and clearly separated.

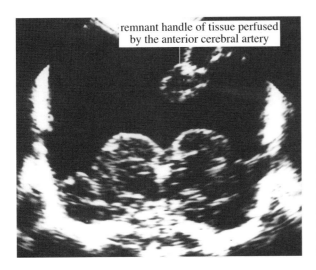

remnant handle of tissue perfused by the anterior cerebral artery

Fig. III.3.b. Preterm infant with apnoea: coronal 7.5 MHz section illustrating the 'basket brain' phenomenon. The left anterior cerebral artery is still perfused and maintains a bridge of tissue around the remnants of a complete infarction in the left middle cerebral artery. On the right there has been necrosis of the areas perfused by the internal carotid artery.

III.4 PORENCEPHALY

Comparing definitions proposed by various neuropathologists one finds strongly divergent descriptions of 'porencephaly'. We believe that three major entities can be distinguished:

• *Embryonic porencephaly*. Schizencephaly ('developmental porencephaly'): generally a bilateral defect in the brain parenchyma with contact between the ventricle and the arachnoid mater over a cleft bordered by neuronal heterotopia; often thought to be acquired; presumably the result of vascular damage to one ray of glioneuronal matrix products.

• *Early fetal porencephaly* (<24 weeks of gestation). Soft-walled defects with well defined, regular margins, often with involvement of both cortex and white matter and with ventricular connection; the superficial borders are lined by polymicrogyric cortex.

• *Perinatal porencephaly*. Clastic lesions, often vascular but sometimes infective, generate multiple or isolated cavities, generally with irregular walls due to the reactive gliosis which becomes apparent only after the 20th gestational week in response to necrosis; examples of these lesions can be seen after leukomalacia and following parenchymal extension of germinal matrix haemorrhage.

Schizencephaly

This anomaly belongs in the list of early fetal disturbances of neuronal migration (see section II.8). Quite often one encounters a bilateral, sometimes asymmetric cleft in the region of the lateral fissure. Direct contact between the ventricular ependyma and the arachnoid space ('pial–ependymal seam') is typical. The seam may be slit-shaped and only recognizable in life by MRI. Wider clefts coincide with ventricular widening and can be traced echographically. Usually there is microcephaly in spite of ventriculomegaly. Along the borders of the cortical defect the arteries bend into the slit, a phenomenon not seen in late fetal clastic porencephaly. A microscopically abnormal vascular rete may exist in the adjacent polymicrogyric cortex. The walls of the slit are lined by abnormally thick grey matter, neuronal heterotopia possibly indenting the lateral ventricular wall. Schizencephaly is usually sporadic but may be seen in association with agenesis of the septum pellucidum (the explanation for which is unclear) and neuro-endocrine anomalies. We thus end up in a nosological overlap with septo-optic dysplasia. A clear cause was reported in a situation where repeated attempts at abortion with intramuscular benzol failed in the first trimester. Less explicit comparable episodes might give rise to perisylvian polymicrogyria.

Simple porencephaly

The frequent association of porencephaly with agenesis of the corpus callosum or septum pellucidum, with heterotopia or with polymicrogyria, suggests a second trimester lesion. Its presentation is accompanied by spastic hemi- or quadriparesis and infantile spasms. Both microcephaly and macrocephaly (via hydrocephalus) are possible. We usually find a cavity at the frontal or parietal horns, communicating with the often dilated ipsilateral ventricle (Fig. III.4.b). A border of cortex and white matter remains between the cavity and the pia mater. Its external wall is often corrugated. Bilaterality is not exceptional. While generally sporadic, the phenomenon may find a place in the wider framework of a syndrome. Rare cases of autosomally dominant familial types of simple porencephaly have been described.

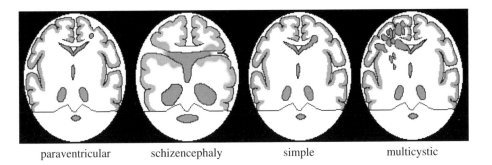

| paraventricular | schizencephaly | simple | multicystic |

Fig. III.4.a. Some variants of antenatal porencephaly.

Porencephaly following ventricular puncture

Exceptionally, transfontanelle ventricular punctures are still necessary during intensive care of preterm infants with acute symptomatic posthaemorrhagic hydrocephalus. Inevitably the lateral ventricle will communicate with the puncture path even after a carefully performed tap with echographic assistance (Figs. III.4.c, III.4.d). Should raised intracranial pressure persist, this path may widen and generate irregular cavitations communicating with the ventricle via a small opening. We are in the environment of the (pre)motor cortex and thus at risk of contralateral motor disturbances. This type of porencephaly can also be seen after endoscopic neurosurgery.

Porencephaly after posthaemorrhagic hydrocephalus

This form is described in the sections on matrix haemorrhage (IV.1) and posthaemorrhagic hydrocephalus (IV.2).

Paraventricular porencephaly

In a rare case a cavity is found in white matter, separated from the lateral ventricle, and towards the leptomeninges it may be bordered by a small arachnoid cyst. Often this cavity is found in the region irrigated by the middle cerebral artery, and infarction caused by occlusion of one of the vessels may be involved. We came across such a cavity in a baby with severe intrauterine growth retardation but without neonatal problems (Fig. III.4.e). Parenchymal remnants may for a while remain visible in the cavity.

Expansive porencephaly

Focal paraventricular necrosis may develop *in utero* following matrix haemorrhage, leuko-malacia or arterial infarction. Especially in the latter instance the cyst may expand by itself (see unilateral hydrocephalus, section II.10). Quite often it is located in an area irrigated by the middle cerebral artery. If occurring between the 16th and 20th week of gestation, the lesion will be bordered by four-layered polymicrogyria. If occurring in the third trimester, the cortex overlying such a porencephalic cavity may be ulegyric. Any further growth of the cyst calls for shunting.

127

Polyporencephaly: multicystic encephalopathy (clastic porencephaly)

Following fetal asphyxia, the death of a member of a monozygotic twin pregnancy, fetal or neonatal encephalitis (*e.g.* due to CMV, toxoplasmosis, HSV, mumps or enterovirus), brain abcess or birth asphyxia, bilateral cavities may form in white matter. They do not communicate with the ventricle. They are often a mixture of large and small juxtaposed cysts, with irregular borders and shapes. They are usually found in the area of the middle cerebral artery. This may constitute an intermediary stage towards hydranencephaly. The cysts may reach as far as the cortex but do not include the molecular layer, which is thickened by gliosis. Sometimes cavities can be found in the striatum and brainstem. Then they are typically symmetric as expected after asphyxia with asystole or profound bradycardia. A strange form of polyporencephaly can be found after antenatal subpial and cerebral haemorrhage in alloimmune thrombocytopenia, most often temporal in location (Figs. III.1.h, III.4.g).

Dorsal porencephaly

In certain instances of congenital hydrocephalus with agenesis of the corpus callosum, a cystic expansion starting at the third or a lateral ventricle may reach up to the pia mater, along the midline. The falx being present and a separation between the basal ganglia having come about, this picture differs from that of holoprosencephalies with dorsal pouch (see median prosencephalic dysgenesis, section II.3).

REFERENCES

Berg, R.A., Aleck, K.A., Kaplan, A.M. (1983) 'Familial porencephaly.' *Archives of Neurology*, **40**, 567–569.

Bordarier, C., Robain, O., Ponsot, G. (1991) 'Bilateral porencephalic defect in a newborn after injection of benzol during pregnancy.' *Brain and Development*, **13**, 126–129.

Hunter, A.G.W. (1993) 'Brain.' *In:* Stevenson, R.E., Hall, J.G., Goodman, R.M. (Eds.) *Human Malformations and Related Anomalies. Vol. II, Oxford Monographs on Medical Genetics, No. 27.* Oxford: Oxford University Press, pp. 78–82.

Lauras, B., Damon, G., Allard, D., Claudy, A., Chavrier, Y. (1990) 'Syndrome oculo-cérébrocutané ou syndrome de Delleman et Oorthuys.' *Pédiatrie*, **45**, 193–196.

Lyen, K.R., Lingam, S., Butterfill, A.M., Marshall, W.C., Dobbing, C.J., Lee, D.S.C. (1981) 'Multicystic encephalomalacia due to fetal viral encephalitis.' *European Journal of Pediatrics*, **137**, 11–16.

Lyon, G., Van Coster, R. (1987) 'Porencephaly and arachnoid cysts.' *In:* Johnson, R.T. (Ed.) *Current Therapy in Neurologic Diseases, 2nd Edn.* Toronto: Decker, B.C., pp. 77–82.

Rahman, N., Adam, K.A.R. (1986) 'Congenital polycystic disease of the brain: report of an unusual case.' *Developmental Medicine and Child Neurology*, **28**, 72–76.

Schmitt, H.P. (1984) 'Multicystic encephalopathy—a polyetiologic condition in early infancy: morphologic, pathogenetic and clinical aspects.' *Brain and Development*, **6**, 1–9.

Smith, J.F., Rodeck, C. (1975) 'Multiple cystic and focal encephalomalacia in infancy and childhood with brain stem damage.' *Journal of the Neurological Sciences*, **25**, 377–388.

Tardieu, M., Evrard, P., Lyon, G. (1981) 'Progressive expanding congenital porencephalies: a treatable cause of progressive encephalopathy.' *Pediatrics*, **68**, 198–202.

Yokota, A., Oota, T., Matsukado, Y. (1984) 'Dorsal cyst malformations. Part I: Clinical study and critical review on the definition of holoprosencephaly.' *Child's Brain*, 11, 320–341.

Zonana, J., Adornato, B.T., Glass, S.T., Webb, M.J. (1986) 'Familial porencephaly and congenital hemiplegia.' *Journal of Pediatrics*, **109**, 671–674.

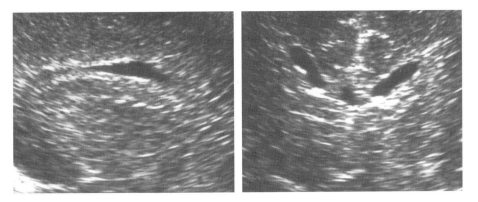

Fig. III.4.b. Ventilated preterm infant (30 weeks gestation), one of dizygotic twins: detail from first day 7.5 MHz scans (*left*, parasagittal; *right*, coronal). On the parasagittal section subtle diverticulation of the lateral ventricles in their parietal parts was noticeable. Focal tissue loss in the periventricular area might have caused this unusual type of minimal porencephaly

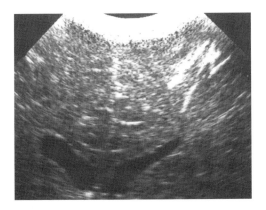

Fig. III.4.c. Coronal 7.5 MHz detail of the parietal area in an infant with spina bifida who had unsuccessful ventricular punctures prior to shunting. In the early stage these needle tracts show as echogenic lines from cortex to ventricle.

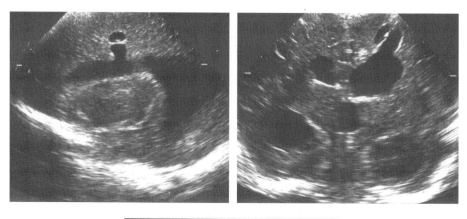

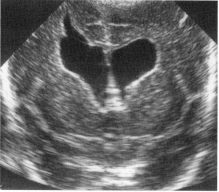

Fig. III.4.d. Two preterm infants with posthaemorrhagic hydrocephalus: 7.5 MHz sections (*top left*, parasagittal; the others coronal near the foramen of Monro).

Top. Baby treated with ventricular punctures for acute intracranial hypertension with severe apnoea.

Bottom. Baby treated with ventriculoscopic neurosurgery (plexus coagulation and perforation of the floor of the third ventricle) because of aqueductal stenosis.

Both cases show dilated puncture paths, so-called trajectory porencephaly. Pressure is guided from the ventricles into the artificially connected paths; this may lead to compression of surrounding tissue in and under the (pre)motor cortex.

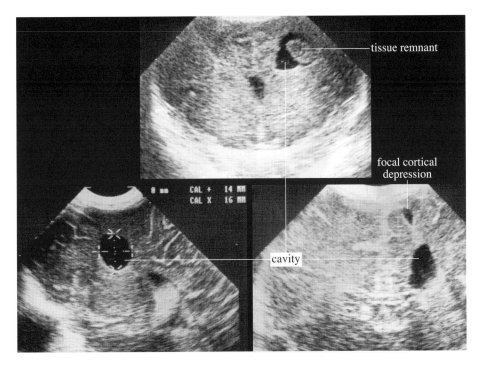

Fig. III.4.e. Growth retarded preterm infant: 7.5 MHz sections showing paraventricular porencephaly. The image at *bottom left* is parasagittal, the others coronal; the *top* image was taken on the first day of life, the others on day 53. In the initial pictures a cavity is seen with tissue remnants hanging on its outer wall; later on there is just a cavity, joined by an adjacent superficial arachnoid cyst where the cortex seems to be focally absent. The whole suggests focal infarction on a vascular, most likely arterial, basis.

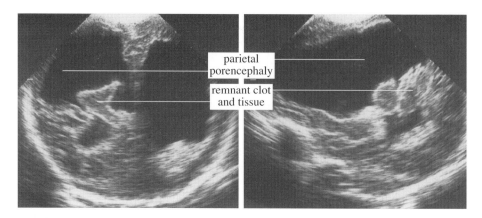

parietal
porencephaly

remnant clot
and tissue

Fig. III.4.g. Infant with *in utero* intracranial haemorrhage due to HPA1 alloimmunization: 7.5 MHz sections (*left*, coronal posterior; *right*, parasagittal). There is severe hydrocephalus, with a huge porencephalic cavity in the right parietal area. A mixture of tissue and clot is sculpting irregular intraluminal figures.

III.5 CHOROID PLEXUS CYST

It is estimated that in the course of the second trimester 0.3–0.6% of all fetuses develop echographically detectable cysts in the plexus of one or both lateral ventricles. Microcysts are most frequent (Fig. III.5.a). In fact plexus cyst formation is a normal histological phenomenon between the 17th and 28th gestational weeks. One should register cysts whenever their diameter exceeds 3 mm. They consist of CSF and cell debris surrounded by a connective tissue membrane, and are of neuro-epithelial origin. As a rule they are not the consequence of an antecedent plexus haemorrhage and they are not bordered by ependyma. They naturally evolve toward regression before the end of the second trimester, which explains why they are rarey found in the living baby. In some cases they are big enough to bulge into the lateral ventricle where they may rarely cause obstructive hydrocephalus. In the tela choroidea of the third ventricle similar cysts may be observed.

If a plexus cyst persists after 22–24 gestational weeks, or if it is exceptionally big (>1 cm), and above all if in combination with another anomaly, an underlying condition such as a chromosomal disorder should be carefully sought (Figs. III.5.b, III.5.c). The existence of smaller cysts, however, does not exclude an anomaly of the karyotype. Isolated plexus cysts predict karyotypic disorders only once in 150 instances, and their recognition therefore does not warrant amniocentesis.

Plexus cysts have been described in association with cysts of the germinal matrix at the foramen of Monro. Differentiation between those two using ultrasound is in some cases difficult, not to say impossible (Fig. III.5.d). Cysts identified in the perinatal period, even if their diameter is less than 7 mm, may remain visible for more than a year.

REFERENCES

Chitkara, U., Cogswell, C., Norton, K., Wilkins, I.A., Mehalek, K., Berkowitz, R.L. (1988) 'Choroid plexus cysts in the fetus: a benign anatomic variant or pathologic entity? Report of 41 cases and review of the literature.' *Obstetrics and Gynecology*, **72**, 185–189.

Fakhry, J., Schechter, A., Tenner, M.S., Reale, M. (1985) 'Cysts of the choroid plexus in neonates: documentation and review of the literature.' *Journal of Ultrasound Medicine*, **4**, 561–563.

Gupta, J.K., Cave, M., Lilford, R.J., Farrell, T.A., Irving, H.C., Mason, G., Hau, C.M. (1995) 'Clinical significance of fetal choroid plexus cysts.' *Lancet*, **346**, 724–729.

Heibel, M., Heber, R., Bechinger, D., Kornhuber, H.H. (1993) 'Early diagnosis of perinatal cerebral lesions in apparently normal full-term newborns by ultrasound of the brain.' *Neuroradiology*, **35**, 85–91.

Hertzberg, B.S., Kay, H.H., Bowie, J.D. (1989) 'Fetal choroid plexus lesions. Relationship of antenatal sonographic appearance to clinical outcome.' *Journal of Ultrasound Medicine*, **8**, 77–82.

Nakase, H., Hisanaga, M., Hashimoto, S., Imanishi, M., Utsumi, S. (1988) 'Intraventricular arachnoid cyst. Report of two cases.' *Journal of Neurosurgery*, **68**, 482–486.

Riebel, T., Nasir, R., Weber, K. (1992) 'Choroid plexus cysts: a normal finding on ultrasound.' *Pediatric Radiology*, **22**, 410–412.

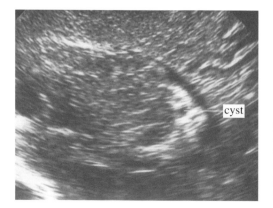

Fig. III.5.a. Term infant born after difficult vacuum extraction: first day parasagittal 7.5 MHz section. The small choroid plexus 'cyst' as observed here is a not uncommon incidental finding, without significance as to aetiology or prognosis.

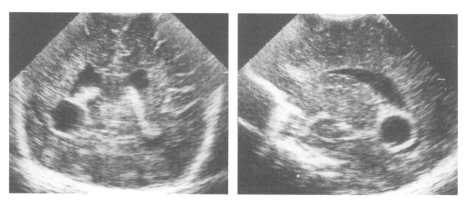

Fig. III.5.b. Term infant, small for gestational age: first day 7.5 MHz sections (*left*, coronal; *right*, parasagittal) of an anomaly detected antenatally in the third trimester. A large cyst can be seen in the glomus of the choroid plexus of the right lateral ventricle. This child had trisomy 18.

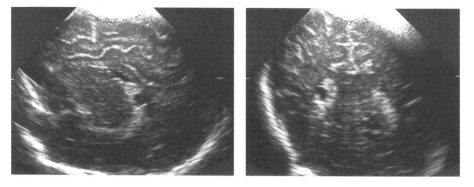

Fig. III.5.c. Term infant with triploidy: first day 7.5 MHz sections (*left*, parasagittal; *right*, coronal). An intermediate size cyst can be seen in the right choroid plexus. The association with other anomalies outweighs size in predicting an underlying chromosomal disorder.

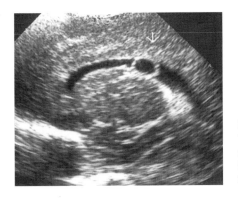

Fig. III.5.d. Preterm infant (29 weeks gestation): 7.5 MHz parasagittal section. Differentiating a germinolytic cyst from a cyst within the choroid plexus is not always easy, although the former may bulge into the lateral ventricle.

III.6 GERMINOLYSIS

Antenatal cystic matrix regression

Germinal matrix is abundantly present in the wall of the lateral ventricle during the second trimester, but in the third it regresses, persisting mostly in the region around the foramina of Monro—the caudothalamic groove—and along the temporal horn lateral wall (Fig. III.6.a). Haemorrhage and/or micro-infarction of this matrix, both *in* and *ex utero*, will often lead to cyst formation in the affected area in the second and third week after the event. As we are dealing with cysts with glial walls encircled by germinal cells but not by ependyma, the term pseudocyst is used. Unlike sonography, CT identifies only major cysts.

A connatal cyst in germinal matrix can be caused by a number of factors, including infective non-bacterial fetopathy (*e.g.* caused by CMV, rubella virus or *Toxoplasma gondii*), prenatal asphyxia, fetofetal transfusion, excessive uterolytic use of indomethacin, peroxisomal disorder, congenital lactacidemia or organic aciduria, intrauterine growth retardation, disorders with fetal convulsions, and anomaly of the karyotype.

It has not yet been shown that an echographic distinction can be made between germinolysis following haemorrhage or pure infarction. Usually one single round cyst is found after bleeding (Figs. III.6.b, III.6.c). The distinction may be irrelevant if one thinks of matrix haemorrhage as the consequence of an infarction as well. The cysts associated with a viral infection are often multiloculated. Sometimes there may be a spherical honeycomb cyst spilling over into the ventricle from the groove upwards. Often pseudocysts are present bilaterally though not entirely symmetrically. The collapsed cyst cannot be distinguished from the encircling echogenic structures in matrix and plexus.

Recently an antenatal variant of *frontal germinolysis* has been described originating around the mid-second to early third trimester (Figs. III.6.d–g). This type of germinolysis is not rare. We are confronted here with an often symmetric cyst under the lateral wall of the frontal horn. It is located medially to and lower than (cystic) periventricular leukomalacia and more laterally than the classic germinolytic cyst at the foramen of Monro. It is thus to be found in front of these foramina and separated from the lateral ventricle by a single membrane. On a parasagittal section it is elongated and often formed into two or three sections separated by thin septa (like a string of beads). Some cysts are almost 2 cm long. On a coronal section they mimic a widened frontal horn, although a distinction can be made using 7.5 MHz sonography. At around 4 months after term nearly all cysts of this type have been integrated into the ventricle. As an isolated finding these germinolytic changes are most often not associated with developmental problems, but exceptions may exist (Fig. III.6.j).

Postnatal cystic matrix regression

Postnatal cyst formation at the rear end of the head of the caudate nucleus is mainly found after a perinatal subependymal haemorrhage. Often one finds one or several rounded cysts, sometimes with trabeculation from the walls. During the following few months those cysts are gradually integrated into surrounding tissue. Although such cysts are often rounded, they may sometimes appear flattened.

Recently we have noted a possible association between bronchopulmonary dysplasia treated by dexamethasone and slow postnatal matrix regression with multilocular character

(Fig. III.6.h). After a period of slow triangular densification of the matrix, this tissue disappears, with or without an intermediate cystic stage. Such changes in matrix density have been registered in infants with proven CMV fetopathy, but we have found no evidence of this. Further studies are needed.

We had the opportunity to see germinolysis develop after acute birth asphyxia in two term newborn infants. In the course of the second week the part of the caudate nucleus just anterior to the caudothalamic groove disappeared, being replaced by an insufflated multilocular cyst with trabecula from wall to wall (Fig. III.6.i). These two clinical pictures (germinolysis after asphyxia and in association with bronchopulmonary dysplasia) suggest the existence of microvascular infarction of the striatal arteries coursing to this zone. In both cases germinolysis is not accompanied by striatal vasculopathy in the sense of echogenic striatal arteries, a phenomenon which may manifest itself after matrix haemorrhage.

Increased echodensity of some tissue bordering the floor of the lateral ventricle at the foramen of Monro was noticed in a case of congenital myelogenous leukaemia and in a newborn infant with fetomaternal transfusion and cutaneous extramedullary haematopoiesis (Fig. III.6.k). In both situations we thought we were dealing with matrix change, coloured as if with a soft white pencil. The distinction with germinolysis in the caudothalamic groove is best made via coronal sections.

REFERENCES

Beltinger, C., Saule, H., (1988) 'Sonography of subependymal cysts in congenital rubella syndrome.' *European Journal of Pediatrics*, **148**, 206–207.

Heibel, M., Heber, R., Bechinger, D., Kornhuber, H.H. (1993) 'Early diagnosis of perinatal cerebral lesions in apparently normal full-term newborns by ultrasound of the brain.' *Neuroradiology*, **35**, 85–91.

Lu, J.H., Emons, D., Kowalewski, S. (1992) 'Connatal periventricular pseudocysts in the neonate.' *Pediatric Radiology*, **22**, 55–58.

Larroche, J-C. (1972) 'Sub-ependymal pseudo-cysts in the newborn.' *Biology of the Neonate*, **21**, 170–183.

Mito, T., Ando, Y., Takeshita, K., Takada, K., Takashima, S. (1989) 'Ultrasonographical and morphological examination of subependymal cystic lesions in maturely born infants.' *Neuropediatrics*, **20**, 211–214.

Rademaker, K.J., de Vries, L.S., Barth, P.G. (1993) 'Subependymal pseudocysts: ultrasound diagnosis and findings at follow-up.' *Acta Paediatrica*, **82**, 394–399.

Russel, I.M.B., van Sonderen, L., van Straaten, H.L.M., Barth, P.G. (1994) 'Subependymal germinolytic cysts in Zellweger syndrome.' *Pediatric Radiology*, **25**, 254–255.

Shackelford, G.D., Fulling, K.H., Glasier, C.M. (1983) 'Cysts of the subependymal germinal matrix: sonographic demonstration with pathologic correlation.' *Radiology*, **149**, 117–121.

Shen, E-Y., Huang, F-Y. (1985) 'Subependymal cysts in normal neonates.' *Archives of Disease in Childhood*, **60**, 1072–1074.

Thun-Hohenstein, L., Forster, I., Kunzle, C., Martin, E., Boltshauser, E. (1994) 'Transient bifrontal solitary periventricular cysts in term neonates.' *Neuroradiology*, **36**, 241–244.

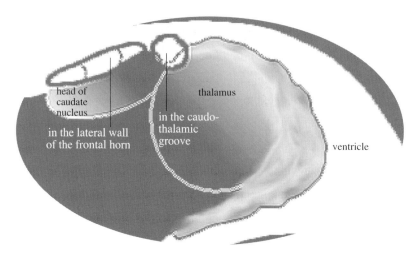

Fig. III.6.a. Two variants of antenatal cystic matrix regression, depicted in a parasagittal section.

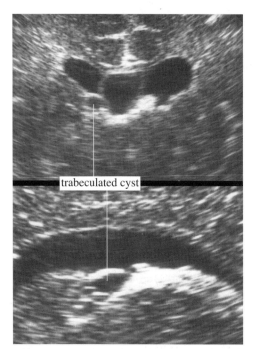

Fig. III.6.b. Preterm infant recovering from hyaline membrane disease: third week 7.5 MHz scans (*top*, coronal; *bottom*, parasagittal). Note moderate bilateral ventriculomegaly. Previous matrix haemorrhage in the caudothalamic groove has undergone cystic regression, the cyst being not quite round and multilocular.

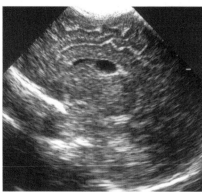

Fig. III.6.c. Term infant with seizures and recent focal thalamic infarction: first day parasagittal 7.5 MHz section. This coincident caudothalamic groove cyst is a longstanding antenatal lesion.

138

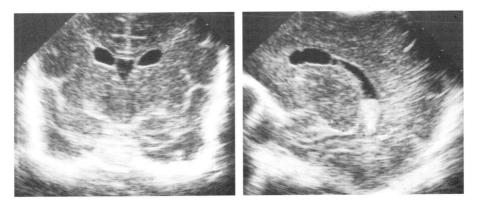

Fig. III.6.d. First day 7.5 MHz sonograms (*left*, coronal; *right*, parasagittal) of a 26 week gestation infant.

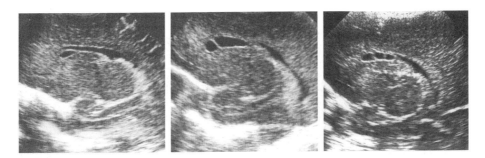

Fig. III.6.e. Frontal germinolysis from uni- to triloculated type in three different babies (all 7.5 MHz parasagittal scans).

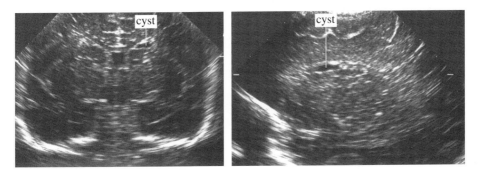

Fig. III.6.f. Day 5 scans of a term infant with urosepsis (*left*, coronal; *right*, parasagittal). Note flat frontal germinolytic cyst on the left.

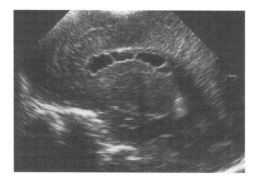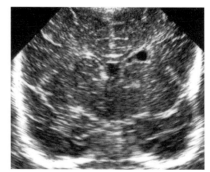

Fig. III.6.g. Two infants from different monozygotic twin pregnancies: *(left)* multilocular cysts giving 'string of beads' appearance (7.5 MHz parasagittal); *(right)* isolated cyst (7.5 MHz coronal). (Reproduced by permission from Rademaker *et al.* 1993.)

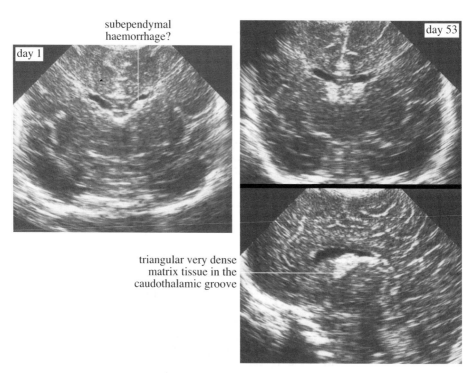

subependymal haemorrhage?

day 1

day 53

triangular very dense matrix tissue in the caudothalamic groove

Fig. III.6.h. *(Above and opposite)* Two preterm infants with severe chronic lung disease and prolonged treatment with oxygen, diuretics and dexamethasone; in both cases congenital and acquired CMV infection was excluded. (7.5 MHz sections). In both infants a triangular area bilateral and almost symmetric in the caudothalamic groove became hyperechogenic in the fourth to sixth weeks of life.

In the infant opposite, cystic regression of these presumed matrix areas started around day 40. There is usually no link with striatal arterial hyperechogenicity. The end result is a deep empty genuine caudothalamic groove. The significance of this type of matrix regression for development is unknown; given the resemblance with posthaemorrhagic or postvasculitic cystic germinolysis, one is tempted to see it as changes due to slow ischaemia. The contribution of steroids is not yet clear.

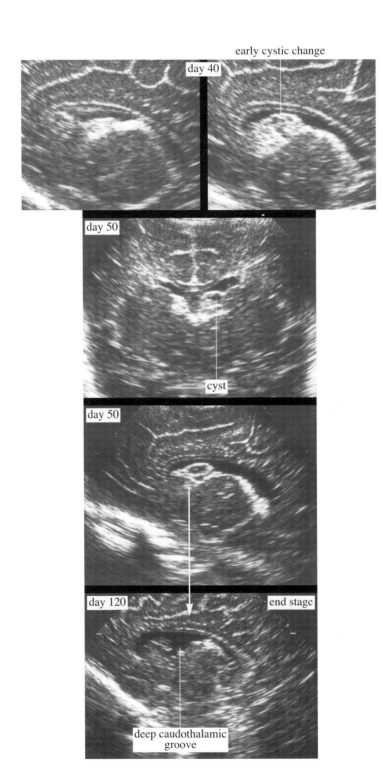

early cystic change

day 40

day 50

cyst

day 50

day 120

end stage

deep caudothalamic groove

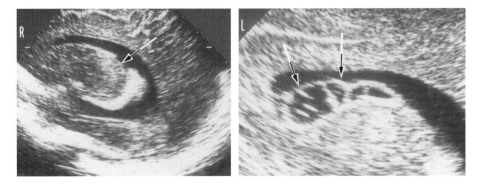

Fig. III.6.i. Parasagittal 7.5 MHz sections in the second week of a term infant with intrapartum hypovolaemic shock due to fetoplacental haemorrhage. The baby developed tremors in the late neonatal period. Dense thalami betray diencephalic damage due to excitotoxic neuronal injury. On the other hand asymmetric left cystic germinolysis in the caudate area is indicative of microvascular striatal hypoperfusion. Necrosis of part of the caudate head itself cannot be excluded. The boy developed within normal limits up to 2 years of age when mild mental retardation became obvious.

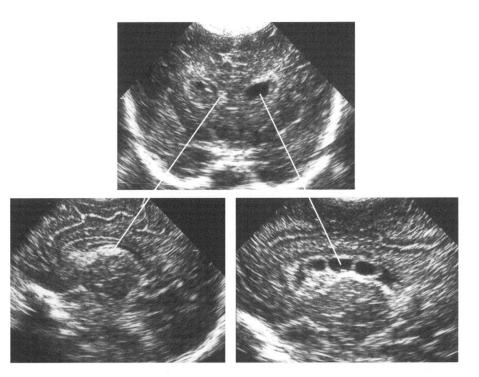

Fig. III.6.j. Preterm infant with fetal distress during labour: 7.5 MHz sections (*top*, coronal; *bottom*, parasagittal). Germinal matrix lesions of different timing are present: (*bottom left*) the echogenicity of the lesions suggests recent ischaemic or haemorrhagic damage; (*bottom right*) the cystic nature and multilocular aspect indicate long-standing ischaemic damage. At 1 year of age there was developmental retardation but no signs of cerebral palsy.

142

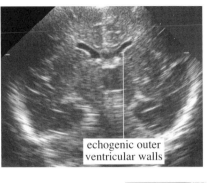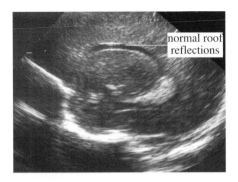

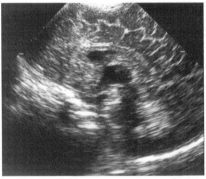

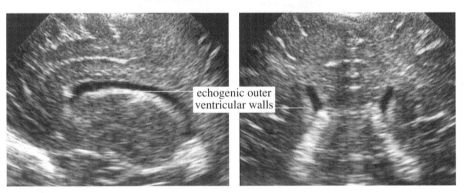

Fig. III.6.k. Term infant with chronic fetomaternal transfusion and cutaneous extramedullary haemato-poiesis (with the 'blueberry muffin rash'); all sections 7.5 MHz (*top left*, coronal; *top right*, parasagittal; *centre*, sagittal; *bottom left*, parasagittal; *bottom right*, coronal). It is not unusual to see bright reflections from the roof of the lateral ventricle directly beneath the angle of insonation; in this case, however, reflections were brighter from its floor. The outer lateral ventricular walls next to the caudate nucleus were softly hyperechogenic in a perfectly symmetric manner. There is dilatation of the third ventricle. From the context a plausible explanation could be haematopoiesis within matrix remnants at term.

III.7 MOEBIUS SEQUENCE AND CHARGE ASSOCIATION

The combination of persisting congenital facial paralysis and external ophthalmoplegia is called the Moebius sequence. The diagnosis of Moebius *syndrome* is in our view best set aside for the entity with late embryonic or early fetal infarction of the tegmentum of the hindbrain, probably due to occlusion of a branch of the primitive trigeminal artery in the second month after conception. The histopathological findings may include calcification, neuronal loss, gliosis and/or focal hypervascularity. Several disorders with congenital facial diplegia may cause or mimic the sequence.

Although it has yet to be shown that the brainstem lesion of Moebius syndrome can be picked up by MRI, one can sometimes diagnose the condition *in vivo* with CT scanning by recognition of calcification in front of the fourth ventricle. Recently we have also been able to show this zone of infarction echographically (Figs. III.7.a–c). Especially on a sagittal section, a region of hyperechogenicity without acoustic shadow is noticeable in the floor of the fourth ventricle. Axial sections can confirm this focus. Consequently, ultrasound by itself ought to make possible the diagnosis of Moebius syndrome, although in two infants with Moebius syndrome but preserved eye abduction we did not see the infarct with sonography.

In the CHARGE association with cranial pareses, one will find a slender brainstem with a dilated, often square fourth ventricle (Fig. III.7.d). Rarely, hemicerebellar atrophy will be found in children with Moebius sequence: one should search for an empty space unilaterally in the posterior fossa. There are isolated reports of total absence of the pons with congenital cranial paralyses or of severe atrophy of the medulla oblongata and the inferior surface of the pons with global cerebellar atrophy. In arthrogrypoid syndromes due to muscular or spinobulbar pathology, normal brain echograms may be expected in children with a normal head circumference (Fig. III.7.e).

REFERENCES

Bavinck, J.N.B., Weaver, D.D. (1986) 'Subclavian artery supply disruption sequence: hypothesis of a vascular etiology for Poland, Klippel–Feil and Möbius anomalies.' *American Journal of Medical Genetics*, **23**, 903–918.

Byerly, K.A., Pauli, R.M. (1993) 'Cranial nerve abnormalities in CHARGE association.' *American Journal of Medical Genetics*, **45**, 751–757.

D'Cruz, O.F., Swisher, C.N., Jaradeh, S., Tang, T., Konkol, R.J. (1993) 'Möbius syndrome: evidence for a vascular etiology.' *Journal of Child Neurology*, **8**, 260–265.

Govaert, P., Vanhaesebrouck, P., De Praeter, C., Fränkel, U., Leroy, J. (1989) 'Moebius sequence and prenatal brainstem ischemia.' *Pediatrics*, **84**, 570–573.

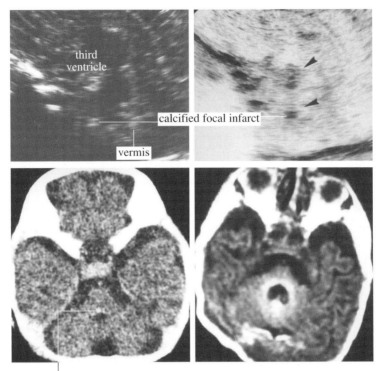

third
ventricle

calcified focal infarct

vermis

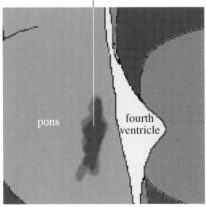

pons

fourth
ventricle

Fig. III.7.a. Term infant with Moebius syndrome: sagittal echograms compared with axial CT *(left)* and MR *(right)* images.

Genuine Moebius syndrome combines congenital facial diplegia with external ophthalmoplegia, both resulting from a focal infarct in the medullopontine tegmentum, the origin of which lies in the second month *in utero*. The area, histologically a zone with neuronal loss and gliosis, may show on CT due to calcification. We confirmed the focus of damage with ultrasound in two of four recent cases; the focus is in the floor of the fourth ventricle and may descend into the medulla oblongata. Conventional MR imaging may miss the lesion. Notice the absence of acoustic shadow underneath the hyperechogenic nodule.

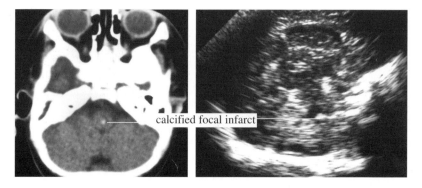

Fig. III.7.b. Axial CT and sagittal 5 MHz scans of a term infant with genuine Moebius syndrome. The calcified focus corresponds to a focal infarct.

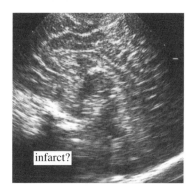

Fig. III.7.c. Sagittal 7.5 MHz sonogram of a term infant with Moebius syndrome and ophthalmoplegia of non-abducens type. A focal infarct is indistinctly seen in front of the fourth ventricle.

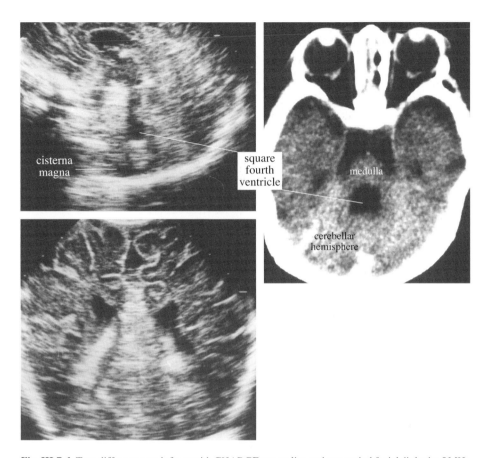

Fig. III.7.d. Two different term infants with CHARGE anomalies and congenital facial diplegia: 5 MHz sonograms (*top*, sagittal; *bottom*, coronal) compared with CT *(above right, below left)* and MR *(below right)* images. The fourth ventricle appears enlarged, with a square shape on sagittal section. The cisterna magna and basal cisterns are larger than expected. Low axial sonographic sections show a wide communication between fourth ventricle and cisterna magna (wrongly referred to as Dandy–Walker variant; see Fig. II.9.g, p. 86).

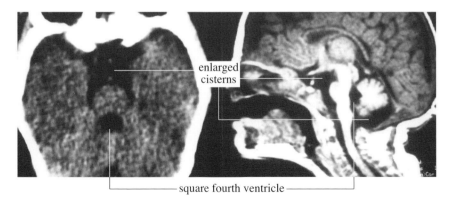

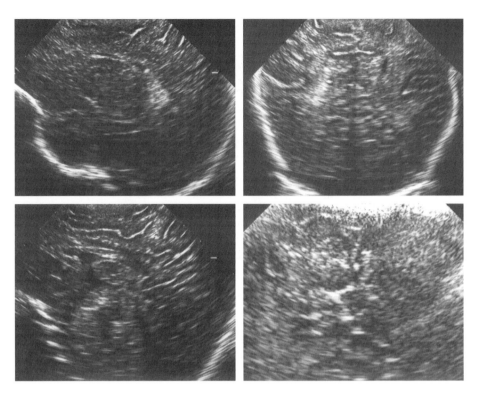

Fig. III.7.e. Term infant with lethal pulmonary hypoplasia due to Pena–Shokeir syndrome type I, a presentation that included facial diplegia and micrognathia: all 7.5 MHz images [*left*, (para)sagittal; *right*, coronal]. Fetal akinesia may be caused by several disorders involving neuromuscular pathways. In this case the postmortem findings corroborated the *in vivo* diagnosis of spinal neurogenic muscular atrophy with akinesia and arthrogryposis. Muscle histology excluded primary muscle disease, and the sonographic findings were entirely normal: there was no brain shrinkage, the ventricles were not dilated, and the midline structures were present. Histological findings included anterior spinal horn gliosis and atrophy of unknown cause. The mother, an alcoholic, reported physical abuse in pregnancy.

III.8 INFECTIVE FETOPATHY

Numerous patterns of antenatal brain injury exist within the framework of an infective fetopathy. In the neonatal period it may be possible to demonstrate the following entities by means of cranial ultrasound.

• *Vasculitis*. Shows as ramified dense lines along striatal arteries (see striatal vasculopathy, section III.9) (Figs. III.8.a–e). Microglial nodules around capillaries do not show echographically.

• *Leukomalacia*. Shows as increased echodensity of white matter, not necessarily only periventricular but stretching into gyral cores and the corpus callosum (Fig. III.8.k). This pattern gives rise to ventriculomegaly and cysts in white matter.

• *Calcification*. Shows as extra dense zones, often punctate in brain matter and 'en plaque' along ventricular walls (Figs. III.8.a–e, III.8.i). As an acoustic shadow is not a prerequisite, the calcified nature of these lesions must be confirmed with CT (MRI does not permit differentiation). As a rule, CMV infection will come to mind where calcification is located periventricularly; however, calcification near the ventricle wall also occurs in congenital rubella syndrome and HSV infection. We encountered CMV fetopathy with calcification in subcortical white matter (CT confirmed), a location habitually linked with toxoplasmosis. The periaqueductal region is preferentially affected by *Toxoplasma gondii*.

• *Ventriculitis*. Shows as dense ependymal borders (ependymitis); intraventricular debris with strand formation; periventricular venous and arterial infarction with or without cavitation (possibly porencephalic) (Fig. III.8.j); hydrocephalus due to aqueductal stenosis (Figs. III.8.h, III.8.i) or atresia of the outlet foramina of the fourth ventricle; or unilateral hydrocephalus from occlusion at the foramen of Monro.

• *Cyst formation in germinal matrix*, especially near the caudothalamic groove (Figs. III.8.e–g). These are often referred to as germinolytic cysts and are preceded not by haemorrhage but by microinfarction (see germinolysis, section III.6). Often this cystic change is honeycomb-like. When of third trimester onset, the initial neonatal scans may show germinal matrix disease in its echogenic stage, preceding a cystic phase.

• *Hydranencephaly*.

• *Subdural hygroma*.

• *Global cerebellar atrophy*.

• *Cerebral abcess and calcification*.

In postnatal encephalitis due to HSV, a marked neuropathologic evolution can be seen: after an interval of a few days the affected—especially parietotemporal—zones become hyperechogenic, thus producing pictures resembling infarction in the middle cerebral artery (Fig. III.8.k). Yet, the basal ganglia and internal capsule are not affected by this process which starts at the brain surface. Later one notices hydrocephalus *ex vacuo*, bilateral temporal necrosis with gyriform calcifications in the subcortex and periventricular calcification. In the worst cases, moving through a stage of multicystic encephalopathy one eventually ends with postnatal hydranencephaly.

Asymmetric lesions in periventricular white matter have been reported in echovirus encephalitis caused by transplacental infection just before birth. Parenchymal cysts and calcification may be seen in association with antenatal brain infection with nematodes (filariasis).

149

REFERENCES

Altshuler, G. (1973) 'Toxoplasmosis as a cause of hydranencephaly.' *American Journal of Diseases of Children*, **125**, 251–252.

Boesch, C., Issakainen, J., Kewitz, G., Kikini, R., Martin, E., Boltshauser, E. (1989) 'Magnetic resonance imaging of the brain in congenital cytomegaolovirus infection.' *Pediatric Radiology*, **19**, 91–93.

Carey, B.M., Arthur, R.J., Houlsby, W.T. (1987) 'Ventriculitis in congenital rubella: ultrasound demonstration.' *Pediatric Radiology*, **17**, 415–416.

Cleveland, R.H., Herman, T.E., Oot, R.F., Kushner, D.C. (1987) 'The evolution of neonatal herpes encephalitis as demonstrated by cranial ultrasound with CT correlation.' *American Journal of Perinatology*, **4**, 215–219.

Dykes, F.D., Ahmann, P.A., Lazzara, A. (1982) 'Cranial ultrasound in the detection of intracranial calcifications.' *Journal of Pediatrics*, **100**, 406–408.

Fonticiella, M., Lopez-Negrete, L., Prieto, A., Garcia-Hernandez, J.B., Orense, M., Fernandez-Diego, J., Gomez, J.L. (1995) 'Congenital intracranial filariasis: a case report.' *Pediatric Radiology*, **25**, 171–172.

Grant, E.G., Williams, A.L., Schellinger, D., Slovis, T.L. (1985) 'Intracranial calcification in the infant and neonate: evaluation by sonography and CT.' *Radiology*, **157**, 63–68.

Gray, P.H., Tudehope, D.I., Masel, J. (1992) 'Cystic encephalomalacia and intrauterine herpes simplex virus infection.' *Pediatric Radiology*, **22**, 529–532.

Haddad, J., Messer, J., Gut, J.P., Chaigne, D., Christmann, D., Willard, D.. (1990) 'Neonatal echovirus encephalitis with white matter necrosis.' *Neuropediatrics*, **21**, 215–217.

Matsumoto, N., Yano, S., Miyao, M., Kamoshita, S., Itoh, K. (1983) 'Two-dimensional ultrasonography of the brain: its diagnostic usefulness in herpes simplex encephalitis and cytomegalic inclusion disease.' *Brain and Development*, **5**, 327–333.

Parisot, S., Droulle, P., Feldmann, M., Pinaud, P., Marchal, C. (1991) 'Unusual encephaloclastic lesions with periventricular calcification in congenital rubella.' *Pediatric Radiology*, **21**, 229–230.

Shaw, D.W.W., Cohen, W.A. (1993) 'Viral infections of the CNS in children: imaging features.' *American Journal of Roentgenology*, **160**, 125–133.

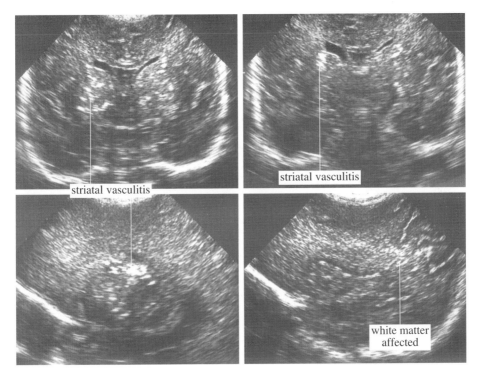

Fig. III.8.a. Term infant with hepatosplenomegaly, thrombocytopenia and apnoea due to fatal fetal infection with CMV: 7.5 MHz sections (*top*, coronal; *bottom*, parasagittal). There are foci of periventricular echogenicity in the heads of the caudate nuclei. Short linear and punctate hyper-echogenicities mark the striatal arteries in the globus pallidus. On the parasagittal sections these vasculitic patterns have induced an echogenic plaque in the rear end of the caudate head. Occipital periventricular white matter is also altered by echogenic punctate foci. Ventricular dilatation is minimal and present only on the right.

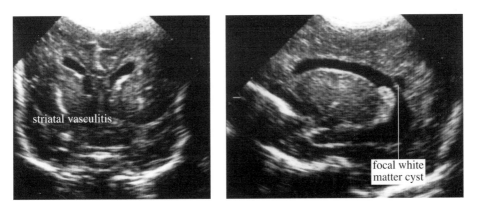

Fig. III.8.b. Preterm infant: 7.5 MHz sections (*left*, coronal; *right*, parasagittal) reveal striatal vasculopathy and periventricular calcification caused by fetal CMV infection. There is mild ventriculomegaly. Note the small porencephalic cyst at the parieto-occipital transition area, possibly the result of focal infarction.

151

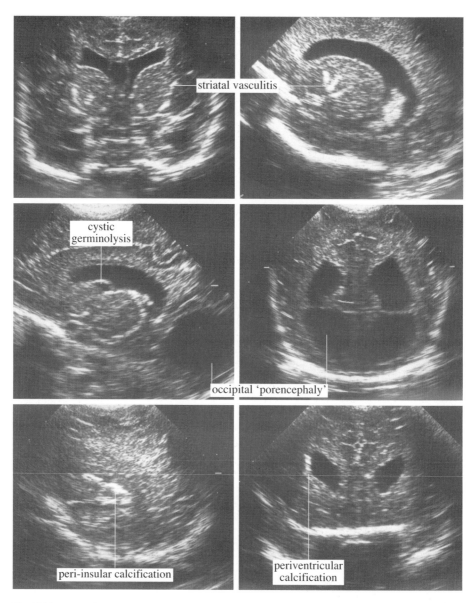

Fig. III.8.c. Term infant with microcephaly and seizures due to intrauterine infection with CMV in the latter part of the second trimester: 7.5 MHz sections (*top left*, coronal; *top right*, parasagittal; *middle left*, parasagittal; *middle right*, coronal; *bottom left*, outward parasagittal; *bottom right*, anterior coronal). There are linear echogenicities along striatal arteries. Cystic germinolysis is seen within the caudothalamic groove. There is moderate ventriculomegaly, with striking porencephalic prolongation of the occipital horns behind symmetric horizontal septae. A periventricular calcium deposit is seen along the right frontal horn. These are all features typical of long-standing fetal brain infection.

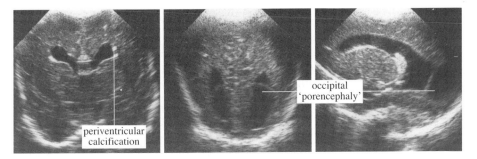

Fig. III.8.d. Preterm infant (36 weeks gestation) with fatal CMV fetopathy: 7.5 MHz sections (*left* and *centre*, coronal; *right*, parasagittal). Note occipital sequestration analogous to that seen in Fig. III.8.c. (This girl was one of triplets; her two sisters were also infected, with one of them showing germinolysis on ultrasound)

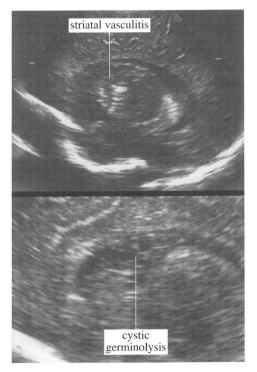

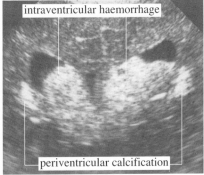

Fig. III.8.e. Two term infants with congenital CMV infection: 7.5 MHz images (*left*, parasagittal; *right*, coronal). Typical features are striatal vasculitis, multicystic germinolysis and periventricular calcification. IVH due to haemostatic defects was a neonatal complication.

153

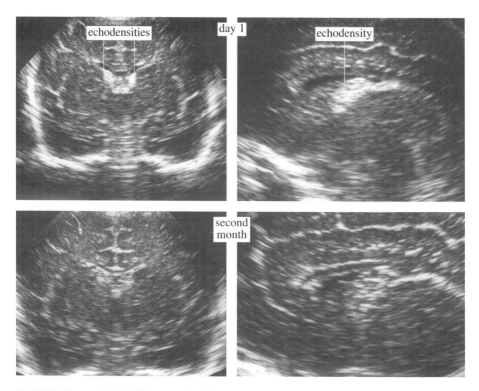

Fig. III.8.f. Parasagittal 7.5 MHz scans of an infant who presented with thrombocytopenia and splenomegaly due to third trimester CMV infection. Triangular areas of echodensity in both caudothalamic grooves were seen for weeks, after which fine cysts formed an intermediate stage before eventual disappearance of these echodense areas. Microvasculitis or direct matrix tissue infection are possible causes for this slow matrix regression.

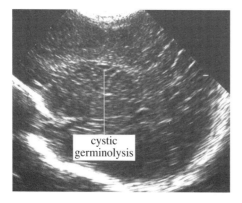

Fig. III.8.g. Asymptomatic term infant whose mother had third trimester CMV infection: 7.5 MHz parasagittal section. Whether the isolated paraventricular frontal germinolysis was an incidental finding or associated with CMV is unclear.

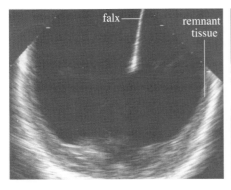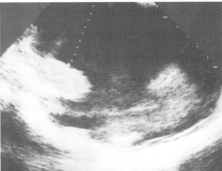

Fig. III.8.h. Term infant with extreme macrocephaly: 5 MHz sections (*left*, coronal; *right*, parasagittal). The mother had clinical varicella around the 10th week of pregnancy. The extreme hydrocephalus was presumably due to aqueductal stenosis. Note persistence of a layer of brain tissue against the bone. The presence of a falx excludes holoprosencephaly. No VZV-specific IgM was found and the virus was not isolated.

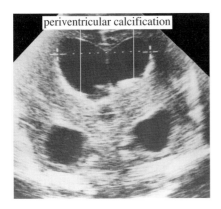

Fig. III.8.i. Congenital toxoplasmosis in a child with seizures and diabetes insipidus: 5 MHz coronal scan demonstrates severe encephalitis and ventriculitis.

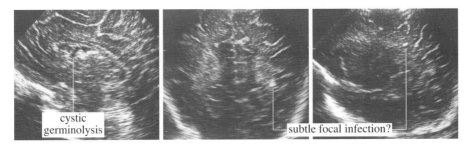

Fig. III.8.j. Asymptomatic *Toxoplasma* infection in a term infant: 7.5 MHz scans (*left*, sagittal; *centre*, coronal; *right*, parasagittal). Maternal pregnancy seroconversion was known to have occurred. The infant had raised *Toxoplasma*-specific IgM and a retinal lesion. Subtle changes such as germinolysis in the caudothalamic groove and focal echodense areas in white matter may indicate *Toxoplasma* brain infection. Striatal vasculopathy is probably uncommon.

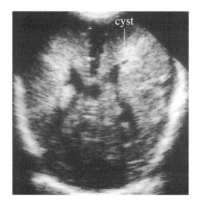

cyst

Fig. III.8.k. Term infant with neonatal HSV encephalitis developing in the second week of life: 5 MHz posterior coronal view. There is white matter inflammation and necrosis, resulting in severe generalized hyperechogenicity, not sparing periventricular or subcortical areas. An early cyst is seen on top of the left lateral ventricle.

III.9 STRIATAL VASCULOPATHY

In recent years high frequency (7.5 MHz) echography has 'discovered' a pathological entity that is surprisingly frequent in the neonatal period. Perforating striatal arteries, branches of the middle cerebral artery, originate in the lateral sulcus and climb upwards to the scanhead in the anterior fontanelle. These vessels are quite prominent in fetal life because they ensure perfusion of the germinal matrix, persisting in the third trimester mainly around the caudothalamic groove (Fig. III.9.a). Whether and why those vessels are preferentially affected or whether they merely catch our attention, is unclear. In about one out of every four instances with striatal vasculopathy intrathalamic arteries are also affected. One of the possible explanations might be found in the normal dynamics of cerebral angiogenesis: in the third trimester a muscular coat is formed around striatal arteries, whereas in arteries in white matter this does not happen until term.

As well as those conditions listed in Table III.1 we have observed striatal vasculopathy in congenital toxoplasmosis, neurosialidosis type II and leukodystrophy of unknown cause. The finding is consequently non-specific.

The fact that genuine infarction in the vessel area of a major striatal artery is a quite different entity, is illustrated in the section on arterial infarction.

Affected striatal arteries show up as unusual *linear echodensities* (Figs. III.9.b, III.9.d–f, III.9.j). They may seem ramified, especially visible in parasagittal sections, and form a branching, often bi- or trifurcated pattern. Generally the lesions are pulsatile. They almost never produce an acoustic shadow unless densely calcified—calling for CT confirmation. Non-calcified lesions will only be seen echographically. On a parasagittal section a string of dense nodules may show up as transverse sections of thalamostriatal arteries just below the outer wall of the lateral ventricle. In many cases the artery can be traced to its origin in the middle cerebral artery in a less echodense form. Doppler imaging reveals the arterial nature of those densities. Flow velocities do not differ from those in normal brains (striatal branches can always be made visible with colour Doppler imaging). In normal infants one can also see softer reflections from these vessels. The transition to pathology resides in an increased density that is particularly difficult to prove objectively, and in the impression that reflections are wider and, in certain places, nodularly thickened when pathological. True striatal vasculopathy is nearly always bilateral, but often asymmetric.

Pointed hyperdensities are often found in these regions, and their pathological nature is dubious (Fig. III.9.c). In such cases they are often located under the head of the caudate nucleus. We suspect that these are tangentially sectioned Virchow–Robin spaces around a normal artery.

We have also observed dense striatal vessel trajectories develop *postnatally* in association with densities in the germinal matrix of sick preterm infants (Figs. III.9.g, III.9.h). They occur following a haemorrhage or infarct in the matrix, in the late neonatal period. We postulate that these involve a vascular reaction to haemorrhage or are the visible expression of a striatal arterial insult also inducing matrix haemorrhage and/or infarction. In those cases the echogenic branches point towards the lesion in the matrix. The fact that this vasculopathy is not seen with classic leukomalacia probably confirms that the latter type of lesion affects a border zone and may not be understood as necrosis within an arterial

157

TABLE III.1
Clinical conditions producing echodense striatal arteries

1. Infective fetopathy: CMV, rubella virus, HSV, *Treponema pallidum*, VZV, *Toxoplasma gondii*, HIV
2. Asphyxia: fetal, perinatal and postnatal
3. Chromosomal anomaly: trisomy 21, trisomy 13, del 5q
4. Storage disease: neonatal sialidosis
5. Bacterial meningitis
6. Other: leukodystrophy, Zellweger syndrome, Lowe syndrome, Weaver syndrome, Smith–Lemli–Opitz syndrome, glutaric aciduria type II, linear naevus sebaceus, maternal heroin abuse, galactosaemia, leukaemia, maternal diabetes mellitus
7. In association with haemorrhage in germinal matrix
8. Recipient twin in fetofetal transfusion syndrome

vessel area. Analogous to hydranencephaly and focal arterial infarction, one might expect intimal hypertrophy and splitting and calcification of the tunica elastica of arteries that used to perfuse an infarcted area. This hypothesis awaits histological confirmation.

The observation of striatal linear densities in children with unexplained neonatal hepatitis or hepatosplenomegaly (Fig. III.9.i) remains as yet unclarified, but suggests the existence of a fetal encephalitis.

REFERENCES

Ben-Ami, T., Yousefzadeh, D., Backus, M., Reichman, B., Kessler, A., Hammerman-Rozenberg, C. (1990) 'Lenticulostriate vasculopathy in infants with infections of the central nervous system: sonographic and Doppler findings.' *Pediatric Radiology*, **20**, 575–579.

Bode, H., Rudin, C. (1995) 'Calcifying arteriopathy in the basal ganglia in human immunodeficiency virus infection.' *Pediatric Radiology*, **25**, 72–73.

Cabañas, F., Pellicer, A., Morales, C., García-Alix, A., Stiris, T.A., Quero, J. (1994) 'New pattern of hyperechogenicity in thalamus and basal ganglia studied by color Doppler flow imaging.' *Pediatric Neurology*, **10**, 109–116.

de Vries, L.S., Beek, F.J.A., Stoutenbeek, P. (1995) 'Lenticulostriate vasculopathy in twin to twin transfusion syndrome: sonographic and CT findings.' *Pediatric Radiology*, **25**, 541–542.

Hughes, P., Weinberger, E., Shaw, D.W.W. (1991) 'Linear areas of echogenicity in the thalami and basal ganglia of neonates: an expanded association. Work in progress.' *Radiology*, **179**, 103–105.

Kuban, K.C.K., Gilles, F.H. (1985) 'Human telencephalic angiogenesis.' *Annals of Neurology*, **17**, 539–548.

Ries, M., Deeg, K-H., Heininger, U. (1990) 'Demonstration of perivascular echogenicities in congenital cytomegalovirus infection by colour Doppler imaging.' *European Journal of Pediatrics*, **150**, 34–36.

Teele, R.L., Hernanz-Schulman, M., Sotrel, A. (1988) 'Echogenic vasculature in the basal ganglia of neonates: a sonographic sign of vasculopathy.' *Radiology*, **169**, 423–427.

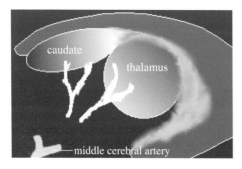

Fig. III.9.a. Localization of linear striatal vasculopathy between the lateral sulcus (with the middle cerebral artery), the head of the caudate nucleus and the caudothalamic groove.

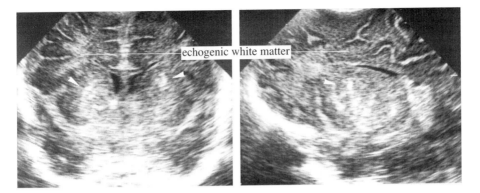
echogenic white matter

Fig. III.9.b. Term infant with thrombocytopenia and hepatosplenomegaly: 7.5 MHz sections (*left*, coronal; *right*, parasagittal). There is a marked increase in echogenicity along striatal and thalamic arteries *(arrowheads)*. White matter is strongly echogenic from the periventricular area well into the gyral cores; this induces a clear contrast between white matter (softly bright), cortex (almost black) and sulcus (very bright), an observation we refer to as 'railway track appearance'. This cortico-medullary contrast is seen in subcortical leukomalacia, with marked venous congestion (as following difficult delivery or with certain congenital cardiac disorders) and in leukodystrophies as here. This child had vacuolated circulating lymphocytes and biochemical proof was found for sialidosis type II, a lysosomal storage disorder.

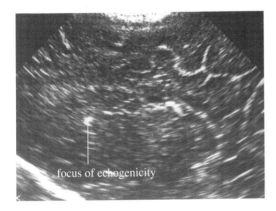
focus of echogenicity

Fig. III.9.c. Term infant with trisomy 21: parasagittal 7.5 MHz section. There is a short linear hyperechogenic focus in the anterior limb of the internal capsule. Doppler examination showed this to be part of a striatal artery.

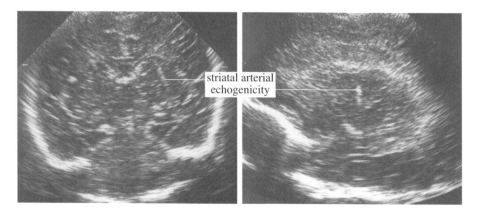

Fig. III.9.d. Term infant with cyanotic heart disease and deletion of part of the long arm of chromosome 5: 7.5 MHz sections (*left*, coronal; *right*, parasagittal). A streak of echogenicity is seen along a striatal artery on the left.

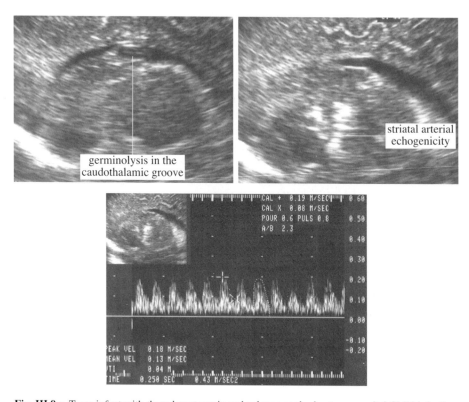

Fig. III.9.e. Term infant with thrombocytopenia and splenomegaly due to congenital CMV infection: parasagittal 7.5 MHz sections and Doppler registration of an involved striatal artery. The combined occurrence of cystic germinolysis and marked striatal vasculopathy is characteristic of fetal brain infection with CMV. The Doppler examination shows normal flow in such hyperechogenic striatal vessels.

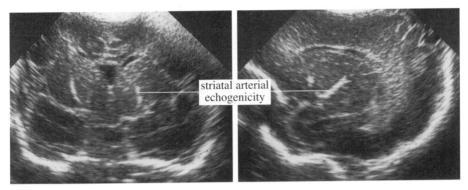

Fig. III.9.f. Preterm infant, the recipient in a fetofetal transfusion syndrome: 7.5 MHz sections (*left*, coronal; *right*, parasagittal). For an unknown reason there is a broad band of echogenicity along a substantial part of a few striatal arteries, without clear indication of matrix haemorrhage or infarction. (Reproduced by permission from de Vries *et al.* 1995.)

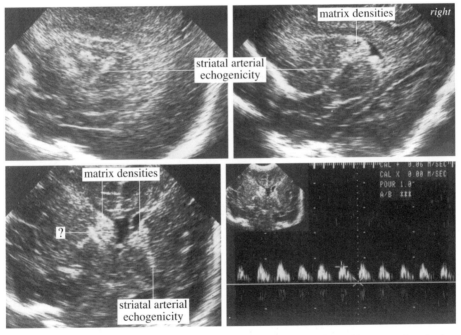

Fig. III.9.g. Preterm infant with bronchopulmonary dysplasia and prolonged hypoxaemic episodes, finally leading to late neonatal death: 7.5 MHz sections (*top*, parasagittal; *bottom left*, coronal) and Doppler examination. Whereas the initial sonograms had been normal, following deterioration there was an increase in echogenicity of both matrix areas in the caudothalamic groove. Underneath these densities, patent striatal arteries (see Doppler trace) pointed to the sick areas. Although unsubstantiated by postmortem findings, the likely diagnosis in this case was bilateral arterial matrix infarction due to hypoxaemia. It is not possible to differentiate with certainty from haemorrhage with sonography, but CT examination had excluded haemorrhage. On the right a density of unknown nature is seen between the matrix density and the striatal artery pointing towards it (see Fig. III.2.d).

161

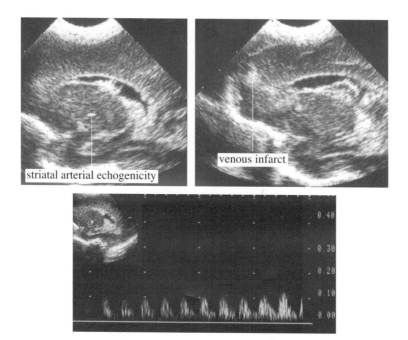

Fig. III.9.h. Preterm (27 weeks) infant, one of dizygotic twins, with severe hyaline membrane disease: second week 7.5 MHz right parasagittal sections and corresponding striatal artery flow signals. There is a right grade II intraventricular haemorrhage, with irregular clot on the choroid plexus and a dense ependymal lining. A frontal parenchymal venous infarction is associated with the subependymal haemorrhage in the caudothalamic groove. Following initial normal appearance a striatal artery (see flow profile) became echodense after the event.

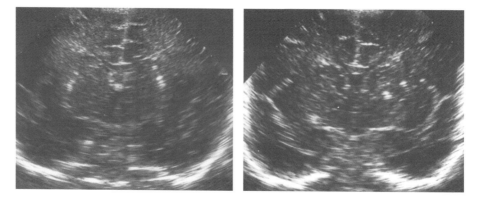

Fig. III.9.i. Coronal 7.5 MHz sections of two term infants: *(left)* with hepatocellular necrosis, splenomegaly and raised total serum IgM; and *(right)* with hepatosplenomegaly. Both show bilateral, almost symmetric, striatal vasculopathy. Screening tests for *Toxoplasma*, rubella virus, CMV and HSV infections were negative. A diagnosis of an unknown viral infection with striatal vasculitis is mooted.

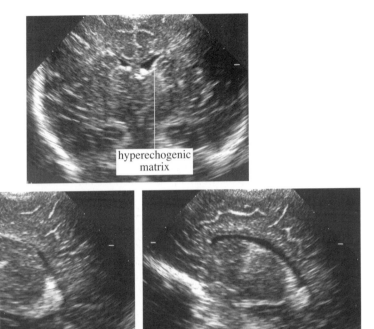

Fig. III.9.j. Term infant with hepatosplenomegaly due to congenital myelogenous leukaemia: 7.5 MHz sections (*top*, coronal; *bottom*, parasagittal). There was soft matrix echogenicity from the start (see Fig. III.6.k). Following a course of chemotherapy striatal arteries became mildly hyperechogenic.

SECTION IV
PATHOLOGY: INTRACRANIAL
HAEMORRHAGE

Three major aspects can be distinguished: (1) antenatal haemorrhage, as described in section III.1; (2) germinal matrix haemorrhage (GMH) and its consequences, seen in sick preterm infants; and (3) intracranial haemorrhage of the term neonate [for details of a personal study and comprehensive references, see Govaert, P. (1993) *Cranial Haemorrhage in the Term Newborn Infant. Clinics in Developmental Medicine No. 129*. London: Mac Keith Press].

IV.1 BLEEDING INTO GERMINAL MATRIX AND VENTRICLE

After the majority of telencephalic cortical neurons have formed (by the 16th gestational week), a network of microsize blood vessels (without a muscular wall) and (sub)ventricular neuroepithelial cells persists in the wall of the lateral ventricle. This is referred to as 'germinal matrix'. Vascular rupture inherent to GMH occurs at those microvessels or their capillaro-venous transition. Pape and Wigglesworth (1979), to whom the reader is referred, describe in detail the anatomical development of arteries, capillaries and veins forming the cerebral and cerebellar vascular beds. The matrix zone widens up to the 34th gestational week, its presence becoming more prominent in the frontal horns and in the body of the lateral ventricle (Fig. IV.1.q). After the 34th week pockets of germinal matrix remain present in the caudothalamic groove, the lateral wall of the occipital horn, the roof of the temporal and the tip of the frontal horn (Fig. IV.1.a). Matrix also resides in the roof of the fourth ventricle, where autopsies reveal primary haemorrhage in one in ten cases of intraventricular haemorrhage (IVH).

Manifest hypoxia or abrupt fluctuations in arterial or venous blood pressure may cause mechanical rupture of those frail vessel walls. Asphyxia and respiratory problems are the two main risk factors for GMH. In a number of babies venous congestion during labour may contribute to the phenomenon. Vaginal breech delivery is an accepted risk factor in preterm infants of less than 34 weeks gestation, and sometimes explains early GMH (onset within six hours after birth).

Video recording has established two variants: (1) the rapidly progressive type, maturing within ten seconds in deeper matrix layers, is immediately echodense and usually presents with a catastrophic clinical picture; (2) the slowly progressive variant, which is less frequent, takes minutes to become visible in the surface layers of the matrix and is initially hypodense. In the first type one may find an island of parenchyma surrounded by blood. The on-line observation of bleeding into germinal matrix has illustrated an arterial jet to the lesion, suggesting the bleeding vessel cannot be distant from striatal arteries. Recent studies appear to show the origin is not in sinusoidal matrix rete, but rather in the small venules of the exterior matrix stratum, where the medullary veins converge (first variant). Having been provoked, haemorrhage may grow due to a disturbance of clot formation, or due to

164

cerebral hyperperfusion accompanying pneumothorax, seizures or hypercarbia. Although it is not exceptional to find thrombosis in the smaller veins around and inside a matrix bleed, this no longer appears to be the primary event. After bleeding, tissue reaction takes place with invasion by macrophages and gliosis. The primary haemorrhage (with a blood pool of 2–30 mm diameter) will regress with cyst formation and/or gliosis.

GMH/IVH occurs in 30–40% of liveborn infants weighing <1500 g. More than two-thirds suffer from ventricular bleeding. In 75% and 90% of cases respectively it occurs within 48 and 72 hours after birth. It is not exceptional within the first two hours of life. A weak preference for the left side (as also found with arterial infarction and subarachnoid haematoma) remains unexplained. IVH at term mostly originates in choroid plexus and not germinal matrix. In the preterm baby the opposite applies, about 90% starting in the matrix.

With the advent of CT scanning, and later ultrasound, differences in severity of GMH/IVH became apparent, leading to a classification in four grades:

- Grade I   — limited to subependymal matrix;
- Grade II   — clear spill-over to the ventricle, but filling less than 50% of the lateral vent-ricle and consequently without acute ventriculomegaly;
- Grade III — spill-over to the ventricle, with acute dilatation because of flooding of 50% or more of one or both lateral ventricles;
- Grade IV   — grades 1, 2 or 3 with haemorrhage in a more or less large part of the perivent-ricular parenchyma.

It is not a simple matter to make a distinction between a subependymal haemorrhage amidst normal anatomic variations on the one hand and a limited IVH or a matrix infarct on the other (Figs. IV.1.c–e). The principal reason to suspect haemorrhage is a dense, often rounded thickening of the plexus near the foramen of Monro at the caudothalamic groove. Normal plexus, not present in the frontal and occipital horns, should be sharply delineated, contain micropulsations and produce a symmetric picture with the head in the midline. Certain findings suggest the recent occurrence of IVH: densities in front of the foramina of Monro, irregular luminal plexus borders, and densities in the occipital horn (Figs. IV.1.f, IV.1.g). A vast subependymal haemorrhage may spill over into the ventricle, while conversely, a large ventricular bleed may hide a subependymal lesion due to the pressure it exerts (Fig. IV.1.h). When blood from the ventricular system passes through the foramina of the fourth ventricle, one can see on a sagittal or frontal section an additional shadow against the bone and under the cerebellar vermis in the cisterna magna's arachnoid membranes.

With ultrasound recent haemorrhages show as echodensities provided there has been fibrin deposition. In the case of a coagulation disorder, the haemorrhage may remain hypo- or isodense for a longer time before turning denser.

The diagnosis of *haemorrhage into choroid plexus* will be made only if one comes across a predominantly asymmetric and clear hyperdensity, undergoing cystic regression at a later stage (Fig. IV.1.i). This asymmetry shows best in a posterior coronal section. In certain cases, especially with an extremely immature baby, it may be impossible to differentiate between a haemorrhage in the germinal matrix of the body of the lateral ventricle or in its plexus. Secondary cysts in the plexus may become quite large, but even

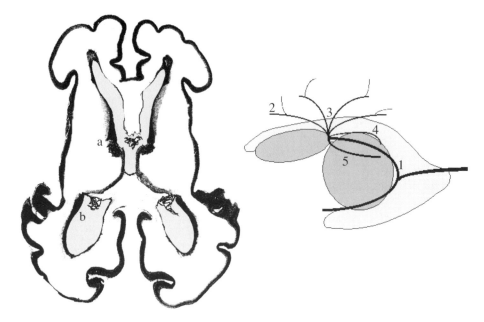

Fig. IV.1.a. *(Left)* At 28 weeks of gestation matrix remnants are most abundant around the caudothalamic groove (a) near the foramen of Monro and (b) in the lateral wall of the temporal and occipital horns, but other sites remain also. [Adapted from Feess-Higgins, A., Larroche, J-C. (1987) *Le Développement du Cerveau Foetal Humain. Atlas Anatomique.* Paris: Masson.]

   (Right) The venous anatomy near the caudothalamic groove may predispose to small vessel rupture: the internal cerebral vein (1) makes a U-turn at the point of collection of the collateral septal (2), trans-caudate (3) and superior choroidal veins (4), before ending as the terminal or thalamostriate vein (5).

then it is not always possible to make a distinction between a germinolytic cyst and an anterior plexus cyst. We suppose that very large cysts exceptionally occur in the matrix and seem to indicate the initial event was a plexus haemorrhage.

   After two or three weeks the ependyma of a ventricle that contained blood becomes denser, a process that may persist for several weeks (Fig. IV.1.g). This observation may suffice to identify a preceding IVH. Clot becomes progressively isodense from the centre outwards, leaving behind a jumble of clot fragments in the cavity. Occasionally one comes across the picture of a 'ventricle within the ventricle': central lysis carves out a cast of the ventricle that was filled with blood. When these organizing clots have become iso- or hypo-dense on CT (in the second and third week), their dense aspect may continue to show up on ultrasound for a while longer, thus sustaining a diagnosis in retrospect. Septation and isolation of a ventricle or a compartment are possible although they are more indicative of ventriculitis. The ventricular fluid remains cloudy as long as there is a haematocrit of at least 0.5% and/or as soon as there is a manifest increase of the protein content (Fig. IV.1.p). Sometimes levels show at the junction of CSF and protein-rich clot residue. Often the original matrix haemorrhage gives rise to a cyst caught in the caudothalamic groove behind the foramen of Monro (Fig. IV.1.l). Mostly this cyst has a single compartment. In other cases

166

only an echogenic strip in the ventricle will remain visible for a time near this groove. Regression does not have to cause visible cyst formation.

Small clot fragments and protein-rich conglomerates may, together with circulating CSF, end up in distal irrigation areas and generate occlusion of the aqueduct, the outlet foramina of the fourth ventricle, pericerebellar cisterns, pericerebral arachnoid spaces or arachnoid villi in venous sinuses. The incidence of *posthaemorrhagic hydrocephalus* is estimated at about 40% in case of grade III haemorrhage, whereas it is less than 20% with grade II. In a rare instance (part of) a ventricle is loculated by glial bands, inducing local hydrocephalus.

Grade IV haemorrhagic involvement of the parenchyma is commonly referred to as either *intraparenchymatous echodensity* (IPE) or *periventricular venous infarction*. Instead of calling it grade IV haemorrhage, some groups prefer a three grade classification system with a separate notation for the haemorrhagic parenchymal component (Volpe 1990).

A venous infarction occurs from a few hours up to a few days after the initial matrix bleeding, and location and size will vary. A venous lesion was first postulated (see Schmidt 1965); later conflicting views about *parenchymal extension* and *parenchymal infarction* have been reviewed in detail by Paneth *et al.* (1994) and will not be repeated here. Postmortem studies by Gould *et al.* (1986) and Takashima *et al.* (1986) strongly suggest that the parenchymal lesion is one of venous infarction.

On ultrasound it is first recognized as a triangular density hardly touching the ventricle. In a second stage the lesion grows and joins up with the ventricle, finally merging into a single globular density together with the original matrix lesion. The process may stabilize at each of those stages (Figs. IV.1.b, IV.1.k). The manifest IPE or parenchymal component that belongs to a large subependymal or intraventricular haemorrhage is extremely echodense, shows irregular borders with the cortex and allows no separation between density and ventricular clot (Fig. IV.1.j). 7.5 and 10 MHz scanning provide a reliable tool for investigating IPEs. Quite often an IPE originally appears to be large, but in the course of the second week the size of the zonal hyperdensity slightly decreases, the genuine infarct becoming better delineated and smaller than expected (Fig. IV.1.r). Three variants of focal IPE can be isolated: (1) a focal parietal infarct associated with a haemorrhage in the caudothalamic matrix; (2) a focal temporal infarct above the dorsal part of the temporal horn, whereby the initial matrix lesion cannot be distinguished from the IPE; (3) a focal frontal infarct (Fig. IV.1.l).

A necrotic IPE evolves with cystic degeneration not unlike purely ischaemic leukomalacia. Those zones are integrated in a curved, dilated lateral ventricle in the second month of life, unlike the self-resorbing cysts of periventricular leukomalacia (Fig. IV.1.l). In many cases a major IPE later shows as a porencephalic cyst: a smooth-walled cavity in the parenchyma communicating with the ventricle through a wide porus. The cavity takes the shape of the infarcted area and will become round when submitted to increased pressure ('*porencéphalie soufflante*').

On a sonogram a secondary *subarachnoid haemorrhage* may be suspected when a normally echopoor cistern or sulcus—*i.e.* the cisterna magna, quadrigeminal cistern, ambient cistern, prepontine cistern, lateral fissure or parieto-occipital sulcus—is filled

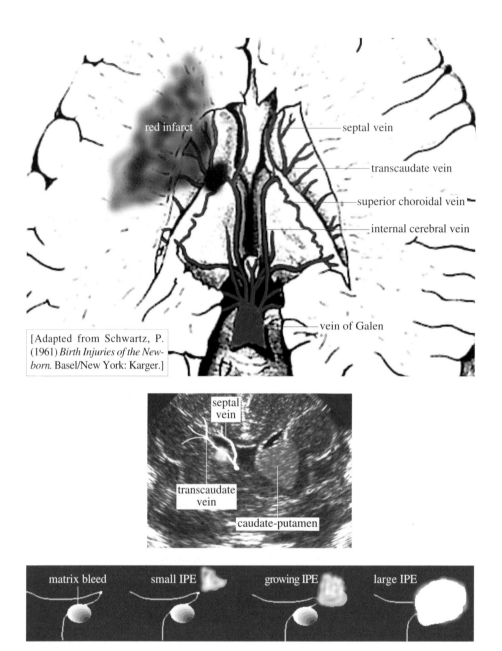

red infarct

septal vein

transcaudate vein

superior choroidal vein ➤

internal cerebral vein

vein of Galen

[Adapted from Schwartz, P. (1961) *Birth Injuries of the Newborn*. Basel/New York: Karger.]

septal vein

transcaudate vein

caudate-putamen

matrix bleed   small IPE   growing IPE   large IPE

Fig. IV.1.b. A large haemorrhage in caudothalamic germinal matrix can exert pressure on a subependymal collector vein (*e.g.* the transcaudate vein) that drains several transmedullary veins to the internal cerebral vein at its U-turn. It is now known that a parenchymal component (IPE or intraparenchymatous echodensity) in matrix bleeding is a venous infarct in the area drained by such an occluded and possibly thrombosed vessel. Growth is not by mechanical expansion but by recruitment of adjacent venous areas with red softening: the more veins obstructed, the larger the IPE. The growing IPE, at first triangular, merges with the matrix lesion into one globular mass.

with reflections (Fig. IV.1.n). In particular the cisterna magna and the prepontine and interpeduncular cisterns are nearly always echo-free under normal circumstances and may consequently be referred to for the interpretation of subarachnoid extravasation of blood. Although echographic identification of subarachnoid haemorrhage by persons familiar with anatomo-pathologic correlation has proved reliable, most authors believe this to be particularly difficult in routine practice. Differentiation from a subdural haematoma is difficult but sometimes possible. Normal variations in meningeal echogenicity and venous congestion also render interpretation tricky. It goes without saying that serial echography is important: changes in echogenicity of a subarachnoid space raise suspicion of a tissue reaction to preceding haemorrhage. As far as prognosis is concerned, the theoretical predictive power of measuring the extent of subarachnoid haemorrhage as far as later hydrocephalus is concerned, has not been shown in clinical practice.

Hypoechogenic zones may occur in the arachnoid space after subarachnoid haemorrhage and, in a sagittal section, they show up best in the supracerebellar and quadrigeminal cisterns (Fig. IV.1.n).

Quite exceptionally mechanical rupture may occur in the parenchyma under pressure from a major ventricular haemorrhage (Fig. IV.1.m). Neonates nursed supine while ventilated will then show a ventricular bleed nearly completely replaced by an extracerebral density in the occipital region after rupture.

A temporal or frontal horn may be isolated from the rest of the ventricular system by active intraluminal clots.

A haemorrhage may start from the plexus of the third ventricle and spread into the cavum veli interpositi (Fig. IV.1.n). It is difficult to distinguish a clot posteriorly in the third ventricle from a secondary subarachnoid hemorrhage in the quadrigeminal cistern or a haemorrhage in the cavum veli interpositi.

In association with a venous infarct around the frontal part of the lateral ventricle, lesions may be seen in the corpus callosum (Fig. IV.1.o).

In the subacute and chronic stage after a matrix haemorrhage it is possible to find linear densities under the head of the caudate nucleus (see striatal vasculopathy, section III.9). The arterial character of those densities will show in a Doppler analysis. The explanation for this observation is unknown to us (limited striatal infarct?). It follows that an arterial component can be echographically shown in some infants with a caudothalamic matrix density.

REFERENCES

Bejar, R., Coen, R.W., Ekpoudia, I., James, H.E., Gluck, L. (1985) 'Real time ultrasound diagnosis of hemorrhagic pathological conditions in the posterior fossa of preterm infants.' *Neurosurgery*, **16**, 281–289.

Brown, W.D., Gerfen, G.W., Vachon, L.A., Nelson, M.D. (1994) 'Real-time ultrasonography of arterial IVH in preterm infants.' *Pediatric Neurology*, **11**, 325–327.

Fleischer, A.C., Hutchison, A.A., Allen, J.H., Stahlman, M., Meacham, W.F., James, A.E. (1981) 'The role of sonography and the radiologist–ultrasonologist in the detection and follow-up of intracranial hemorrhage in the preterm neonate.' *Radiology*, **139**, 733–736.

Funato, M., Tamai, H., Takeda, Z. (1994) 'Moment of intraventricular hemorrhage—clinical pathogenic events.' *In:* Lou, H.C., Greisen, G., Larsen, J.F. (Eds.) *Brain Lesions in the Newborn. Hypoxic and Haemodynamic Pathogenesis. Alfred Benzon Symposium No. 37.* Munksgaard, pp. 456–469.

Gould, S.J., Howard, S., Hope, P.L., Reynolds, E.O.R. (1986) 'Periventricular intraparenchymal cerebral haemorrhage in preterm infants: the role of venous infarction.' *Journal of Pathology*, **151**, 197–202.

Grant, E.G., White, E.M. (1986) 'Pediatric neurosonography.' *Journal of Child Neurology*, **1**, 319–337.

Kirks, D.R., Bowie, J.D. (1986) 'Cranial ultrasonography of neonatal periventricular/intraventricular hemorrhage: who, how, why and when?' *Pediatric Radiology*, **16**, 114–119.

Kuban, K., Teele, R.L. (1984) 'Rationale for grading intracranial hemorrhage in premature infants.' *Pediatrics*, **74**, 358–363.

Paneth, N., Rudelli, R., Kazam, E., Monte, W. (1994) *Brain Damage in the Preterm Infant. Clinics in Developmental Medicine No. 131.* London: Mac Keith Press.

Pape, K.E., Wigglesworth, J.S. (1979) *Haemorrhage, Ischaemia and the Perinatal Brain. Clinics in Developmental Medicine No. 69/70.* London: Spastics International Medical Publications.

Perlman, J.M., Rollins, N., Burns, D, Risser, R. (1993) 'Relationship between periventricular intraparenchymal echodensities and germinal matrix–intraventricular hemorrhage in the very low birth weight neonate.' *Pediatrics*, **91**, 474–480.

Rademaker, K.J., Groenendaal, F., Jansen, G.H., Eken, P., de Vries, L.S. (1994) 'Unilateral haemorrhagic parenchymal lesions in the preterm infant: shape, site and prognosis.' *Acta Paediatrica*, **83**, 602–608.

Reeder, J.D., Kaude, J.V., Setzer, E.S. (1982) 'Choroid plexus hemorrhage in premature neonates: recognition by sonography.' *American Journal of Neuroradiology*, **3**, 619–622.

Rushton, D.I., Preston, P.R., Durbin, G.M. (1985) 'Structure and evolution of echo dense lesions in the neonatal brain. A combined ultrasound and necropsy study.' *Archives of Disease in Childhood*, **60**, 798–808.

Schmidt, H. (1965) *Untersuchungen zur Pathogenese und Ätiologie der geburtstraumatischen Hirnschädigungen Früh- und Reifgeborener.* Jena: Gustav Fisher Verlag.

Slovis, T.L., Shankaran, S. (1984) 'Ultrasound in the evaluation of hypoxic–ischemic injury and intracranial hemorrhage in neonates: the state of the art.' *Pediatric Radiology*, **14**, 67–75.

Takashima, S., Mito, T., Ando, Y. (1986) 'Pathogenesis of periventricular white matter hemorrhages in preterm infants.' *Brain and Development*, **8**, 25–30.

Volpe, J.J. (1989) 'Intraventricular hemorrhage and brain injury in the premature infant. Neuropathology and pathogenesis.' *Clinics in Perinatology*, **16**, 361–411.

— — (1990) 'Brain injury in the premature infant: is it preventable?' *Pediatric Research*, **27**, S28–S33.

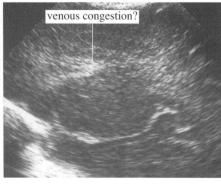

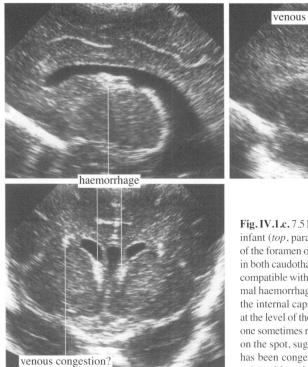

Fig. IV.1.c. 7.5 MHz scans of a ventilated preterm infant (*top*, parasagittal; *bottom*, coronal in front of the foramen of Monro). There are echodensities in both caudothalamic grooves (most on the right) compatible with, but not diagnostic of subependymal haemorrhage. In addition the anterior limb of the internal capsule is nodularly hyperechogenic at the level of the outer ventricular tips. At autopsy one sometimes recognizes dilated venous channels on the spot, suggesting that in this survivor there has been congestion of transmedullary collector veins without infarction.

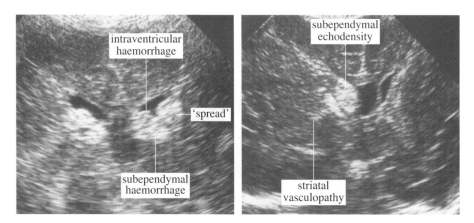

Fig. IV.1.d. Identification of subependymal haemorrhage with ultrasound is by no means straightforward, as illustrated by these coronal 7.5 MHz sonograms of two different preterm infants. (*Left*) Germinal matrix haemorrhage has 'spread' from the caudothalamic groove to cover the entire caudate head, with some blood spilling over into the ventricle. (*Right*) A subependymal density compatible with haemorrhage is supported by an oblique caudate density and an echogenic striatal artery. CT excluded haemorrhage, suggesting the echogenic changes were part of a focal arterial infarct within striate branches of the anterior or middle cerebral artery.

171

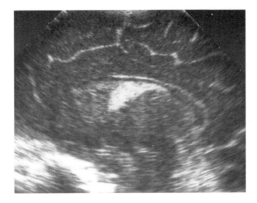

Fig. IV.1.e. Not all matrix echogenicities in the caudothalamic groove are of haemorrhagic nature, as exemplified in this 7.5 MHz para-sagittal section of a preterm infant with broncho-pulmonary dysplasia. Whereas initially there were no lesions, these densities developed from the late neonatal period and are probably slow matrix infarcts. Their triangular and very homo-geneous aspect is striking.

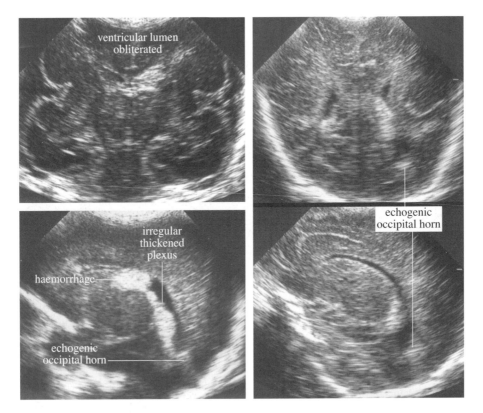

Fig. IV.1.f. 7.5 MHz sections of three different infants with grade II IVH. The presence of blood in a ventricular cavity may fill the cavity on coronal section, or may suggest itself as echogenicity of the floor of the occipital horn or irregular thickening of the choroid plexus.

172

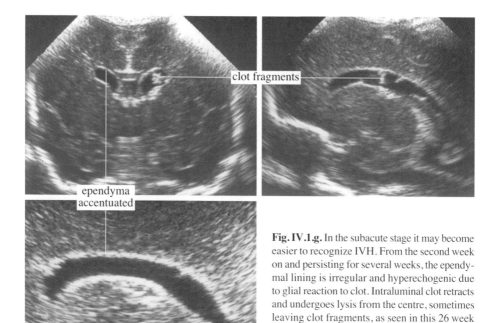

clot fragments

ependyma accentuated

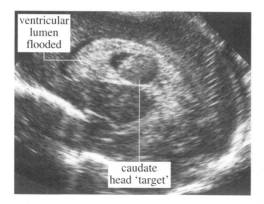

Fig. IV.1.g. In the subacute stage it may become easier to recognize IVH. From the second week on and persisting for several weeks, the ependymal lining is irregular and hyperechogenic due to glial reaction to clot. Intraluminal clot retracts and undergoes lysis from the centre, sometimes leaving clot fragments, as seen in this 26 week gestation preterm infant. (Day 10, 7.5 MHz sections—*top left*, coronal; *top right*, parasagittal; *left*, parasagittal detail.)

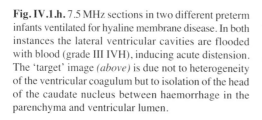

ventricular lumen flooded

caudate head 'target'

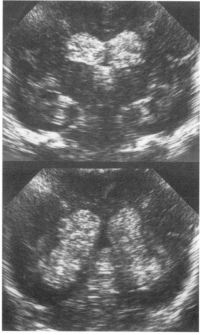

Fig. IV.1.h. 7.5 MHz sections in two different preterm infants ventilated for hyaline membrane disease. In both instances the lateral ventricular cavities are flooded with blood (grade III IVH), inducing acute distension. The 'target' image *(above)* is due not to heterogeneity of the ventricular coagulum but to isolation of the head of the caudate nucleus between haemorrhage in the parenchyma and ventricular lumen.

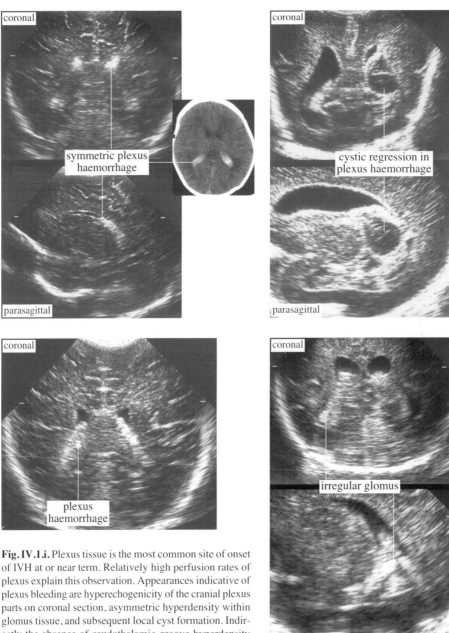

Fig. IV.1.i. Plexus tissue is the most common site of onset of IVH at or near term. Relatively high perfusion rates of plexus explain this observation. Appearances indicative of plexus bleeding are hyperechogenicity of the cranial plexus parts on coronal section, asymmetric hyperdensity within glomus tissue, and subsequent local cyst formation. Indirectly the absence of caudothalamic groove hyperdensity (subependymal haemorrhage) may support this diagnosis.

Here are shown 7.5 MHz sections of four different infants with plexus haemorrhage (confirmed by CT in the term babies): *(top left)* term infant with cardiac failure due to longstanding supraventricular tachycardia; *(top right)* term infant with persistent pulmonary hypertension; *(bottom left)* term infant after difficult ventouse extraction; *(bottom right)* ventilated preterm infant (24 weeks gestation).

174

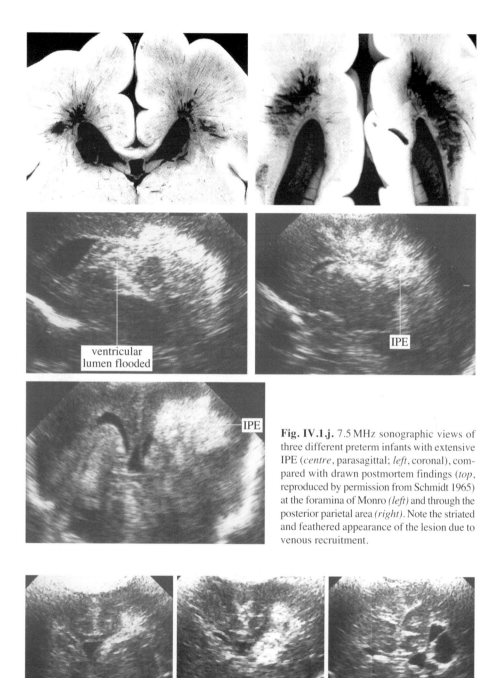

Fig. IV.1.j. 7.5 MHz sonographic views of three different preterm infants with extensive IPE (*centre*, parasagittal; *left*, coronal), compared with drawn postmortem findings (*top*, reproduced by permission from Schmidt 1965) at the foramina of Monro *(left)* and through the posterior parietal area *(right)*. Note the striated and feathered appearance of the lesion due to venous recruitment.

Fig. IV.1.k. Natural history of a venous infarct (frontoparietal IPE): adapted 7.5 MHz details of a 29 weeks gestation infant on days 1, 2 and 20. Growth of both infarct and matrix lesion led to a rounded conglomerate, with subsequent cystic regression of both.

175

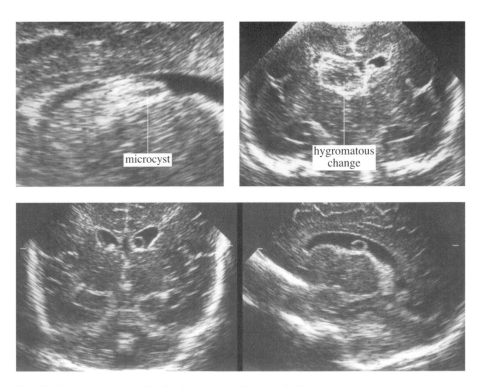

Fig. IV.1.l. Cystic changes following haemorrhage into germinal matrix.

(Above) Most matrix haemorrhages undergo cystic change in the second week after the event. Size and location of the cyst will vary in accord with the original haemorrhage. Cysts in the ventricular lumen probably never originate in the choroid plexus. [7.5 MHz sonograms of three different preterm infants: *top left*, parasagittal image; *top right*, coronal image; *bottom*, coronal *(left)* and parasagittal *(right)* images.]

(Below and opposite) Parenchymal venous infarcts, like the matrix haemorrhages they develop from, change into cysts. Eventually irregular porencephalic cavities gradually disappear into the ventricular lumen, leaving angular, sometimes expansive defects. Whole or parts of ventricles may become isolated by glial strands (loculation)

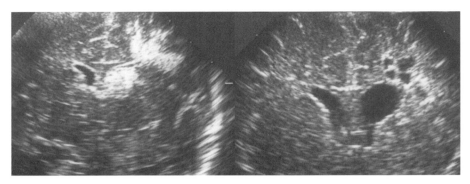

Preterm infant (35 weeks gestation) who presented with episodes of apnoea: coronal 7.5 MHz scans taken in early *(left)* and late *(right)* neonatal period.

176

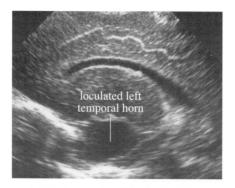

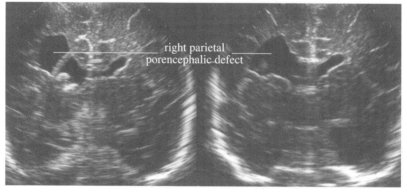

Evolution of a large right-sided parenchymal infarct in a preterm infant (one of twins born at 29 weeks gestation): 7.5 MHz sections (*top*, parasagittal, day 2; *bottom*, coronal, day 21).

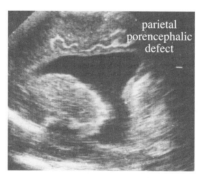

Preterm infant: 5 MHz parasagittal section.

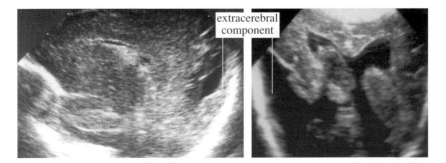

Fig. IV.1.m. Two different preterm infants with grade III IVH that suddenly disappeared because of transparenchymal penetration of the blood into the subarachnoid/subdural space (7.5 MHz images: *left*, parasagittal; *right*, coronal). This mechanical extension of haemorrhage was formerly believed to be the mechanism underlying parenchymal involvement, but it is now known to be exceptional.

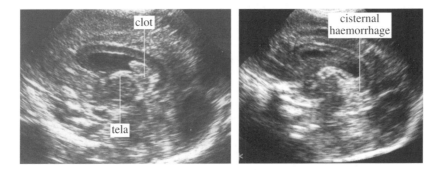

Fig. IV.1.n. Extraventricular haemorrhage in two different preterm infants with matrix bleeding (sagittal 7.5 MHz sections): *(left)* clot in the cavum vergae or cavum veli interpositi, probably an extension of bleeding into the tela choroidea; *(right)* secondary subarachnoid haemorrhage with thickening and hyperechogenicity of the quadrigeminal cistern.

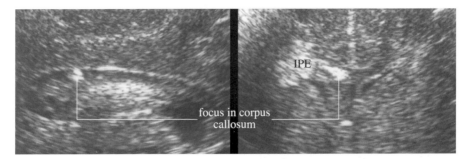

Fig. IV.1.o. Ventilated preterm infant (27 weeks gestation) with grade II IVH and right frontal IPE: 7.5 MHz sections *(left*, sagittal; *right*, coronal). A very dense lesion is seen anteriorly in the body of the corpus callosum, just to the right of the midline. It is probably associated with the frontal venous infarct.

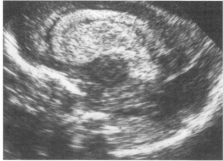

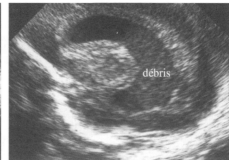
débris

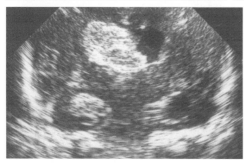

Fig. IV.1.p. 7.5 MHz scans of a ventilated preterm infant before withdrawal of intensive care (*top*, parasagittal right and left views; *left*, coronal view). There is a grade III IVH on the right, with extensive clot in the third ventricle. CSF stasis with increase of protein content and mixture with blood may lead to mild hyperechogenicity of ventricular fluid ('débris').

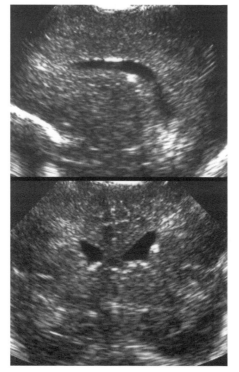

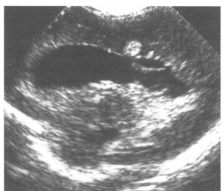

Fig. IV.1.q. 7.5 MHz sections of two different preterm infants (both 25 weeks gestation) with matrix haemorrhage in the caudothalamic groove (*left: top*, parasagittal, *bottom*, coronal behind the foramen of Monro; *right*, parasagittal). Focal nodular echogenicities erratically dispersed along the ventricular wall represent matrix haemorrhage outside the classic foci in the temporo-occipital area or caudothalamic groove.

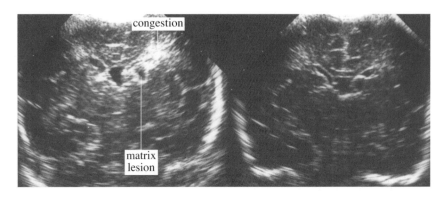

Fig. IV.1.r. Coronal 7.5 MHz scans of a preterm (31 weeks) infant on days 2 and 18. Disappearance of the echogenic focus near a left matrix haemorrhage, in the absence of ventriculomegaly or cystic necrosis, suggests that it was only congestion.

IV.2 POSTHAEMORRHAGIC HYDROCEPHALUS

After the acute event the normal flow of CSF may be hindered by organization of and re-action to blood in the ventricles, leaking secondarily from the fourth ventricle into the peri-cerebellar leptomeninges. In the second week following haemorrhage, ultrasound will show small protein-containing particles floating about in the CSF and most probably contributing to the obliteration of its distal flow. *Obstruction* may be found in the lateral ventricle, near the foramen of Monro, in the cerebral aqueduct, near the foramina of the fourth ventricle, in the pericerebellar cisterns, near the tentorial groove, in the pericerebral arachnoid spaces and in the arachnoid granulations of sinuses. The result varies from unilateral hydrocephalus, through supratentorial or complete internal hydrocephalus, to combined internal and external hydrocephalus (of communicating type).

In four out of five cases we are confronted with the *communicating* variant due to oblit-erative arachnoiditis in the pericerebellar and pericerebral spaces. In some situations both aqueduct and foramina of the fourth ventricle may be obstructed, giving rise to an '*isolated fourth ventricle*': continued CSF production in the plexus of the lateral and fourth ventricles gives rise to hydrocephalus above and below the tentorium despite occlusion of the aqueduct. Isolation of the fourth ventricle is a rare complication of repeated shunt revision. It may be accompanied by transtentorial upward herniation of that ventricle.

The chance of progressive ventricular widening in the weeks after haemorrhage in-creases from 5% in the case of grade II up to 40–80% for grades III and IV. The outlook for children with posthaemorrhagic hydrocephalus is worse than expected on account of haemorrhage alone: factors contributing to this may be subependymal damage from within the ventricular cavity and cerebellar cortical injury from within the leptomeninges. Injury to the inferior olive may follow cerebellar cortical damage. Often one observes a slow first stage of *ventriculomegaly* which in 50% of cases subsequently regresses but in the other 50% persists, evolving towards symptomatic hydrocephalus. Clinical signs may nearly always be anticipated by serial sonography of the cranium.

Cranial ultrasound plays an important role in the detection and follow-up of posthaemor-rhagic complications.

(1) Given sufficient experience, it is possible to *evaluate the severity of ventriculomegaly* via repeated measurements: we obtain (i) the laterolateral diameter of both lateral ventricles together on a coronal section through the foramen of Monro, (ii) the roof to floor diagonal height on the same section, and then (iii) proceed to precise measurement of the third vent-ricular width in an axial section through the sphenoidal fontanelle (Fig. IV.2.a). The latter measurement is facilitated by the existence of dense ependymal lining. As for lateral vent-ricular diameters, normal values have been established for gestational age (*e.g.* Levene and Starte 1981). Treatment will almost certainly be necessary when this value is above the 97th centile. There is a certain amount of controversy regarding where lateral ventricular dilatation may best be traced. Absence of widening of the frontal horns may be falsely re-assuring as neonates tend toward colpocephaly (discrepant overdilatation of the occipital horns). On a coronal section the boomerang-shape of the frontal horns above the caudate nuclei disappears after a while under the influence of pressure. Balloon-shaped frontal horns are usually an indication for treatment. We find measurements on parasagittal sections

particularly sensitive to caliper placement: repeated measurements on the exact same spots are difficult, which is why estimation of the diameter of the third ventricle appears to be at least as reliable. Once again, one must be careful because the third ventricle does not necessarily widen uniformly. Normally the width of the neonatal third ventricle does not exceed 2 mm. When the baby lies on its side the underlying lateral ventricle may widen considerably more than the proximal ventricle. Any follow-up of ventriculomegaly in the case of an infant with an acceptable fontanelle opening should be done with ultrasound: repeated CT scanning is unjustifiable. With manifestly increased pressure the frontal subfontanellar region may present signs of transependymal CSF *resorption*: soft hyperechogenic zones show up radially on both sides of the lateral ventricular horns. Those zones are hypodense on CT.

(2) Sagittal and axial sections reveal whether there is a *discrepancy* between dilatation of the supratentorial ventricles and the fourth ventricle (Figs. IV.2.b–d). They enable one (i) to see the aqueduct running to a slit in the case of stenosis on that particular spot, (ii) to see a discrepant dilatation of the fourth ventricle, and (iii) in the absence of a large cisterna magna, to predict absence of communication between the fourth ventricle and the pericerebellar (and consequently spinal subdural) spaces. In a rare case the aqueduct will be so manifestly dilated that it will show up on a sonogram. When dilating, the normally triangular fourth ventricle will attempt to find the way of least resistance and form a round or more tubular structure in the cerebellar vermis. In some cases this happens suddenly, generating life-threatening pressure on vital centres in the brainstem.

(3) Sonographic measurements before and after lumbar puncture may help to show that the ventricular system communicates with the lumbar subdural space. The shape of the lateral ventricle may have significantly changed as well.

(4) There are various ways of *evaluating the severity* of intracranial hypertension in the case of posthaemorrhagic hydrocephalus: (i) recording the head circumference; (ii) measuring the pressure by means of applanation tonometry over the anterior fontanelle; and (iii) serial measurement of ventricular diameters. Ultrasound will also allow the study of transependymal CSF resorption (Fig. IV.2.e). The measurement of arterial flow rates with calculation of a resistance index is a particularly useful approach. Either on account of mechanical pressure on the arteries under influence of the ventricle contours, or more likely due to intracranial hypertension itself, one will observe that hydrocephalus requiring treatment induces a decrease or even inversion of diastolic flow rates in the anterior, middle and cerebral arteries. Resistance indices above 0.8 (RI = S–D/S, where S = systolic peak rate and D = end diastolic rate) suggest the vessel bed has been affected. Necrosis of the medial part of the occipital lobe is known to occur with hydrocephalus and is probably the result of compression of the posterior cerebral artery.

(5) While installing a *shunt* the neurosurgeon may be guided by ultrasound: in order to avoid early plexus in-growth it is ideally advised to position the shunt tip in the frontal and not in the temporal horn (Fig. IV.2.f).

(6) *Complications* of treatment are discussed in the section on porencephaly (III.4).

REFERENCES

Bejar, R., Curbelo, V., Coen, R.W., Leopold, G., James, H., Gluck, L. (1980) 'Diagnosis and follow-up of intraventricular and intracerebral hemorrhages by ultrasound: studies of infant's brain through the fontanelles and sutures.' *Pediatrics*, **66**, 661–673.

— — Coen, R.W., Ekpoudia, I., James, H.E., Gluck, L. (1985) 'Real time ultrasound diagnosis of hemorrhagic pathological conditions in the posterior fossa of preterm infants.' *Neurosurgery*, **16**, 281–289.

Blumhagen, J.D., Mack, L.A. (1985) 'Abnormalities of the neonatal cerebral ventricles.' *Radiologic Clinics of North America*, **23**, 13–27.

Coker, S.B., Anderson, C.L. (1989) 'Occluded fourth ventricle after multiple shunt revisions for hydrocephalus.' *Pediatrics*, **83**, 981–985.

Deeg, K.H., Rupprecht, T. (1989) 'Pulsed Doppler sonographic measurement of normal values for the flow velocities in the intracranial arteries of healthy newborns.' *Pediatric Radiology*, **19**, 71–78.

Fukumizu, M., Takashima, S., Becker, L.E. (1995) 'Neonatal posthemorrhagic hydrocephalus: neuropathologic and immunohistochemical studies.' *Pediatric Neurology*, **13**, 230–234.

Goodwin, L., Quisling, R.G. (1983) 'The neonatal cisterna magna: ultrasonic evaluation.' *Radiology*, **149**, 691–695.

Hall, T.R., Choi, A., Schellinger, D., Grant, E.G. (1992) 'Isolation of the fourth ventricle causing transtentorial herniation: neurosonographic findings in premature infants.' *American Journal of Roentgenology*, **159**, 811–815.

Hill, A., Volpe, J.J. (1981) 'Normal pressure hydrocephalus in the newborn.' *Pediatrics*, **68**, 623–629.

— — Shackelford, G.D., Volpe, J.J. (1984) 'A potential mechanism of pathogenesis for early posthemorrhagic hydrocephalus in the premature newborn.' *Pediatrics*, **73**, 19–21.

Larroche, J-C. (1972) 'Post-haemorrhagic hydrocephalus in infancy. Anatomical study.' *Biology of the Neonate*, **20**, 287–299.

Levene, M. (1981) 'Measurement of the growth of the lateral ventricles in preterm infants with real-time ultrasound.' *Archives of Disease in Childhood*, **56**, 900–904.

— — Starte, D.R. (1981) 'A longitudinal study of post-haemorrhagic ventricular dilatation in the newborn.' *Archives of Disease in Childhood*, **56**, 905–910.

Rademaker, K.J., Govaert, P., Vandertop, W.P., Gooskens, R., Meiners, L.C., de Vries, L.S. (1995) 'Rapidly progressive enlargement of the fourth ventricle in the preterm infant with post-haemorrhagic ventricular dilatation.' *Acta Paediatrica*, **84**, 1193–1196.

Saliba, E., Pottier, J.M., Chergui, A., Bloc, D., Gold, F., Laugier, J. (1985) 'Surveillance échographique des dilatations ventriculaires post-hémorragiques chez le nouveau-né prématuré. Intérêt de la détermination d'un index ventriculaire.' *Archives Françaises de Pédiatrie*, **42**, 281–284.

Sauerbrei, E.E., Digney, M., Harrison, P.B., Cooperberg, P.L. (1981) 'Ultrasonic evaluation of neonatal intracranial hemorrhage and its complications.' *Radiology*, **139**, 677–685.

Shankaran, S., Slovis, T.L., Bedard, M.P., Poland, R.L. (1982) 'Sonographic classification of intracranial hemorrhage. A prognostic indicator of mortality, morbidity, and short-term neurologic outcome.' *Journal of Pediatrics*, **100**, 469–475.

Veyrac, C., Couture, A., Baud, C. (1994) 'Les lésions hémorragiques cérébrales.' *In:* Couture, A., Veyrac, C., Baud, C. (Eds.) *Echographie Cérébrale du Foetus au Nouveau-né*. Montpellier: Sauramps Médical, pp. 133–166.

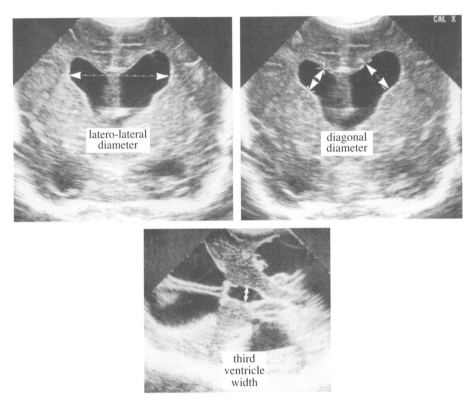

Fig. IV.2.a. Three measures for serial follow-up of ventricular dilatation: the latero-lateral diameter of both lateral ventricles at the foramen of Monro; the diagonal floor to roof diameter in the same section; and the width of the third ventricle in an axial section.

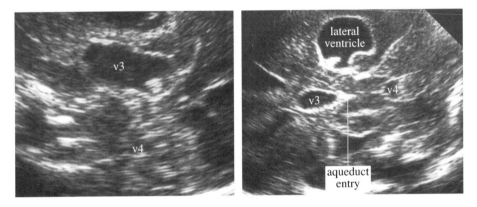

Fig. IV.2.b. Preterm infant with severe grade II IVH: 7.5 MHz sections (*left*, sagittal; *right*, axial). Some observations argue in favour of aqueductal obstruction: the third and lateral ventricles are more dilated than the fourth; and the third ventricle, containing clot near the pineal recess, is tapered in the direction of the aqueduct.

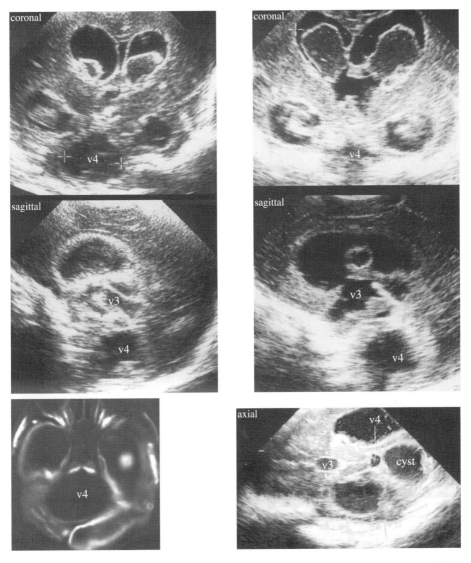

Fig. IV.2.c. Three different preterm infants (all with birthweight <1000 g) suffering from grade III IVH with subsequent posterior fossa 'cavitation'. In those at *left* and *top right*, intensive care was withdrawn because of brainstem compression and isolation of the fourth ventricle in the second week of life. All sonograms are 7.5 MHz images; a corresponding axial T$_1$-weighted MRI is given for the infant at *left*. In the scan at *bottom right*, a peritentorial arachnoid cyst is identified behind the upper part of the fourth ventricle at mesencephalic level.

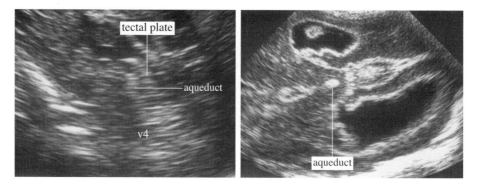

Fig. IV.2.d. 7.5 MHz sections (*left*, sagittal; *right*, axial) of two different infants with respiratory distress syndrome. Following intraventricular blood collection, the ependyma reacts with nodular gliotic thickening, rosette formation and active subependymal siderophagia. At aqueductal level the echogenicity may increase so that the normal subtle reflections are replaced by a bright focus, longitudinal in sagittal sections.

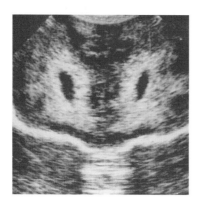

Fig. IV.2.e. Periventricular frontal, immediately subependymal hyperechogenicity in a preterm infant with acute intracranial hypertension following IVH (coronal 5 MHz section): transependymal CSF shift?

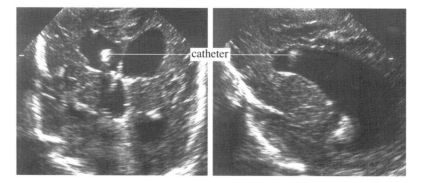

Fig. IV.2.f. Intraoperative 7.5 MHz sections through the anterior fontanelle (*left*, coronal; *right*, parasagittal). The advancing catheter tip is easily seen at the correct site, lodging above the plexus in the right frontal horn.

IV.3 EPIDURAL HAEMATOMA

Except in the rare case of a primary coagulation disorder, neonatal epidural haemorrhage is an irrefutable sign of mechanical trauma. The lesion has been described following complicated breech delivery and after cephalic delivery with instrumental traction. The bleeding is nearly always located underneath a linear cranial fracture. Very often a cephalhaematoma will be found on top of the injured bone (Fig. IV.3.a). Reports on ultrasound diagnosis are very rare. The diagnosis is best verified with CT. One will typically find an extracerebral density with biconvex contours (Fig. IV.3.b). Early liquefaction of the clot (within 24–48 hours) is typical for this lesion (Figs. IV.3.b, IV.3.c), CT scans of which may indicate the relative fluid levels. Major haemorrhage may give rise to uncal herniation, intracranial hypertension and hypoperfusion of the ipsilateral middle cerebral artery or its branches. In the case of a mass effect the ipsilateral ventricle may be compressed, with a shift of the interhemispheric fissure and third ventricle.

REFERENCES

Aoki, N. (1990) 'Epidural haematoma in the newborn infants: therapeutic consequences from the correlation between haematoma content and computed tomography features.' *Acta Neurochirurgica*, **106**, 65–67.
Lam, A., Cruz, G.B., Johnson, I. (1991) 'Extradural hematoma in neonates.' *Journal of Ultrasound Medicine*, **10**, 205–209.

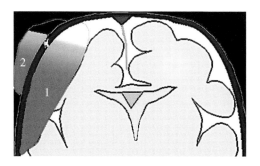

Fig. IV.3.a. Very often an epidural haematoma or internal cephalhaematoma (1) is covered by a fractured bone with a genuine external cephalhaematoma (2) on top of it. The bleeding has a tendency toward early (within 24 hours) liquefaction. If large enough it may be recognized with ultrasound. The haematoma may be hypodense due to liquefaction but characteristically remains a biconvex, lentiform lesion.

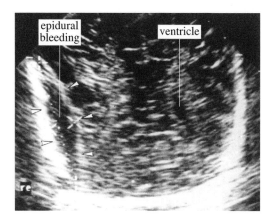

Fig. IV.3.b. Term infant born by the breech and presenting at 24 hours with right uncal herniation: coronal 5 MHz section. Because of midline shift and compression the ipsilateral ventricle is invisible.

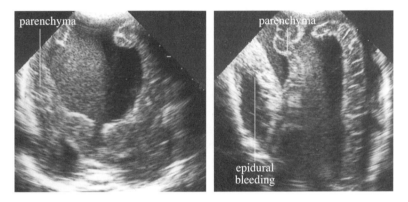

Fig. IV.3.c. Term infant with fetal ventriculomegaly, absence of corpus callosum and a midline dorsal cyst; during parturition ventricular puncture was necessary to allow delivery of the large head. On day 2 the child presented with hypovolaemia due to a large right extracerebral haemorrhage, subsequently shown to be extradural during surgical intervention. The child succumbed several days after the operation. Both images are coronal 7.5 MHz sections before surgery (*left*, anterior; *right*, posterior).

IV.4 SUBDURAL HAEMATOMA
Tentorial tear
Some clinical and echographic entities exist with tentorial injury following birth trauma (Fig. IV.4.a). The most frequent and well-known entity is traumatic birth with sufficient compression of the cranium to cause a partial or complete tear of the free tentorial margin. The site of least resistance is located next to the insertion of the straight sinus and its transition towards the great cerebral vein. Haemorrhage around the laceration will extend from the quadrigeminal cistern to the interhemispheric fissure above and behind the corpus callosum, in the transverse fissure under the corpus callosum, in the space above the cerebellar vermis and above the tentorium itself, and under and between the occipital lobes. In our experience those lesions are almost always related to difficult instrumental traction or breech delivery. Excessive pressure on the base of the occipital bone, whether manual or instrumental, may displace it inwards towards the posterior fossa, at the fibrous junction between its squamous and lateral portions, a phenomenon called occipital osteodiastasis (Figs. IV.4.c, IV.4.d).

The centrotentorial tear cannot be directly identified echographically. However, a perilesional haemorrhage of sufficient size will show up in coronal section as a density between the echogenic strips of choroid plexus (Fig. IV.4.b). Sagittal sections in particular allow diagnosis of a tentorial tear if, after 'difficult' birth, a density is found behind the usual retrotectal white echo line of the quadrigeminal cistern. The latter forms a bridge between vermal reflections and the tela choroidea of the third ventricle. The centrotentorial clot rests on the cerebellar vermis and appears to penetrate into cerebellar substance. Axial sections through a sphenoidal fontanelle may confirm this assumption provided dense reflections are found behind the cerebral peduncles. Even partial tears with limited perilesional haemorrhage (fraying) may be identified echographically as an asymmetric linear peritentorial echodensity on coronal sections.

The differential diagnosis should envisage the possibility of abundant subarachnoid haemorrhage, secondary for instance to ventricular haemorrhage. Blood may rise from the fourth ventricle along the posterior fossa to fill the quadrigeminal cistern around the tentorial groove.

Although radiographic confirmation is advised, occipital osteodiastasis can be identified on sagittal sonograms: the squamous part of the occipital bone has been anteposed some millimetres in comparison to the basal and lateral parts (Fig. IV.4.d).

At least two stages of hydrocephalus are known following severe tentorial trauma (Fig. IV.4.e). In the first days after birth clots may obstruct CSF flow: the *obstructive* stage. Due to a mass effect of the haemorrhage in the posterior cranial fossa, compression of the aqueduct or fourth ventricle may also occur. Later, after an interval of weeks or even months, hydrocephalus will often occur due to disturbed *resorption*, and in our practice we have come across a two-stage event with a neonatal peak of ventricular dilatation and another in infancy. Mechanisms here are obstruction to the CSF circulation in the peritentorial arachnoid spaces and obturation of the villi in the arachnoid granulations. The severity of late hydrocephalus correlates with the degree of subarachnoid haemorrhage associated with the tentorial lesion.

189

During recovery some babies consequently go through a temporary stage of hygroma in the posterior fossa (Fig. IV.4.e). The pericerebellar spaces are so dilated that the vermis 'floats' in CSF with possible clot remnants in the cisterna magna. This may later lead to arachnoid cyst formation in the posterior fossa or quadrigeminal cistern.

Supratentorial subdural haemorrhage

A subdural haemorrhage above the cerebellar tentorium may be found with a *central tentorial tear*, even though the epicentre of bleeding will in reality be situated in the ambient and quadrigeminal cisterns and above and around the cerebellum.

Convexity subdural haematoma starts from a torn bridging vein near the superior sagittal sinus or from an anastomosing vein along the parietal hemispheric convexity: in this case the bulk of clot will be located above the insula, often centred around the superior sagittal sinus. A tear in the non-central part of the tentorium or a rupture of an anchor vein of the transverse sinus will produce accumulation of blood under and along the temporal lobe, often with posterior interhemispheric extension: *basal subdural haematoma*, the location of which is beneath the insula. Such subdural haemorrhage is nearly always the consequence of birth trauma, although vascular anomalies and coagulation disturbances must be excluded in certain situations. Subdural haemorrhage may also follow rupture of an anchor vein after insertion of a shunt. CT scanning remains the best technique to diagnose these lesions so long as they are of significant size.

Both types of haemorrhage may be identified with sonography but this remains difficult due to their eccentric location, under bone and on the edge of the sector. A basal subdural haematoma may look like a lobar temporal haemorrhage and it may be confused with a subarachnoid haematoma (Fig. IV.4.i). We could trace no data in the literature on the ultrasound diagnosis of those haemorrhages. 10 MHz scanning may sometimes reveal a subdural clot under the superior sagittal sinus (Fig. IV.4.f). Quite often there is subarachnoid CSF retention under a subdural haematoma producing a neat picture of the arachnoid membrane between collections of different echogenicity (see external hydrocephalus, section II.10). Fresh subdural haemorrhage may initially remain hypodense before fibrin formation (as during heparinization for extracorporeal membrane oxygenation [ECMO]) (Fig. IV.4.g). It is impossible to differentiate with certainty between minor subdural bleeding and *contusion* of parenchyma under bony margins moved during excessive moulding (Fig. IV.4.h).

REFERENCES

de Vries, L.S., Eken, P., Beek, E., Groenendaal, F., Meiners, F.C. (1996) 'The posterior fontanelle: a neglected acoustic window.' *Neuropediatrics*, **27**, 101–104.
Huang, C-C., Shen, E-Y. (1991) 'Tentorial subdural hemorrhage in term newborns: ultrasonographic diagnosis and clinical correlates.' *Pediatric Neurology*, **7**, 171–177.

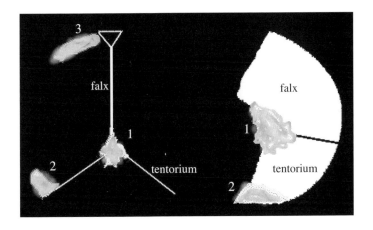

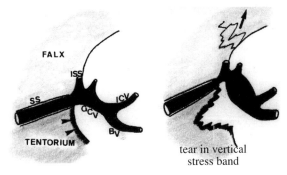

Fig. IV.4.a. Several types of subdural haematoma may be found in the newborn infant: if the epicentre is the vertical tentorial stress band, bleeding is centrotentorial (1); with a laterotentorial epicentre we use the term basal subdural haematoma, with bleeding under and along the temporal lobe up to the insula (2); with the epicentre near the superior sagittal sinus or above the insula we use the term convexity subdural haematoma (3). (SS = straight sinus; ISS = inferior sagittal sinus; GCV = great cerebral vein; BV = basal vein; ICV = internal cerebral vein.)

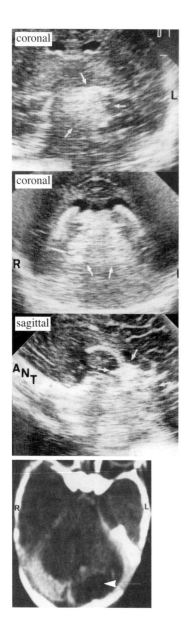

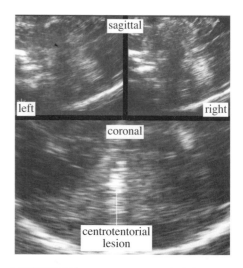

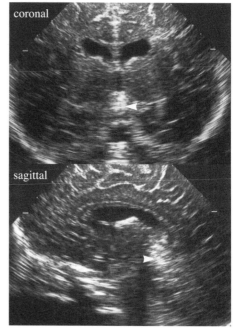

Fig. IV.4.b. Three infants with centrotentorial haematoma of different degrees of severity.

(Left) Sonograms and CT of a term infant presenting with intracranial hypertension within four hours of breech delivery. Part of the large retrocerebellar clot *(arrows)* was removed during posterior fossa craniotomy. The only consequence at 5 years was strabismus.

(Top right) Sonograms of a term infant who died of hypoplastic left heart syndrome. The dense area right of the midline along the tentorial leaflet was shown at postmortem examination to be a superficial tear with minimal subdural bleeding, due to difficult ventouse extraction.

(Bottom right) CT confirmed peritentorial haematoma of moderate size *(arrow)* in a term infant delivered by ventouse extraction.

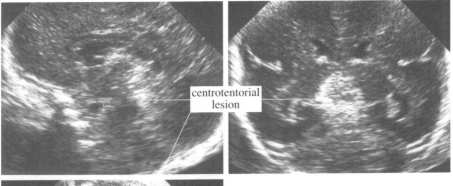

centrotentorial
lesion

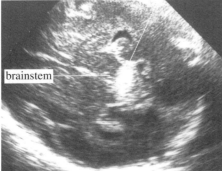

brainstem

Fig. IV.4.c. 7.5 MHz sections (*top left*, sagittal; *top right*, coronal; *left*, axial) of a 25 week gestation infant delivered by the breech; he later succumbed to grade III IVH. The centrotentorial haemorrhage shown here on day 1 is suggestive of tentorial tear, even though the obstetrician did not judge delivery as difficult. Usually, in breech delivery it will be occipital osteodiastasis that causes structural changes in the posterior fossa.

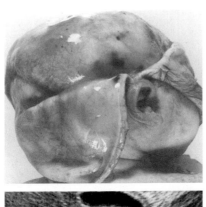

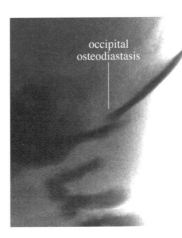

occipital
osteodiastasis

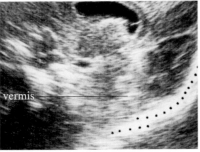

vermis

Fig. IV.4.d. Occipital osteodiastasis, inward displacement of the occipital squama at the hinge with the basal parts of the occipital bone (*upper left*), can often be diagnosed with lateral skull X rays (*upper right*) (unless pressure returned the bone to its initial position), but also with sagittal sonography (*left*). (Upper pictures reproduced from Govaert 1993.)

193

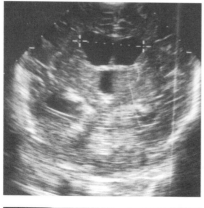
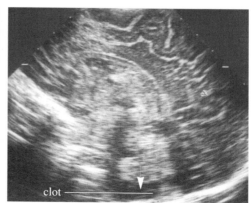

clot

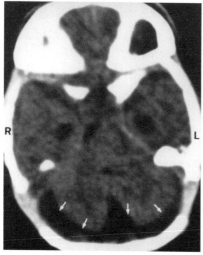

R L

Fig. IV.4.e. Term boy, a difficult ventouse delivery, who had a huge peritentorial haematoma, not operated on: 7.5 MHz echograms (*top left*, coronal; *top right*, sagittal) and axial CT on day 20. A posterior fossa hygroma *(arrows)* shows as an echofree area encircling the cerebellum, and a clot rests on the occipital squama. Hydrocephalus was stabilized with serial lumbar punctures and acetazolamide + furosemide at 5 months of age.

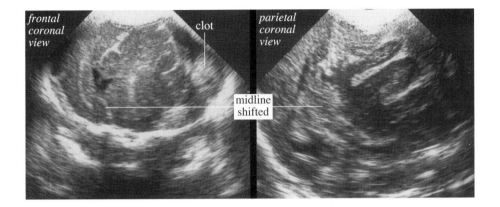

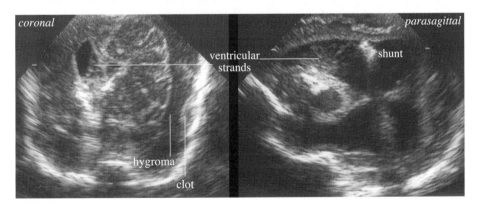

Fig. IV.4.f. Convexity subdural haematoma: the bulk of the clot lies between the insula and superior sagittal sinus.

(Top) Maternal coumarin treatment until delivery at 30 weeks.

(Centre) Infantile subdural haematoma in the subacute (CT isodense) stage.

(Bottom) Shunting for hydrocephalus due to toxoplasmosis was complicated by ventriculitis and subdural haematoma in this term infant.

195

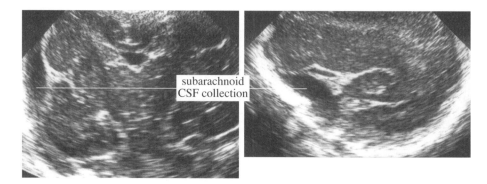

Fig. IV.4.g. Preterm infant (24 weeks gestation) with unexplained anaemia: 7.5 MHz sonograms (*left*, coronal; *right*, parasagittal). The partially echodense, but mainly hypodense collection around the right insula was not due to subdural haematoma. Postmortem examination revealed only local meningeal oedema.

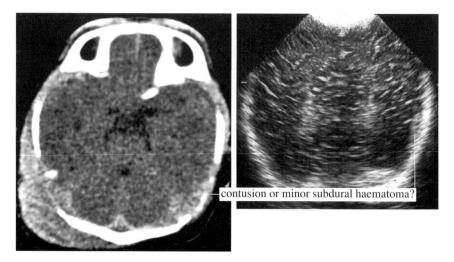

Fig. IV.4.h. Axial CT and coronal 7.5 MHz sonogram of a term infant with focal seizures following difficult ventouse delivery. Both CT and ultrasound may not suffice to correctly diagnose a minor subdural haematoma and differentiate it from contusion due to bone displacement. The occurrence of seizures in the absence of asphyxia would suggest that some cortical damage must be present.

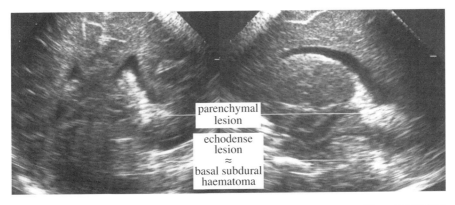

parenchymal
lesion

echodense
lesion
≈
basal subdural
haematoma

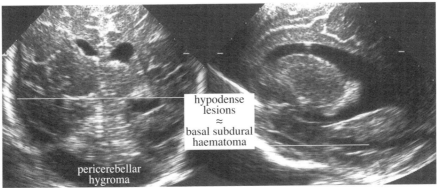

hypodense
lesions
≈
basal subdural
haematoma

pericerebellar
hygroma

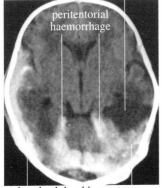

arterial hypo-
perfusion?

peritentorial
haemorrhage

basal subdural haematoma

Fig. IV.4.i. Term infant, delivered by caesarean section, admitted on day 2 with umbilical and cutaneous bleeding; a primary defect of haemostasis was not documented. The sonograms are 7.5 MHz sections (*left*, coronal; *right*, parasagittal through the left hemisphere). In the acute stage blood was seen around both tentorial leaflets and a parenchymal echodense lesion lodged in the left posterior temporal area. Subsequently a hypodense collection formed where a juxtatemporal subdural clot had been on the right, a posterior fossa hygroma developed, and the lesion in the left temporal lobe gave rise to parenchymal cystic changes. The whole picture suggests bilateral tentorial injury with supra- and infratentorial bleeding. Left parietal posterior hypodensity on CT may correspond with arterial hypoperfusion. (Reproduced by permission from de Vries *et al.* 1996.)

IV.5 LOBAR CEREBRAL HAEMORRHAGE

In a limited number of newborn infants and in the absence of major ventricular bleeding, one may find haemorrhage in one or more brain lobes. Lesions in each region of the cerebrum have already been described, albeit exclusively with CT. The presenting sign has often been (multi)focal convulsive activity. In most instances the exact mode of genesis remains unknown.

Such haemorrhage in the *frontal* lobe generally goes hand in hand with an extracerebral haematoma against the falx and/or in the sylvian fissure. In some cases a vascular malformation has been angiographically excluded. Although trauma was mooted as one of the causes, there was no conclusive evidence, *e.g.* in the way of associated bone damage. In two personal observations fetal asphyxia and coagulation disorder, and enteroviral sepsis with intravascular coagulation and liver failure (Fig. IV.5.a), were considered respectively as probable causes.

Lobar haematomas have been observed in the *parietal* (Fig. IV.5.b) and *temporal* (Fig. IV.5.c) lobes of several infants. In one case we were confronted with IVH due to germinal matrix bleeding and associated venous infarction. We came across this variant a few times with clear prenatal origin (see fetal intracranial haemorrhage, section III.2). In another case we were primarily dealing with a total or partial middle cerebral artery infarction with secondary haemorrhagic conversion, due to, *inter alia*, reperfusion damage and coagulation disorder. Haemostatic failure, especially thrombocytopenia, is by itself sufficient as a cause for haemorrhage of the temporal lobe. This must be distinguished from subarachnoid haematoma and from basal subdural haematoma with contusion of the temporal lobe. Should the clinical history not explain the event, one will have to search for a vascular malformation.

Lobar haemorrhage has been rarely described in the *occipital* lobe (Fig. IV.5.d). Its pathogenesis is as mysterious as it is for the frontal variant. This type of haemorrhage is probably caused by haemostatic failure together with asphyxia and/or congestion.

Echographically these lobar haematomas show as round or elliptic, hyperdense and often clearly delineated zones. Where haematoma borders are irregular, one may be dealing with haemorrhagic conversion of an ischaemic area. Rarely echography will indicate whether there is still parenchyma between the lesion and the adjacent cranial bone: this allows for a distinction from temporal subarachnoid haematoma. After a few weeks cystic regression occurs of part (often most) of the affected lobe. The overlying cortex is often necrotic. We were sometimes struck by the absence of mass effect, which one might have expected in case of extracerebral haemorrhage of similar size.

REFERENCES

Bergman, I., Bauer, R.E., Barmada, M.A., Latchaw, R.E., Taylor, H.G., David, R., Painter, M.J. (1985) 'Intra-cerebral hemorrhage in the full-term neonatal infant.' *Pediatrics*, **75**, 488–496.

Hanigan, W.C., Powell, F.C., Palagallo, G., Miller, T.C. (1995) 'Lobar hemorrhages in full-term neonates.' *Child's Nervous System*, **11**, 276–280.

Hayashi, T., Harada, K., Honda, E., Utsunomiya, H., Hashimoto, T. (1987) 'Rare neonatal intracerebral hemorrhage. Two cases in full-term infants.' *Child's Nervous System*, **3**, 161–164.

Pierre-Kahn, A., Renier, D., Sainte-Rose, C., Flandin, C., Hirsch, J-F. (1985) 'Les hématomes intracrâniens aigus du nouveau-né à terme. A propos de dix-sept cas.' *Annales de Pédiatrie*, **32**, 419–425.

Ries, M., Wölfel, D., Maier-Brandt, B. (1995) 'Severe intracranial hemorrhage in a newborn infant with transplacental transfer of an acquired factor VIII:C inhibitor.' *Journal of Pediatrics*, **127**, 649–650.

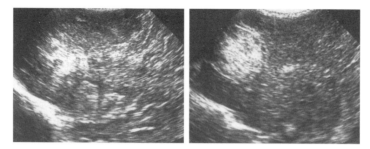

Above: **Fig. IV.5.a.** Term infant with non-immune hydrops and antepartum asphyxia: day 1, 7.5 MHz sections, both parasagittal. The *frontal* nodular lesion with feathered outer margins above and in front of the right insula was hyperdense on CT, suggesting recent haemorrhage of unknown cause.

Below: **Fig. IV.5.b.** Three haemorrhagic lesions in the *parietal* area (all 7.5 MHz sonograms).

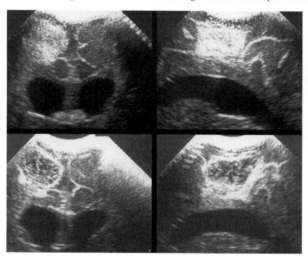

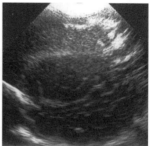

Term infant with difficult ventouse delivery: parasagittal image. Clouds of density high in the posterior parietal area suggested contusion, subsequently confirmed by CT.

Term infant treated with ECMO: *left*, coronal images; *right*, parasagittal; the *top* images were taken on day 10, the *bottom* ones one month later. A quadrangular hyperdense area undergoes cystic change in the ensuing weeks: haemorrhagic infarct?

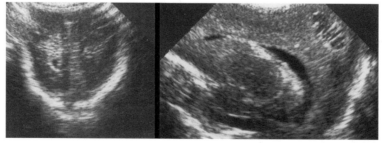

Preterm infant (25 weeks gestation) who was dropped onto the floor following delivery. The cystic appearance of the posterior parietal lobe may be due to previous contusion.

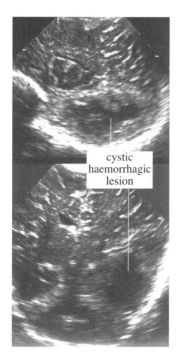

cystic
haemorrhagic
lesion

Fig. IV.5.c. Bleeding into the parenchyma of the *temporal* lobe is quite often a consequence of haemostatic dysfunction. With ultrasound it is difficult or even impossible to distinguish between genuine lobar bleeding and extensive subarachnoid haematoma. Four examples are shown on this page and opposite

(Left) Second week 7.5 MHz sections *(top,* parasagittal; *bottom,* coronal) in a term infant following operation for transposition of great vessels. (Probable cause: excessive heparinization?)

(Below) 7.5 MHz images *(left,* coronal; *right,* parasagittal) of a near-term growth retarded infant with perinatal intracranial haemorrhage due to alloimmune thrombocytopenia. With CT blood was found in the cerebellum as well. Cystic periventricular leukomalacia can also be seen *(arrows).*

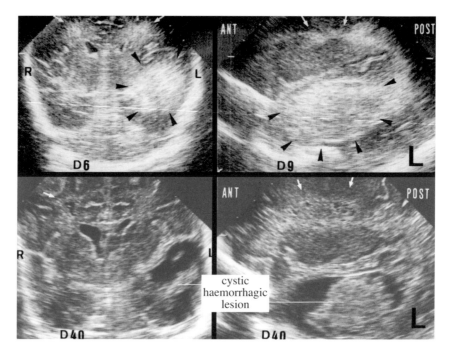

cystic
haemorrhagic
lesion

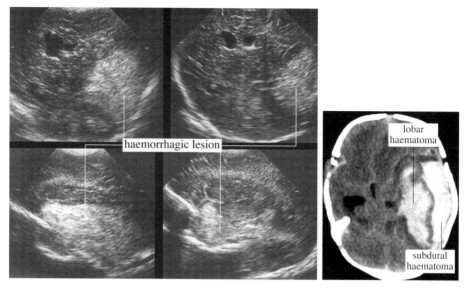

7.5 MHz images (*top*, coronal; *bottom*, parasagittal; *left*, day 2, *right*, day 8) of a term infant presenting with apnoea, vomiting, unilateral left mydriasis and anaemia on day 2 following uneventful spontaneous vaginal delivery. Coagulation screen, platelet count and bleeding time were repeatedly within normal limits. MRI at 6 months of age did not suggest the existence of a vascular anomaly; the corresponding CT shows lobar clot separated from subdural blood by a rim of cortex. The non-festooning of sulci militates against a diagnosis of subarachnoid haematoma.

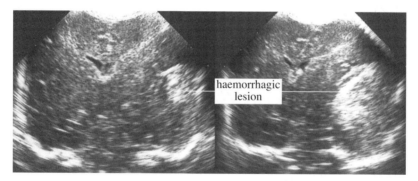

Growth retarded preterm infant (33 weeks gestation) with thrombocytopenia: 7.5 MHz coronal sections (*left*, day 1; *right*, day 3). Fatal outcome. (Also cf. Fig. IV.8.a.)

Fig. IV.5.d. *Occipital* lobar haemorrhage may not be as rare as current literature suggests it to be. Four examples are given on this page and opposite.

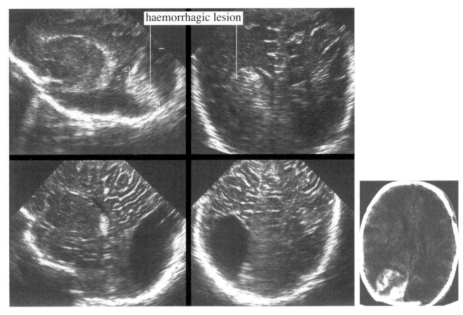

Term growth retarded infant with fetal distress during labour and evidence of disseminated intravascular coagulation after birth: 7.5 MHz sections (*left*, parasagittal; *right*, occipital coronal; *top*, day 2; *bottom*, day 30) and CT (day 3). Additional parietal haemorrhage was observed on the left.

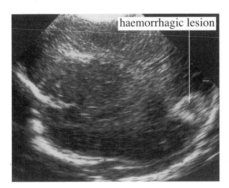

Growth retarded preterm infant (30 weeks gestation) with thrombocytopenia: parasagittal 7.5 MHz section.

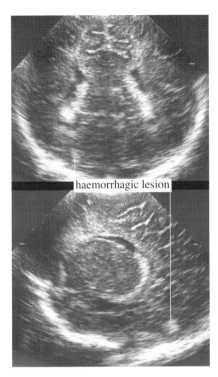

haemorrhagic lesion

Term infant with apnoea and macroscopic haematuria (haemostatic failure was appropriately excluded): 7.5 MHz sections (*top*, coronal; others parasagittal) and axial CT scan. Ventricular and right occipital lobar haemorrhage are evident.

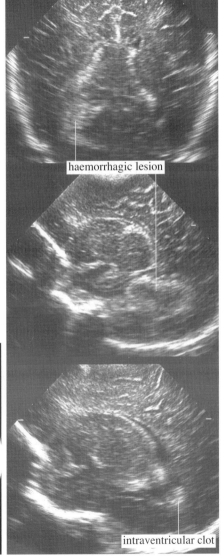

haemorrhagic lesion

intraventricular clot

Term infant with pulmonary hypertension, who had had well documented fetal distress one week prior to delivery (the mother, a farmer's wife, had sustained an injury when hit on the thigh by a bull). 7.5 MHz sections (*top*, coronal; *bottom*, parasagittal).

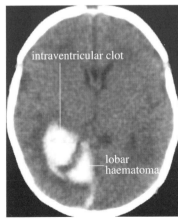

intraventricular clot

lobar haematoma

203

IV.6 CEREBELLAR HAEMORRHAGE

In preterm infants one can observe cerebellar haemorrhage under the same circumstances as those provoking GMH, the latter dominating the clinical picture. A handful of associated causes can be recognized in the term neonate. In the case of occipital osteodiastasis, haemorrhage is provoked by contusion of the caudal and dorsal cerebellum. When a tentorial tear occurs with rupture of a major vessel, the haematoma will expand in the rostral part of the cerebellar vermis. With a haemostatic or metabolic disorder, we may be facing one or more (confluent) parenchymal haemorrhages without anatomic predilection.

Cerebellar haemorrhage was sonographically identified in the preterm infant as early as the beginning of the 1980s. It must be said, however, that the distance to the fontanelle and the spontaneous heterogeneous hyperdensity of the cerebellar vermis make interpretation particularly difficult. Vague round hyperdensities in (para)sagittal or coronal sections can be visualized more clearly in preterm babies by means of axial sonography through the sphenoidal fontanelle. Haemorrhage around the tentorial groove or along a tentorial leaflet is echographically difficult to distinguish from a large haemorrhage in the superior vermis. Hemispheric haemorrhage may be best shown on a parasagittal section immediately adjacent to the midline, having first noticed asymmetry in cerebellar echoreflections in the coronal plane. A parenchymal haemorrhage may regress after a few weeks with cyst formation, which is exceptional following peritentorial subdural haematoma.

Due to heparinization (*e.g.* during ECMO), or with underlying haemorrhagic diathesis, the haemorrhage may remain hypodense initially and yet grow at a surprisingly fast rate.

REFERENCES

Bulas, D.I., Taylor, G.A., Fitz, C.R., Revenis, M.E., Glass, P., Ingram, J.D. (1991) 'Posterior fossa intracranial hemorrhage in infants treated with extracorporeal membrane oxygenation: sonographic findings.' *American Journal of Roentgenology*, **156**, 571–575.

De Campo, M. (1989) 'Neonatal posterior fossa haemorrhage: a difficult ultrasound diagnosis.' *Australasian Radiology*, **33**, 150–153.

Foy, P., Dubbins, P.A., Waldroup, L., Graziani, L., Goldberg, B.B., Berry, R. (1982) 'Ultrasound demonstration of cerebellar hemorrhage in a neonate.' *Journal of Clinical Ultrasound*, **10**, 196–198.

Huang, C-C., Shen, E-Y. (1991) 'Tentorial subdural hemorrhage in term newborns: ultrasonographic diagnosis and clinical correlates.' *Pediatric Neurology*, **7**, 171–177.

Perlman, J.M., Nelson, J.S., McAlister, W.H., Volpe, J.J. (1983) 'Intracerebellar hemorrhage in a premature newborn: diagnosis by real-time ultrasound and correlation with autopsy findings.' *Pediatrics*, **71**, 159–162.

Peterson, C.M., Smith, W.L., Franken, E.A. (1984) 'Neonatal intracerebellar hemorrhage: detection by real-time ultrasound.' *Radiology*, **150**, 391–392.

Reeder, J.D., Setzer, E.E., Kaude, J.V. (1982) 'Ultrasonographic detection of perinatal intracerebellar hemorrhage.' *Pediatrics*, **70**, 385–386.

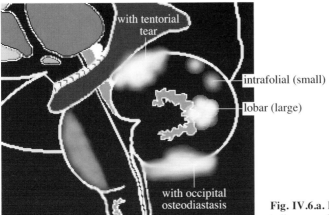

Fig. IV.6.a. Four main variants of cerebellar parenchymal haemorrhage.

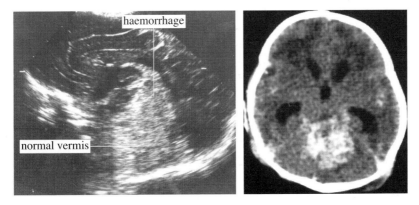

Fig. IV.6.b. Term infant with apnoea and tense fontanelle on the second day following uneventful vaginal delivery: *(left)* sagittal 7.5 MHz sonogram; *(right)* axial CT scan on the same day. The upper vermis is completely obscured by haemorrhage, exploding as it were from the parenchyma. On CT the density is heterogeneous due to mixture of blood with parenchyma. The evolution excluded primary haemostatic failure and persistent vascular anomaly. Compression has caused obstructive hydrocephalus.

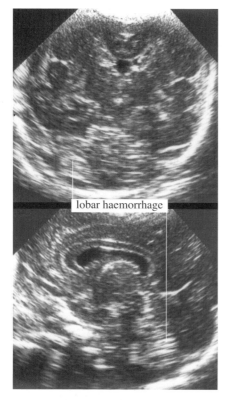

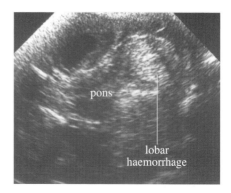

pons

lobar
haemorrhage

lobar haemorrhage

Fig. IV.6.c. Three preterm infants with cerebellar haemorrhage, autopsy-confirmed in each case.

(Left) 25 week gestation baby with respiratory distress syndrome: 7.5 MHz scans.

(Above) 29 weeks gestation, with *Listeria* bacteraemia and disseminated intravascular coagulation (7.5 MHz axial scan).

(Below) 25 weeks gestation, with respiratory distress syndrome and agenesis of the corpus callosum (10 MHz axial scans).

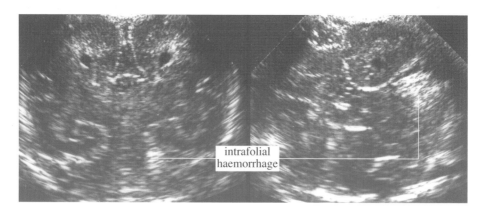

intrafolial
haemorrhage

IV.7 BLEEDING INTO BASAL GANGLIA AND VENTRICLE (DEEP VENOUS INFARCTION)

Manifest congestion, mostly with thrombosis of the great vein of Galen and/or the internal cerebral vein and its branches, will put the fragile vessels under pressure that can be found even in the term baby in the vicinity of residual germinal matrix or in plexus (Fig. IV.7.a).This will lead to deep venous infarction with a haemorrhagic necrotic zone especially in the thalamus but also in the adjoining grey nuclei (caudate nucleus or globus pallidus) when there is extensive injury. The phenomenon is nearly always associated with IVH, mostly grade II. The infarct may stretch as far as the corpus callosum and periventricular white matter, without affecting subcortical areas.

When a single branch of the internal cerebral vein thromboses, the most striking phenomenon may be unilateral haemorrhagic infarction in the thalamus or caudate nucleus (see section VII).

Besides propagation from thrombosis in the superior sagittal sinus, along the straight sinus to the deep venous system, well known other causes of deep venous thrombosis are: excessive congestion, as during long labour; leptomeningitis and ventriculitis; hyperviscosity as with cyanotic heart defect or polycythaemia; asphyxia; and antithrombin III deficiency. Vascular malformations may give rise to deep haemorrhage looking like deep venous thrombosis.

So-called parenchymal extensions of IVH are generally the consequence of venous infarction in medullary veins compressed at the foramen of Monro by an expanding matrix haemorrhage or by a major clot in the lateral ventricle.

Cranial echography will initially show asymmetric or unilateral particularly dense lesions in the thalamus or caudate nucleus, close to the plexus of the lateral ventricle. In the ventricle itself one will often find clot fragments (Figs. IV.7.b, IV.7.c). A coronal section clearly shows a density abutting the midline, immediately under the fornix and the cavity of the septum pellucidum. Associated periventricular white matter infarction shows up as irregular and asymmetric manifest hyperechogenicites in white matter. Veins caught in the process of congestion or thrombosis may appear as short linear echos (Fig. IV.7.d).

REFERENCES

Govaert, P., Achten, E., Vanhaesebrouck, P., De Praeter, C., Van Damme, J. (1992) 'Deep cerebral venous thrombosis in thalamo-ventricular hemorrhage of the term newborn.' *Pediatric Radiology*, **22**, 123–127.

Montoya, F., Couture, A., Frèrebeau, P., Bonnet, H. (1987) 'Hémorragie intraventriculaire chez le nouveau-né à terme: origine thalamique.' *Pédiatrie*, **42**, 205–209.

Trounce, J.Q., Dodd, K.L., Fawer, C-L., Fielder, A.R., Punt, J., Levene, M.I. (1985) 'Primary thalamic haemorrhage in the newborn: a new clinical entity.' *Lancet*, **1**, 190–192.

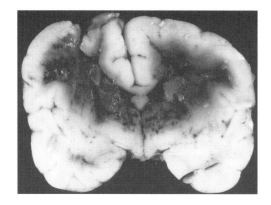

Fig. IV.7.a. Deep venous thrombosis in both internal cerebral vein areas. Red softening involves thalami, caudate nuclei, part of the pallidum and putamen, as well as an area of white matter, sparing subcortical tissue.

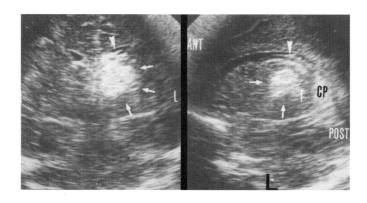

ventricular   white matter
haemorrhage   infarct

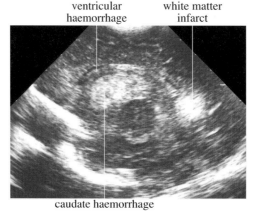

caudate haemorrhage

Fig. IV.7.b. Two examples of bleeding into thalamus and lateral ventricle.

(Top) Term infant with seizures due to group B streptococcal meningitis: 7.5 MHz sections on day 2 (*left*, coronal; *right*, parasagittal; *arrows* = venous infarct; *arrowheads* = IVH).

(Bottom) 34 week gestation baby with minimal respiratory distress who suffered fatal deep venous thrombosis (confirmed by MRI) due to an overtight nuchal collar of a negative pressure chamber, with IVH, caudate and periventricular haemorrhage.

208

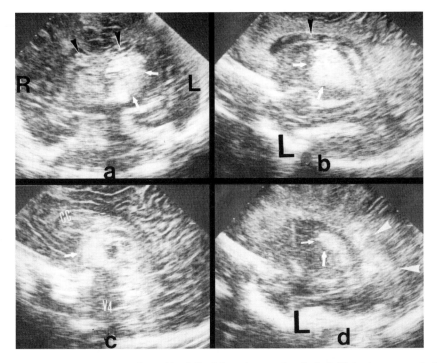

Fig. IV.7.c. Term male infant, delivered by difficult breech extraction (locked chin), who presented with seizures on day 6: 7.5 MHz sections (*top left*, coronal; *bottom left*, sagittal; *right*, parasagittal). CT and MRI confirmed venous thrombosis from the superior sagittal sinus, along the straight sinus and great vein of Galen, into deep veins (left internal cerebral vein, choroidal veins). Note haemorrhagic infarction of left thalamic area *(arrows)*, IVH *(black arrowheads)* and periventricular infarction *(arrowheads)*. At 5 years the boy had mild contralateral hemiplegia and epilepsy.

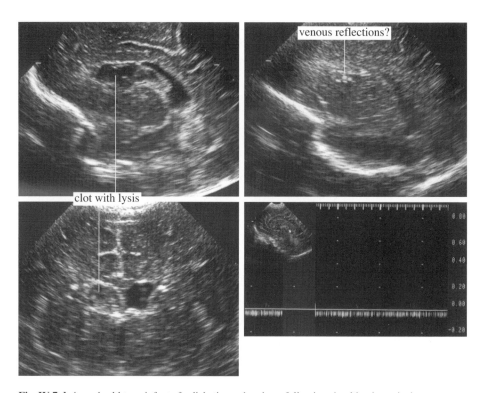

Fig. IV.7.d. 4-week-old term infant of a diabetic mother, born following shoulder dystocia due to macrosomia; the child was referred because of excessive tremors. 7.5 MHz sections (*top*, parasagittal; *bottom left*, coronal) and Doppler registrations. CT had shown haemorrhage in the right lateral ventricle and the head of the caudate nucleus in the early neonatal period. Cystic central regression of the clot is visible in the area of the right caudate head. Short linear hyperechogenicities are clearly seen under the tip of the left lateral ventricle in coronal as well as parasagittal sections, probably representing veins. Doppler registrations are probably from the internal cerebral vein (difficult to be certain with grey-scale imaging only), showing patency of that vessel. Complete thrombosis of the internal cerebral vein would have caused infarction of the thalamus as well. Probably the vessel involved here was a vein draining the caudate area (a transcaudate or septal vein). Given the presence of early round haematoma, focal arterial infarction would be unlikely as a mechanism, but cannot be excluded with certainty. Follow-up excluded tumour and vascular anomaly.

IV.8 SUBARACHNOID HAEMATOMA

This term refers to a space-occupying haemorrhage on the brain surface, but located under the arachnoid membranes. Primarily concerned is a fast growing subarachnoid or subpial haemorrhage. Mostly those lesions are found alongside and under the temporal and parietal lobes, usually on the left. Although the exact mechanism remains unknown, one will often find a context of haemorrhagic diathesis, frequently intravascular coagulation occurring during sepsis. In a few cases involving extremely ill, often preterm neonates, attempts have been made to identify the haemorrhage *in vivo*. A few reports describe the lesion with CT imaging.

Subarachnoid haemorrhage was one of the components of a strange pattern of haemorrhagic necrosis in both parietal lobes of extremely preterm infants, a pattern not yet fully explained (Cross *et al.* 1992). The lesions evolved toward a cystic stage in the parenchyma and eventually turned out to be fatal.

Ultrasound may suggest the diagnosis based on a hyperdensity against the temporoparietal bones, the borders of which irregularly penetrate the parenchyma. This represents sulci and fissures filled with coagulated blood. Subdural haemorrhage will displace rather than penetrate the adjacent parenchyma. The midline may be shifted and the ipsilateral ventricle closed under pressure. Associated haemorrhage may be noticed in the germinal matrix. Rarely, sonographic differentiation from a lobar parietotemporal haematoma is possible after identification on coronal sections of a border of parenchyma embracing a lobar but not a subarachnoid haematoma. Haemorrhagic conversion of an infarct in the region of the middle cerebral artery and subdural haemorrhage may also produce similar sonograms. It will be interesting to see, in the years ahead, what will be the consequences of any such lesion, often causing total cystic regression of a temporal lobe.

REFERENCES

Chessells, J.M., Wigglesworth, J.S.W. (1970) 'Secondary haemorrhagic disease of the newborn.' *Archives of Disease in Childhood*, **45**, 539–543.
Cross, J.H., Harrison, C.J., Preston, P.R., Rushton, D.I., Newell, S.J., Morgan, M.E.I., Durbin, G.M. (1992) 'Postnatal encephaloclastic porencephaly—a new lesion?' *Archives of Disease in Childhood*, **67**, 307–311.
Govaert, P., Leroy, J., Caemaert, J., Wood, B.P. (1992) 'Radiological case of the month. Extensive neonatal subarachnoid hematoma.' *American Journal of Diseases of Children*, **146**, 635–636.
Levene, M., de Vries, L.S. (1995) 'Intracranial haemorrhage.' *In:* Levene, M., Punt, J. (Eds.) *Fetal and Neonatal Neurology and Neurosurgery*. Edinburgh: Churchill Livingstone, pp. 335–366.
Morgan, M.E.I., Hensey, O.J., Cooke, R.W.I. (1983) 'Convexity cerebral haemorrhage in the neonate: *in vivo* ultrasound diagnosis.' *Archives of Disease in Childhood*, **58**, 814–818.

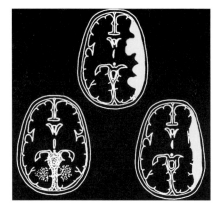

Fig. IV.8.a. Typical of subarachnoid haematoma *(top)* and discriminating it from subdural haematoma *(right)* is the festooned appearance of the inner clot margins, as coagula fill sulci and fissures to penetrate into the parenchyma. The terms subarachnoid or leptomeningeal haemorrhage *(left)* are reserved for minor bleeding into the arachnoid membranes without mass effect.

Fig. IV.8.b. Three infants with left temporal subarachnoid haematoma.

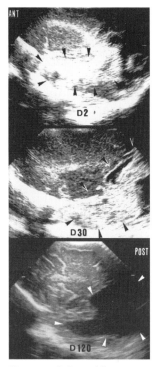

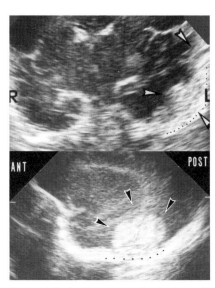

Preterm infant with gram-negative bacteraemia near the end of the first week: 7.5 MHz sections *(top,* coronal; *bottom,* parasagittal). The inner border of the clot is clearly corrugated.

Near-term infant with pneumococcal bacteraemia. On these serial outer parasagittal sections one can observe cystic regression of the entire left temporal lobe.

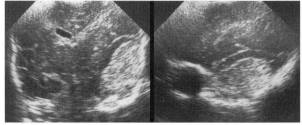

Growth retarded preterm infant (34 weeks gestation) with thrombocytopenia. (Reproduced by permission from Levene and de Vries 1995.)

212

SECTION V
PATHOLOGY: WHITE MATTER DISEASE

Nearly every histological alteration of white matter is accompanied by increased echodensity. Later, cystic change may supervene. In some disease states loss of white matter without cystic change may lead to compensatory replacement by CSF (hydrocephalus *ex vacuo*). An area of moderate hyperechogenicity, appearing somewhat like a flame and radiating out perpendicularly to the cavity, is normal in frontal and parieto-occipital periventricular regions. As neuronal and especially glial migration proceed and myelination increases, those physiological densities disappear in the young infant. In the postnatal period white matter becomes progressively less echogenic.

Gliosis (even without mineralization) and venous *congestion* probably go hand in hand with increased echodensity. Recognition of increased density in white matter is still subjective, and with no reproducible method of registering it objectively yet available, sonographic diagnosis of the spectrum of white matter disease is not easy. We have occasionally seen temporary or even persisting 'flares' (zonal echogenicities in white matter), without ventriculomegaly occurring, the infant's neurological development remaining normal (Fig. V.1.g). There are a number of causes of white matter disease which may be recognized in the neonatal period; some are very rare and cannot be discussed here. Leukomalacia is covered separately in section V.2.

V.1 PERINATAL LEUKODYSTROPHY

Progressive perinatal degeneration of glia undergoing myelination and white matter axons is rare. Faith in MRI has become such that in-depth sonographic analysis has been ignored or at least underestimated. And yet, it is a sensitive means of detecting changes in white matter at an early stage. The problem remains how to distinguish between normal echogenicity and discretely increased pathological hyperechogenicity. Comparison with clinical findings and confirmation with MRI is consequently often indicated.

Changes in white matter that are a consequence of a dystrophic process are very echodense; they are often irregularly shaped, or may be linear or of undulating appearance. A cystic intermediary, as in periventricular leukomalacia, is uncommon.

The typical location of periventricular leukomalacia, against the extreme outer wall of the lateral ventricles, is not necessarily the same as in dystrophic processes: often these densities are located below or above the lateral corner of the lateral ventricle (Fig. V.1.a). By definition they are bilateral but asymmetric, which is unusual with leukomalacia. Lesions that are part of a phakomatosis or gliomatosis may be an exception to the usual asymmetry. Unlike leukomalacia, periventricular leukodystrophic echodensities persist for months. Both lead to ventriculomegaly *ex vacuo*. Intralesional fine granular calcifications may suggest intrauterine infection.

Boltshauser *et al.* (1991) reported ultrasound findings in three infants with a similar clinical picture seen after the neonatal period, in whom damage to periventricular white matter was more apparent than associated lesions of the basal ganglia. Recently we observed a similar pattern in an infant with convulsions and elevated serum IgM, the most usual fetal infections having been excluded (Fig. V.1.b). This clinical picture can be distinguished from Aicardi–Goutières syndrome as the protein and cell content of CSF were normal.

In a child with congenital lactacidosis due to unspecified *mitochondrial* disorder we recognized diffuse involvement of white matter with punctate foci of maximal hyper-echogenicity in periventricular zones (Fig. V.1.d). With Leigh syndrome, it is possible to identify densities in the caudate nucleus and putamen at an early stage, whereas later on hydrocephalus *ex vacuo* follows with persisting characteristic hyperdense striatal areas. Should a mitochondrial encephalopathy be so serious as to cause antenatal brain damage, one may expect ventriculomegaly with calcification in white matter but also polymicrogyria and dysplasia of the corpus callosum.

Although *demyelinating* diseases also belong to this group, a hyperechogenic phase may be lacking. This phenomenon was observed in a child with neonatal progeroid (Wiedemann–Rautenstrauch) syndrome: over a period of weeks, without having observed echodense lesions, we noted progressive and generalized ventriculomegaly due to degeneration of white matter (Fig. V.1.e). Such slow atrophy of white matter may also be expected when neurons (and their axons) disappear due to transsynaptic degeneration. Although the phenomenon has not been reported with ultrasound, little or no hyperdensity would be expected in neuropil between degenerating neuronal nuclei.

If accompanied by subependymal cysts and linear striatal vasculopathy, asymmetric densities in white matter immediately beside the lateral ventricle may point to the Aicardi–Goutières syndrome. This entity comprises leukodystrophy with later striocerebellar calcification. A type of leukomalacia that needs to be distinguished from it is the 'variegata' type described by Leech and Alvord (1974): the ischaemic zone then presents itself as an irregular undulating confluence of echogenic foci parallel to the ventricle (Fig. V.1.f).

Germinolytic cysts, the volume of which increase postnatally, have been reported in children suffering from Alexander's disease. Echogenicity of white matter in *asphyxia* affects not only the centrum semi-ovale but also gyral cores (Fig. V.1.a). In leukomalacia there is usually no involvement of gyral core white matter fibres.

REFERENCES

Aicardi, J., Goutières, F. (1984) 'A progressive familial encephalopathy in infancy with calcifications of the basal ganglia and chronic cerebrospinal fluid lymphocytosis.' *Annals of Neurology*, **15**, 49–54.

Boltshauser, E., Steinlin, M., Boesch, C., Martin, E., Schubiger, G. (1991) 'Magnetic resonance imaging in infantile encephalopathy with cerebral calcification and leukodystrophy.' *Neuropediatrics*, **22**, 33–35.

Bönnemann, C.G., Meinecke, P. (1992) 'Encephalopathy of infancy with intracerebral calcification and chronic spinal fluid lymphocytosis — another case of the Aicardi–Goutières syndrome.' *Neuropediatrics*, **23**, 157–161.

Bošnjak, V., Bešenski, N., Della-Marina, B.M., Polak, J. (1988) 'Ultrasonography in hereditary degenerative diseases of the cerebral white matter in infancy.' *Neuropediatrics*, **19**, 208–211.

Chi, C-S., Mak, S-C., Shian, W-J. (1994) 'Leigh syndrome with progressive ventriculomegaly.' *Pediatric Neurology*, **10**, 244–246.

Hess, D.C., Fischer, A.Q., Yaghmai, F., Figueroa, R., Akamatsu, Y. (1990) 'Comparative neuroimaging with pathologic correlates in Alexander's disease.' *Journal of Child Neurology*, **5**, 248–252.

Leech, R.W., Alvord, E.C. (1974) 'Morphologic variations in periventricular leukomalacia.' *American Journal of Pathology*, 74, 591–602.

Martin, J.J., Ceuterick, C.M., Leroy, J.G., Devos, E.A., Roelens, J.G. (1984) 'The Wiedemann–Rautenstrauch or neonatal progeroid syndrome. Neuropathological study of a case.' *Neuropediatrics*, **15**, 43–48.

Razavi-Encha, F., Larroche, J.C., Gaillard, D. (1988) 'Infantile familial encephalopathy with cerebral calcifications and leukodystrophy.' *Neuropediatrics*, **19**, 72–79.

Sabatino, G., Domizio, S., Verrotti, A., Ramenghi, L.A., Pelliccia, P., Morgese, G. (1994) 'Fetal encephalopathy with cerebral calcifications: a case report.' *Child's Nervous System*, **10**, 195–197.

Samsom, J.F., Barth, P.G., de Vries, J.I.P., Menko, F.H., Ruitenbeek, W., van Oost, B.A., Jakobs, C. (1994) 'Familial mitochondrial encephalopathy with fetal ultrasonographic ventriculomegaly and intracerebral calcifications.' *European Journal of Pediatrics*, **153**, 510–516.

Yamagata, T., Yano, S., Okabe, I., Miyao, M., Momoi, M.Y., Yanagisawa, M., Hirata, H., Komatsu, K. (1990) 'Ultrasonography and magnetic resonance imaging in Leigh disease.' *Pediatric Neurology*, **6**, 326–329.

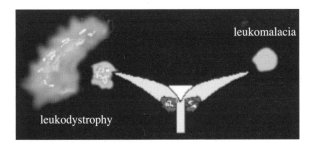

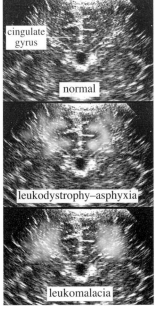

Fig. V.1.a. Leukomalacia, in its typical presentation, spares a rim of immediate periventricular white matter and lies along the long axis of the lateral ventricle. Leukodystrophic areas may be more erratically sited, are almost by definition irregular in echogenicity, asymmetric and persist for weeks to months.

(Left) Congestion as well as white matter ischaemia in asphyxia and some leukodystrophic processes affect gyral cores, whereas in leukomalacia these cores are usually free of echogenicity (depicted here on an adapted coronal detail of the interhemispheric fissure at the foramen of Monro).

215

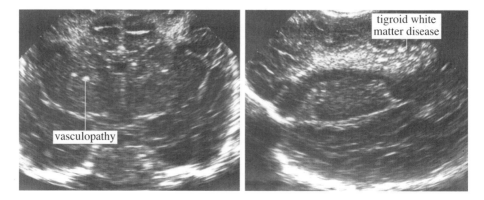

Fig. V.1.b. Infant born at 36 weeks following hydramnios of several weeks duration, who presented with seizures and hypotonia. We found elevated serum IgM (1.5 g/L) in the first week but evidence for the more common intrauterine infections was not found. White matter appears tigroid with regular occipital foci of hyperechogenicity. Diffuse echogenicity was seen in frontal and parietal areas. In addition there was striatal vasculopathy, and areas of subcortical calcification were revealed on CT. (Diagnosis: Boltshauser syndrome or viral fetal encephalitis?)

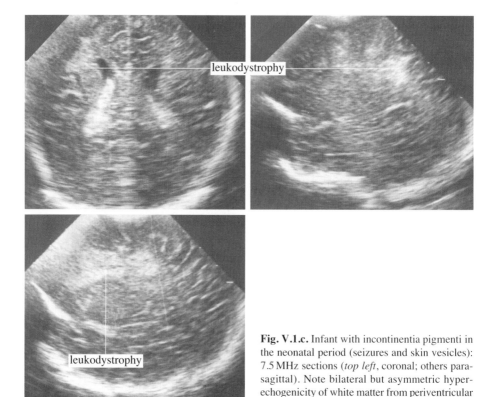

Fig. V.1.c. Infant with incontinentia pigmenti in the neonatal period (seizures and skin vesicles): 7.5 MHz sections (*top left*, coronal; others parasagittal). Note bilateral but asymmetric hyperechogenicity of white matter from periventricular to subcortical areas.

216

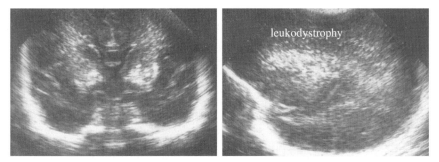

Fig. V.1.d. Term infant with congenital lactacidosis, microcephaly, hypertrophic cardiomyopathy and corneal dystrophy, probably due to an unidentified mitochondrial disorder: 7.5 MHz sections on day 2 (*left*, coronal; *right*, parasagittal). Apart from pallidal hyperechogenicities, there was a diffuse increase of reflections from white matter, especially in the frontal lobe.

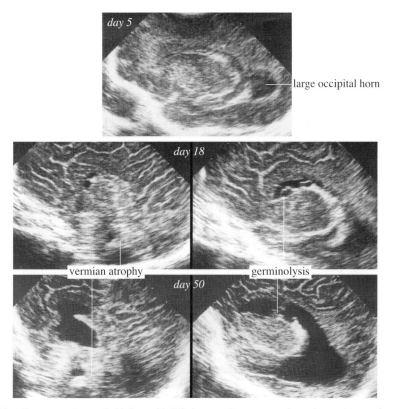

Fig. V.1.e. Term growth retarded infant with Wiedemann–Rautenstrauch syndrome (neonatal progeric features): (para)sagittal 7.5 MHz sections. Histologically a sudanophilic leukodystrophic process was present. Although white matter disease is obvious because of the fast evolution towards hydrocephalus *ex vacuo*, at no stage did it become hyperechogenic. The vermis seemed atrophic from the start, but more cerebellar tissue disappeared over this short period. Small germinolytic cysts in both caudothalamic grooves were first seen in the late neonatal period.

217

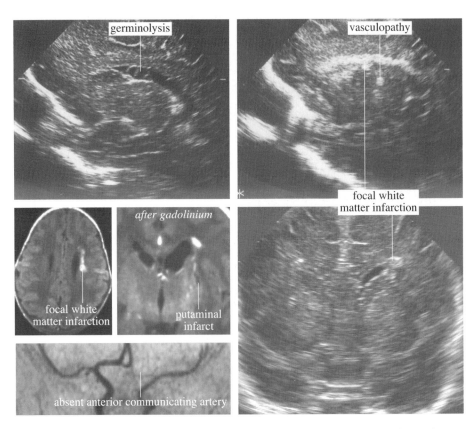

Fig. V.1.f. Day 2 left parasagittal *(top)* and anterior coronal *(bottom right)* 7.5 MHz sections and corresponding MR images of a term hypotonic infant with dysmorphic features and seizures but a normal karyotype. There was a large germinolytic cyst in the left caudothalamic groove. A thick wave of hyperechogenicity was seen immediately along the left outer ventricle margin (no spared rim as in leukomalacia). Striatal vessels were hyperechogenic and a fluffy putaminal dense focus was seen on the affected side (MRI confirmed focal infarct). MR angiography demonstrated anomalous design of the circle of Willis (absent left anterior communicating artery). The subsequent evolution excluded progressive brain disease, and our conclusion was focal infarction of periventricular white matter due to congenital vascular anomaly. Strict unilaterality militated against leukomalacia. The hyperechogenic band persisted for a few months.

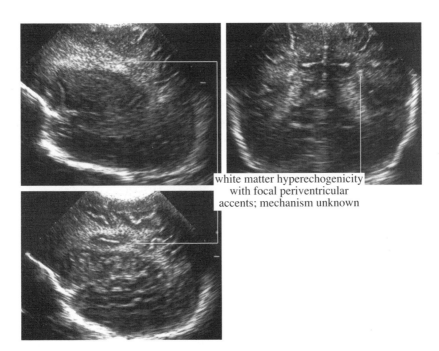

white matter hyperechogenicity with focal periventricular accents; mechanism unknown

Fig. V.1.g. Term infant with congenital heart defect (mother diabetic): neonatal 7.5 MHz sections (*left*, parasagittal; *right*, coronal). The remarkable hyperechogenicity of gyral and periventricular white matter persisted for weeks, without cyst formation and without ensuing ventricular dilatation. Within the periventricular area soft accents of hyperechogenicity with striking symmetry can be seen. Neuromotor development was normal at 12 months.

V.2 LEUKOMALACIA

Damage to white matter in the perinatal period occurs: (i) as an isolated phenomenon due to cerebral hypoperfusion; (ii) in association with haemorrhage in germinal matrix; and (iii) as part of the neuropathological substrate in fetal, intrapartum or neonatal acute asphyxia or chronic hypoxia.

More exceptional forms of white matter injury are dealt with under perinatal leukodystrophy (above), infectious fetopathy (section III.8), postnatal CNS infection (section VIII.1), and sinus thrombosis (section VII.9).

The term *periventricular leukomalacia* was coined in 1962 by Banker and Larroche and literally means softening of the white matter. Although the pathogenesis is not fully understood, the common denominator is hypoperfusion of the brain with ischaemia in the zones between the most important arterial irrigation areas ('border zones'). For the third trimester this area is mainly found between ventriculofugal (striatal) and ventriculopetal (cortical) branches of the middle cerebral artery, showing necrosis in a band of white matter located in the coronal axis of the lateral ventricle at a distance of about 1 cm from its lateral wall (at least 3 mm from the ependyma). Often the most damaged areas are found at the junction between the parietal and the frontal or occipital lobes because those are border zones between major cerebral arteries.

Recently doubts have been cast on the validity of the prevailing interarterial pathogenetic theory (Fig. V.2.b) because with stereomicroscopy proof could not be found of arterial border zones. The arteries from the striatal area that used to be considered ventriculofugal branches, appear to be venous. Whatever the exact pathogenesis may be, necrosis in the centrum semi-ovale in association with a clinical picture compatible with cerebral hypoperfusion is relatively common in preterm babies.

Leukomalacia, in its traditional picture (Fig. V.2.a) evolving toward coagulation and later cystic necrosis, is characteristically located in the periventricular area in the preterm infant. With maturation, the sensitive area moves to the cortex, which explains why leukomalacia in the term asphyxiated neonate is most evident in white matter adjacent to the floor of a sulcus (Fig. V.2.j). Mixed periventricular and subcortical variants are not common. Histological change in subcortical white matter is not exceptional in preterm infants but may show a picture that differs from the traditional presentation at or near term. The fluid within the cysts is eventually absorbed by surrounding white matter, giving rise after some time to a gliotic scar zone with local perturbation of myelination. It is suspected that this is due not to degradation of formed myelin but rather to interference with glial cells containing myelin precursors. Mostly the initial spot is circular, but variants with a linear or undulating appearance have been described.

Ischaemia without necrosis may engender a gliotic, non-cystic type of leukomalacia, referred to by Gilles and Murphy (1969) as *telencephalic leukoencephalopathy*. Although this entity is clinically less well delineated, we do indeed have to acknowledge the existence of a type of white matter damage with an evolution of echodensities toward ventriculomegaly without cystic intermediary. This milder degree of leukomalacia might be quite common. The existence of such a mitigated form may in part explain the variation in published prevalence rates of echographic leukomalacia.

In very low birthweight infants (<1500 g) there is a reported 20–25% overall risk of sonographic leukomalacia. For reasons explained below, the exact prevalence of leukomalacia is not known.

Necrotic white matter, even if it has not been superimposed on germinal matrix haemorrhage, may bleed secondarily (*haemorrhagic conversion*): cerebral hyperperfusion plays a part secondary to microvascular damage due to free radical formation and disturbed haemostasis (Fig. V.2.h). This phenomenon occurs in about one in five cases of leukomalacia. Its prognostic significance is unclear.

In contrast to GMH/IVH, which mostly occurs during the first 72 hours and rarely beyond the first week of life, in preterm infants leukomalacia can occur up till term age. As it can also occur antenatally, an early, preferably first day examination will be of paramount importance in determining the timing of the injury (Fig. V.2.d). It has been shown that there are two ways of clearly establishing the antenatal origin of leukomalacia. The first is when cysts are evident at birth. The alternative is to find abnormal hyperechogenicities evolving to cyst formation within the first week of life. The exact interval between insult and cystic change may depend on gestational age, the severity of the lesion and ongoing secondary damage after birth. Therefore it is unlikely that one could differentiate a very early neonatal insult from one occurring a few hours before birth.

Although there is not one generally accepted classification system for leukomalacia, the following four-grade system, developed by one of the present authors (de Vries *et al.* 1992), has achieved some recognition:

Grade I   — transient periventricular densities (>7 days);
Grade II   — localized cysts in the external angle of the lateral ventricle;
Grade III — extensive cysts in frontoparietal and/or occipital periventricular white matter (cystic periventricular leukomalacia);
Grade IV — extensive cysts in subcortical white matter (cystic subcortical leukomalacia).

It is not a simple matter to make a distinction between grade I leukomalacia and normal anatomic variations, often referred to as venous congestion or 'peritrigonal blush'.

Echoreflections that are (nearly) as dense as choroid plexus, a tissue often used as a reference for diagnosing leukomalacia, are abnormal (Fig. V.2.a). This approach is not without problems: (i) plexus is highly perfused in this age group and furthermore there are varying degrees of congestion or haemorrhage; and (ii) the more preterm the child is, the more prominent and dense the plexus appears to be, and consequently its property as a calibrator is made relatively weak in the very immature baby. In practice, white matter hyperechogenicities are considered important if they match or exceed plexus density.

Soft symmetric radial echodensities are normal around the frontal horns and the parieto-occipital junction of the lateral ventricle (Fig. V.2.a). This 'peritrigonal blush' may (in term babies) be observed to disappear slowly in the course of the second month of life. Perinatal white matter is relatively echogenic due to an increased water content, active late glial migration and early myelination (fat-laden oligodendroglia). In a parasagittal section those normal densities form a conspicuous border of periventricular brain matter. The shorter the gestation, the more pronounced these physiological periventricular echodensities probably are. In case of doubt, insonation through the posterior fontanelle allows for easier differentiation from ischaemia or haemorrhage because the sound beam runs parallel to the axons in the 'blush'.

When echodense zones turn isodense without cyst formation or ventricular dilatation within the first weeks of life, the phenomenon is described as a stage of temporary 'flare'. A persistence of the flares beyond 7–14 days may be considered abnormal and indicative of damage. The duration of flaring corresponds with the severity of injury.

Sometimes thick lines or rounded figures develop in the flares without cystic regression: this suggests gliosis without total necrosis (survival of macrophages and astroglia). We refer to these flares with a nidus of even more echogenicity as clouded or patchy (Fig. V.2.l).

Cyst formation is a process typical for the second week (range 10–40 days) after the insult, whereby subcortical leukomalacia turns cystic slightly earlier than the periventricular form. The cysts represent total tissue necrosis.

The best way to check white matter for ischaemia is with a wide sector angle (≥90°) and a 7.5 MHz scanhead (Fig. V.2.c). Due to slow evolution into cysts one is committed to follow up on the insult for at least four weeks.

The cysts can be very localized and few in number (grade II) and are then usually noted in the frontal or frontoparietal white matter. When they are widespread and extend into the parieto-occipital region, they are referred to as grade III leukomalacia. Such cysts are bundled and sharply delineated. They grow and then gradually disappear leaving an irregularly dilated angular lateral ventricle. Often the interhemispheric fissure widens. The cystic zone is always smaller than the echogenic zone. Sulci may in some manifest cases penetrate as far as the lateral ventricle.

Subcortical cysts remain visible for a longer period (sometimes months) and they are often bigger. Large cysts are a consequence of a merger of smaller ones with, during the active process, a period of irregular cavitation with intraluminal septae ('Swiss cheese pattern').

Cystic leukomalacia strongly correlates with residual neuromotor dysfunction. Often the same child suffers from matrix haemorrhage (Fig. V.2.k). Other associated lesions, difficult or not at all recognizable *in vivo*, are pontosubicular necrosis and cerebellar damage. Extensive bilateral cystic leukomalacia predicts spastic diplegia (especially with periventricular lesions) or even quadriplegia (especially with mixed and subcortical lesions) with visual impairment. The most affected descending axonal routes are those closest to the ventricle, *i.e.* the corticospinal projection fibres associated with the lower limbs. Association fibres, commissural axons and corticobulbar efferents may also be damaged in their crosswise passage through the centrum semi-ovale. Motor dysfunction is also possible after leukomalacia without cyst formation, but usually is less marked than with cystic leukomalacia.

Limited cystic leukomalacia must be distinguished from: (i) paraventricular frontal germinolysis; (ii) paraventricular porencephaly; (iii) cystic regression of a limited venous infarct due to germinal matrix haemorrhage; and (iv) arterial infarct in a terminal branch of a striatal artery.

Objective measurement of echodensity could provide the answer to inherent problems of subjective visual interpretation of lesions in white matter (Fig. V.2.n). Only then will discrepant incidences of 'flares' be explainable. Estimation of the timing of the insult may also become possible. Prediction of subsequent disability is certainly feasible provided one has acquired sufficient experience with leukomalacia in all its sonographic manifestations. In particular, ventriculomegaly and cyst formation are important negative prognostic variables. Although one might gain the impression that everything possible has been written regarding injury to perinatal white matter, we are not of that opinion (Fig. V.2.m). The reader is referred to Paneth *et al.* (1994) for a survey of the literature and for a discussion of related questions.

REFERENCES

Banker, B.Q., Larroche, J-C. (1962) 'Periventricular leukomalacia of infancy. A form of neonatal anoxic encephalopathy.' *Archives of Neurology*, **7**, 386–410.
Costello, A.M.deL, Hamilton, P.A., Baudin, J., Townsend, J., Bradford, B.C., Stewart, A.L., Reynolds, E.O.R. (1988) 'Prediction of neurodevelopmental impairment at four years from brain ultrasound appearance of very preterm infants.' *Developmental Medicine and Child Neurology*, **30**, 711–722.
de Vries, L.S., Wigglesworth, J.S., Regev, R., Dubowitz, L.M.S. (1988) 'Evolution of periventricular leukomalacia during the neonatal period and infancy: correlation of imaging and postmortem findings.' *Early Human Development*, **17**, 205–219.
— — Eken, P., Dubowitz, L.M.S. (1992) 'The spectrum of leukomalacia using cranial ultrasound.' *Behavioural Brain Research*, **49**, 1–6.
— — — Groenendaal, F., van Haastert, I.C., Meiners, L.C. (1993) 'Correlation between the degree of periventricular leukomalacia diagnosed using cranial ultrasound and MRI later in infancy in children with cerebral palsy.' *Neuropediatrics*, **24**, 263–268.
DiPietro, M.A., Brody, B.A., Teele, R.L., (1986) 'Peritrigonal echogenic "blush" on cranial sonography: pathologic correlates.' *American Journal of Roentgenology*, **146**, 1067–1072.
Eken, P., Jansen, G.H., Groenendaal, F., Rademaker, K., de Vries, L.S. (1994) 'Intracranial lesions in the full-term infant with hypoxic–ischaemic encephalopathy: ultrasound and autopsy correlations.' *Neuropediatrics*, **25**, 301–307.
— — de Vries, L.S., van der Graaf, Y., Meiners, L.C., van Nieuwenhuizen, O. (1995) 'Haemorrhagic–ischaemic lesions of the neonatal brain: correlation between cerebral visual impairment, neurodevelopmental outcome and MRI in infancy.' *Developmental Medicine and Child Neurology*, **37**, 41–55.
Fawer, C-L., Calame, A., Perentes, E., Anderegg, A. (1985) 'Periventricular leukomalacia: a correlation study between real-time ultrasound and autopsy findings. Periventricular leukomalacia in the neonate.' *Neuroradiology*, **27**, 292–300.
Fazzi, E., Orcesi, S., Caffi, L., Ometto, A., Rondini, G., Telesca, C., Lanzi, G. (1994) 'Neurodevelopmental outcome at 5–7 years in preterm infants with periventricular leukomalacia.' *Neuropediatrics*, **25**, 134–139.
Gilles, F.H., Murphy, S.F. (1969) 'Perinatal telencephalic leukoencephalopathy.' *Journal of Neurology, Neurosurgery and Psychiatry*, **32**, 404–413.
Grunnet, M. (1982) 'Periventricular leukomalacia complex. Clinical and pathologic correlates.' *Archives of Pathology and Laboratory Medicine*, **106**, 81–82.
Guit, G.L., van de Bor, M., den Ouden, L., Wondergem, J.H.M. (1990) 'Prediction of neurodevelopmental outcome in the preterm infant: MR-staged myelination compared with cranial US.' *Radiology*, **175**, 107–109.
Hope, P.L., Gould, S.J., Howard, S., Hamilton, P.A., Costello, A.M.deL., Reynolds, E.O.R. (1988) 'Precision of ultrasound diagnosis of pathologically verified lesions in the brains of very preterm infants.' *Developmental Medicine and Child Neurology*, **30**, 457–471.
Laub, M.C., Ingrisch, H. (1986) 'Increased periventricular echogenicity (periventricular halos) in neonatal brain: a sonographic study.' *Neuropediatrics*, **17**, 39–43.
Levene, M.I., Wigglesworth, J.S., Dubowitz, V. (1983) 'Hemorrhagic periventricular leukomalacia in the neonate: a real-time ultrasound study.' *Pediatrics*, **71**, 794–797.
Leviton, A., Paneth, N. (1990) 'White matter damage in preterm newborns—an epidemiologic perspective.' *Early Human Development*, **24**, 1–22.

Paneth, N., Rudelli, R., Monte, W., Rodriguez, E., Pinto, J., Kairam, R., Kazam, E. (1990) 'White matter necrosis in very low birth weight infants: neuropathologic and ultrasonographic findings in infants surviving six days or longer.' *Journal of Pediatrics*, **116**, 975–984.

— — — — Kazam, E., Monte, W.(1994) *Brain Damage in the Preterm Infant. Clinics in Developmental Medicine No. 131.* London: Mac Keith Press.

Perlman, J.M., Rollins, N., Burns, D, Risser, R. (1993) 'Relationship between periventricular intraparenchymal echodensities and germinal matrix–intraventricular hemorrhage in the very low birth weight neonate.' *Pediatrics*, **91**, 474–480.

Pidcock, F.S., Graziani, L.J., Stanley, C., Mitchell, D.G., Merton, D. (1990) 'Neurosonographic features of periventricular echodensities associated with cerebral palsy in preterm infants.' *Journal of Pediatrics*, **116**, 417–422.

Ringelberg, J., van de Bor, M. (1993) 'Outcome of transient periventricular echodensities in preterm infants.' *Neuropediatrics*, **24**, 269–273.

Rodriguez, J., Claus, D., Verellen, G., Lyon, G. (1990) 'Periventricular leukomalacia: ultrasonic and neuropathological correlations.' *Developmental Medicine and Child Neurology*, **32**, 347–352.

Rushton, D.I., Preston, P.R., Durbin, G.M. (1985) 'Structure and evolution of echodense lesions in the neonatal brain. A combined ultrasound and necropsy study.' *Archives of Disease in Childhood*, **60**, 798–808.

Tamisari, L., Vigi, V., Fortini, C., Scarpa, P. (1986)' Neonatal periventricular leukomalacia: diagnosis and evolution evaluated by real-time ultrasound.' *Helvetica Paediatrica Acta*, **41**, 399–407.

Trounce, J.Q., Levene, M.I. (1985) 'Diagnosis and outcome of subcortical cystic leucomalacia.' *Archives of Disease in Childhood*, **60**, 1041–1044.

Volpe, J.J. (1990) 'Brain injury in the premature infant: is it preventable?' *Pediatric Research*, **27**, S28–S33.

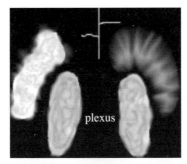

Leukomalacia		*Peritrigonal blush*
bilateral, slightly asymmetric		symmetric
hard		soft
not radial		radial
sharply delineated		vague margins
with nodular accents, clouded	plexus	homogeneous

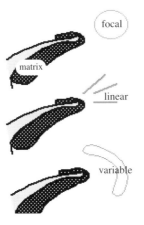

plexus

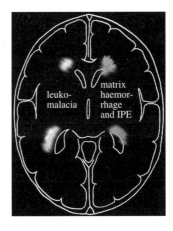

physiologic flares

Fig. V.2.a. *(Top)* In clinical practice, the condition of white matter is judged by its echogenic potential as compared with choroid plexus. This method has proved its strength, but may have limits in the very immature preterm infant.

(Above, left) 7.5 MHz parasagittal scan of a baby born at 23 weeks gestation: choroid plexus is strongly echogenic at this stage. *(Above, right)* 7.5 MHz coronal scan of a healthy infant born at 32 weeks gestation and later shown to have normal development: physiologic flares are symmetric and soft.

(Below, left) Three morphological appearances of leukomalacia are discernible: focal, linear, and variable other ('variegata' type). *(Below, right)* Compared with matrix haemorrhage and venous infarction related to it, the echogenic foci of classical leukomalacia are removed a short distance from the ventricular ependyma. Near the frontal horn they are rounded or elliptical, unlike the triangle of early IPEs (intraparenchymal echodensities). Near the temporal horn leukomalacia is more lateral than matrix haemorrhage, the later being sited on top of the curved outer ventricular wall.

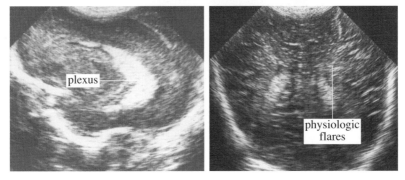

focal

matrix

linear

variable

leuko-malacia

matrix haemor-rhage and IPE

225

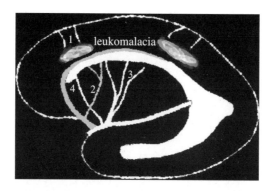

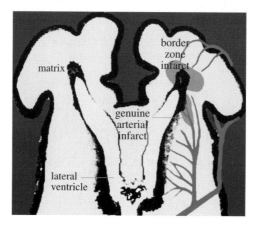

Fig. V.2.b. *(Above)* The interarterial or border zone hypothesis claims that periventricular leukomalacia is the result of infarction between ventriculopetal cortical branches of the middle cerebral artery (1) and ventriculofugal striatal branches of the anterior (2), middle cerebral (3) and anterior choroidal (4) arteries. The presence of proper ventriculofugal striatal end arteries bowing away from the ventricle has been proved wrong but this does not challenge the existence of a vulnerable area between deep striatal arteries and penetrating cortical ones. On the other hand it is conceivable that both matrix lesions (whether haemorrhage or infarction) and periventricular white matter necrosis may follow genuine arterial infarction in a small terminal branch of either perfusion system.

(Opposite) Typical border zone leukomalacia may be limited to one of two or both typical areas at the transition between the middle and anterior cerebral arteries in front, and between the middle and posterior cerebral arteries posteriorly. In that sense leukomalacia is akin to parasagittal cerebral injury of asphyxia at or near term. Extensive types involve more subcortical areas and also encompass the parietal lobe. Asymmetric, focal white matter infarcts more likely represent proper arterial infarction. Given the absence of association between leukomalacia and sonographic striatal vasculopathy, the contribution of striatal arteries to these focal periventricular infarcts must be questioned, or at least be considered unproven.

226

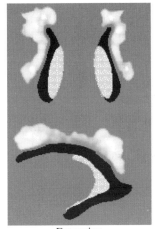

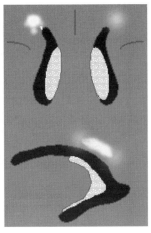

Extensive

Border zone infarct? Genuine arterial infarct?

Limited

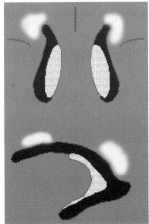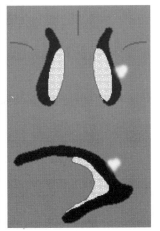

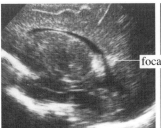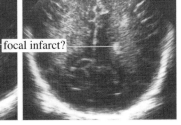

focal infarct?

227

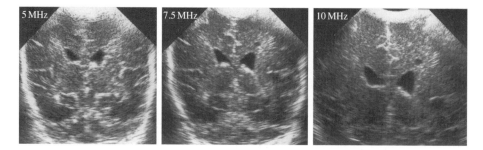

Fig. V.2.c. Coronal images of the same patient taken at the same moment with different sound wave frequencies. To interpret subtle changes in white matter one needs higher frequency 7.5 or 10 MHz scan-heads; literature based on 5 MHz imaging may have missed subtle cystic leukomalacia or overestimated hyperechogenicities. [Reproduced by permission from de Vries, L.S. (1996) 'Neurological assessment of the preterm infant.' *Acta Paediatrica*, **85**, 765–771.]

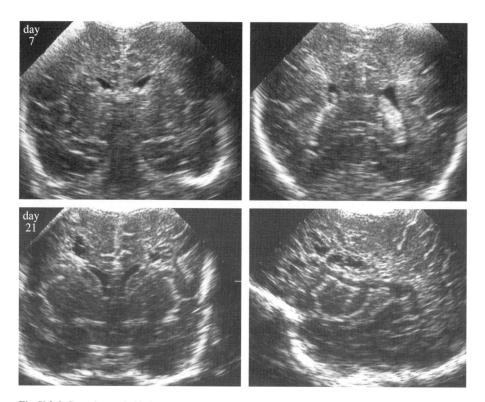

Fig. V.2.d. Growth retarded infant, one of twins born at 35 weeks gestation, with birth asphyxia, referred on day 7: 7.5 MHz sonograms, taken on admission *(top)* and two weeks later *(bottom)* *(lower right, parasagittal; others coronal)*. As no early hyperechogenic stage was recorded, initial interpretation of white matter echogenicity in this infant underestimated the severity of necrosis, later shown by extensive cyst formation. This is an exception to the rule that cystic periventricular leukomalacia of postnatal onset is (almost?) always preceded by a hyperechogenic phase.

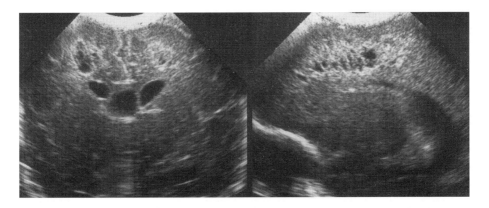

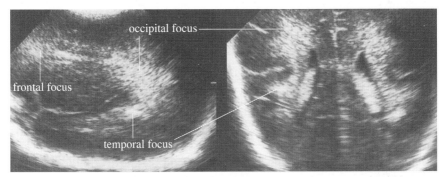

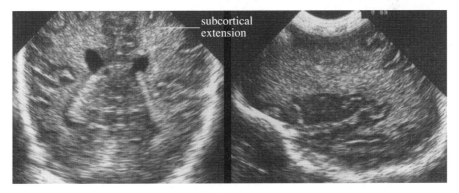

Fig. V.2.e. 7.5 MHz sections of three different infants with the extensive type of cystic leukomalacia. There is maximal involvement of frontal and occipital necrotic areas, and in severe cases subcortical extension. These lesions predict spastic quadriplegia and mental retardation.

(Top) 25 weeks gestation, postnatal shock.

(Middle) 29 weeks gestation, unexplained early neonatal flares and subsequent cyst formation in an infant without postnatal problems.

(Bottom) 34 weeks gestation, growth retarded baby with cardiac failure and pulmonary haemorrhage on the second day.

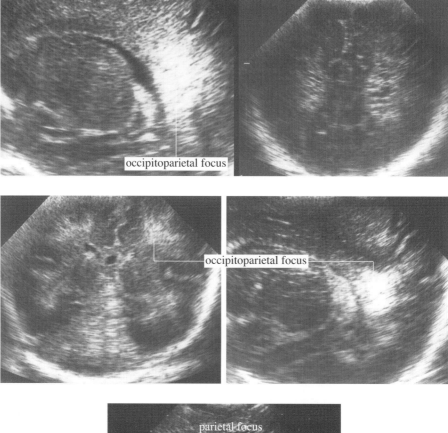

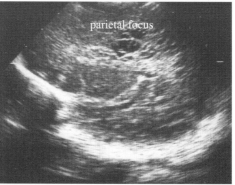

Fig. V.2.f. Focal severe cystic leukomalacia is seen in two preferential areas: in the occipitoparietal border zone and in the parietal area itself. Isolated cystic frontal leukomalacia is exceptional. The 7.5 MHz images shown here are from three different infants.

(Top) 33 weeks gestation; donor twin in chronic fetofetal transfusion (*left*, parasagittal scan, day 1; *right*, coronal scan four weeks later). Spastic diplegia was evident at later follow-up.

(Middle) 35 weeks gestation; meconium peritonitis (day 1 scans: *left*, coronal; *right*, parasagittal).

(Bottom) Term infant who had intrauterine growth retardation: day 20 parasagittal scan.

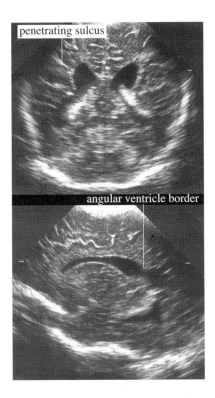

Fig. V.2.g. 7.5 MHz sonograms (*top*, coronal; *bottom*, parasagittal) of a preterm infant with respiratory distress syndrome. The end stage of focal parieto-occipital cystic leukomalacia is marked by two sonographic criteria, recognizable even months later: ventricular dilatation with irregular, angular borders; and deep sulcal penetration (sulci reaching the ventricle wall). MRI may demonstrate impaired myelination and gliosis for years.

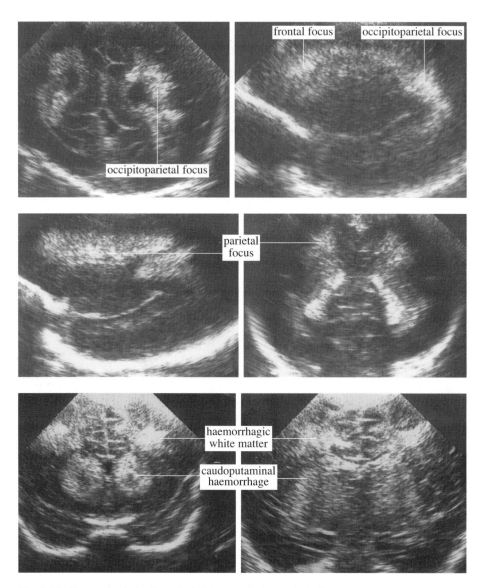

Fig. V.2.h. Haemorrhagic (periventricular) leukomalacia may look like pure white matter necrosis in the early stage. On the other hand haemorrhage can often be suspected due to disseminated nodular foci of even greater hyperechogenicity within pathological flares. In the three infants shown here haemorrhagic leukomalacia was confirmed at postmortem examination.

(Top) Girl stillborn at 28 weeks gestation: 7.5 MHz sonograms taken within an hour of birth. All organs were pale, except for haemorrhagic white matter.

(Centre) Recipient twin in fetofetal transfusion syndrome, born at 28 weeks with non-immune hydrops.

(Bottom) Preterm infant born following maternal eclampsia and fetal asphyxia, succumbing shortly after birth. Ischaemic haemorrhages were identified in the striatum and in white matter at postmortem examination. (Reproduced by permission from Eken *et al.* 1994.)

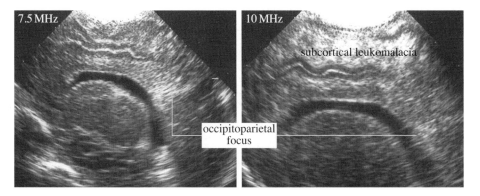

Fig. V.2.i. Subcortical white matter damage can be missed with routine 5 and even 7.5 MHz scanning. One needs 10 MHz sections to estimate subcortical injury under the anterior fontanelle. These two parasagittal sonograms of the same area illustrate further the optimal visualization of periventricular foci with 7.5 MHz imaging: they are day 1 scans from a 37 weeks gestation infant, with fetal hydrops due to atrial flutter *in utero*. Postmortem findings included extensive white matter necrosis. The accentuation of subcortical versus periventricular injury is typical of at or near term babies. One can observe sharp contrast between very bright white matter and hypoechogenic cortex near the cingulate sulcus, probably due to a striking difference in (circulating) blood content.

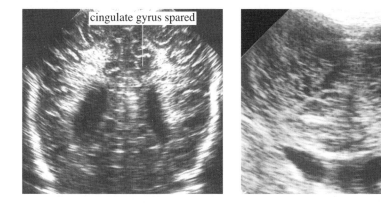

Fig. V.2.j. Examples of different types of subcortical leukomalacia.

(Left) The hyperechogenic stage (day 10) of generalized white matter injury observed in 7.5 MHz coronal sonogram of a growth retarded near-term infant with postnatal cardiac failure. Although fingers of echogenic white matter point from the centrum semi-ovale towards intersulcal white matter, there is no hyperechogenicity of the cingulate gyrus.

(Right) The multicystic stage of subcortical leukomalacia observed in 7.5 MHz coronal sonogram of a 4-week-old term infant who had birth asphyxia. The process of cystic necrosis is not sparing the cingulate gyrus.

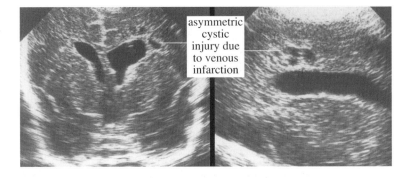

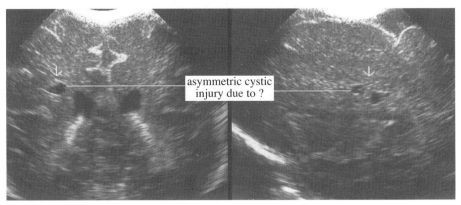

Fig. V.2.k. Leukomalacia, like most ischaemic injury in the perinatal period, is not an isolated finding: it may be associated with neuronal necrosis in cortex or deep grey matter, leukomalacia, cerebellar injury, haemorrhage, matrix infarction or pontosubicular necrosis. The concurrence of such patterns has been referred to as the periventricular leukomalacia complex (Grunnet 1982). The four examples given here show the interplay between matrix lesions and white matter damage. Genuine leukomalacia is almost always bilateral and nearly symmetric.

(Top) 7.5 MHz sections of a left grade II intraventricular with subependymal haemorrhage and parenchymal venous infarct in its cystic stage in an infant born at 30 weeks gestation after partial separation of the placenta.

(Above) 7.5 MHz sonograms of a preterm infant (29 weeks gestation) on day 21, showing cystic white matter changes in the absence of visible matrix injury.

(Opposite) 7.5 MHz sonograms (*top*, coronal; *bottom*, parasagittal) of two different infants in whom cystic germinolysis of antenatal origin went hand in hand with parietal cystic white matter injury. A similar insult caused both, either through genuine arterial infarction and/or via border-zone necrosis.

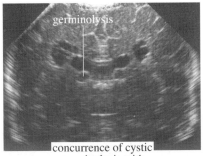

germinolysis

concurrence of cystic
germinolysis with
cystic leukomalacia

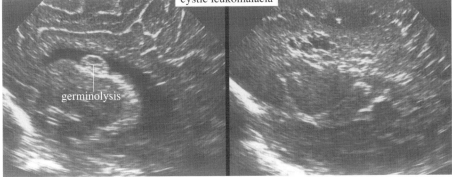

germinolysis

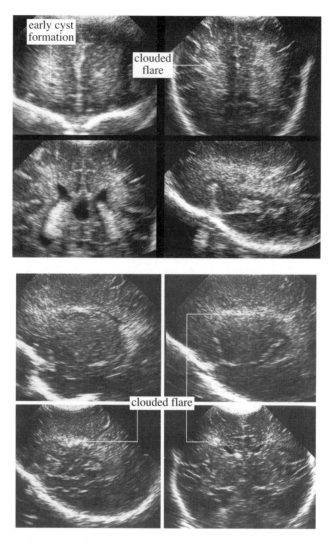

Fig. V.2.l. Grading the severity of hyperechogenic white matter change is usually not done in the initial stage. Only when cysts are appearing or the underlying lateral ventricles dilate can one safely predict neuromotor disability. In combination with IVH, ventriculomegaly may even be misleading, if caused not by tissue loss but by obstructed CSF circulation. If hyperechogenic periventricular areas remain too echodense for too long a period (more than 14 days) one speaks of grade I leukomalacia, in itself increasing the risk of later sequelae.

Subtle leukomalacia may not lead to cyst formation and may only cause very discrete (within normal range) ventriculomegaly. Prediction of a mild form of cerebral palsy—usually mild spastic diplegia—is possible upon recognition of clouded flares, *i.e.* hyperechogenic areas carrying even brighter forms of genuine necrosis within. These accentuated flares involve several predilection areas: usually they are found within the parietal lobe or at the parieto-occipital transition zone. Initially the area is just hyperechogenic, then it becomes clouded, and finally most hyperechogenicity subsides and a small gliotic scar remains for several weeks as a limited very bright focus.

The sonograms (all 7.5 MHz) show prolonged, clouded flares in five different preterm infants.

236

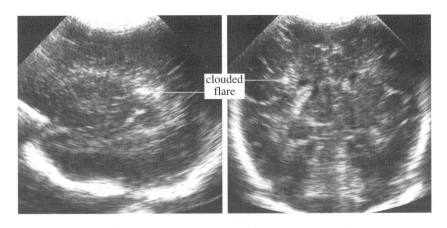

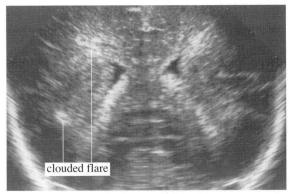

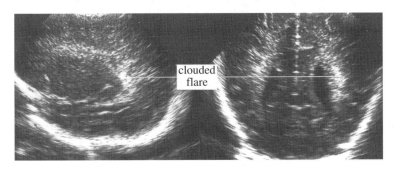

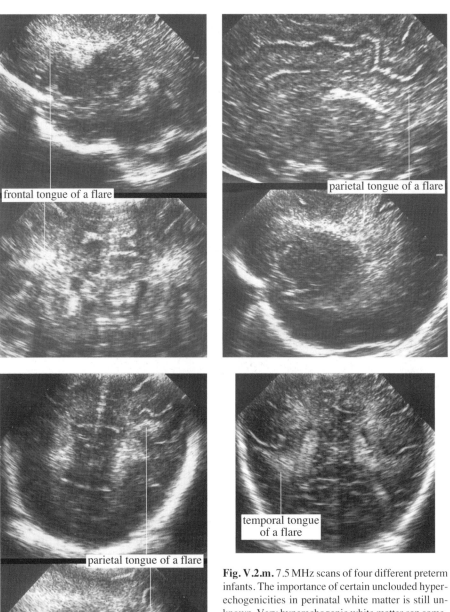

frontal tongue of a flare

parietal tongue of a flare

parietal tongue of a flare

temporal tongue
of a flare

Fig. V.2.m. 7.5 MHz scans of four different preterm infants. The importance of certain unclouded hyperechogenicities in perinatal white matter is still unknown. Very hyperechogenic white matter can sometimes be seen along the frontal horn above the anterior limb of the internal capsule (*top left*). Fairly common are hyperechogenic areas extending from the parietooccipital transition zone or from the temporal horn outer wall into the subcortex. These tongues from periventricular flares do not become very bright like clouded flares and do not leave cysts or ventricular dilatation.

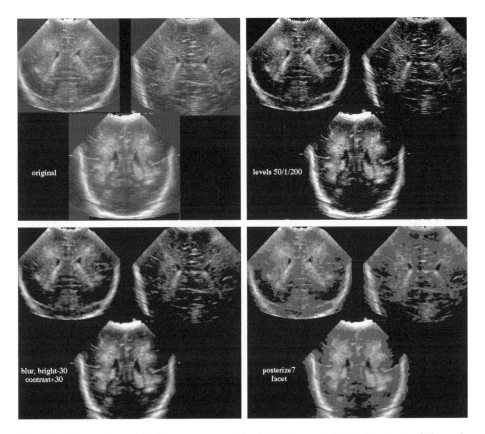

Fig. V.2.n. Even without objective measurement of echodensity, we feel that attempts should be made to present periventricular flares in such a form that comparison with normal structures, such as plexus, bone or CSF-containing cavities, should become easier. Above are shown a few variations of the top left triad of clouded flares obtainable with commercially available photo-editing software. Analysing the analogue signal in the same way might increase the predictive value of ultrasound in case of white matter change.

SECTION VI
PATHOLOGY: INTRAPARTUM ASPHYXIA

Hypoxia and cerebral hypoperfusion, if occurring in isolation, must be marked to provoke neurological damage. In combination they induce anaerobic metabolism in the brain with local acidosis (especially lactic acidosis). An asphyxial insult with acidosis is often accompanied by a period of systemic and cerebral hypotension. Neurons are more susceptible to asphyxia than glia. Selective neuronal necrosis will occur. When followed by endothelial necrosis and disruption of the blood–brain barrier, the whole tissue may necrose and become infarcted. The clinical neurological picture following birth asphyxia is termed hypoxic–ischaemic encephalopathy.

The cerebral and cerebellar neuropathological changes in the term newborn infant may be divided into two groups. *Biochemical* changes present morphologically as immediate cytotoxic oedema, while triggering a chain of reactions provoking in select areas microvascular lesions and delayed neuronal necrosis with ferrugination, the latter spread out over hours to a few days. *Vascular* events, on the other hand, alter cerebral perfusion in four stages: (1) initial hyperaemia (minutes); (2) lack of reflow (lasting hours), with lowered brain activity and low voltage EEG; (3) luxury perfusion (for a few days); and (4) late hypoperfusion.

Loss of cerebrovascular autoregulation and simultaneous hypotension are the probable causes of genuine arterial infarcts and border zone infarction as in parasagittal cerebral injury and leukomalacia. Episodic hyperperfusion transforms certain ischaemic areas in haemorrhagic infarcts. In spite of abundant data in the literature on asphyxia in all its aspects, it is as yet unclear how the two components of hypoperfusion and excitotoxicity relate to each other in each region (Fig. VI.a). This double lesion pattern creates a number of neuropathological entities, not necessarily limited to the neonatal setting (Fig. VI.k).

The extent of damage may depend on the following factors: (1) cause, extent and duration of the insult; (2) gestational age (the intensity of ongoing metabolic activities codetermines which zones are sensitive and this sensitivity varies with maturation of the nervous system); (3) the preexistence of growth retardation; (4) the repetitive character of an insult (often the lesions become worse when a hypoxic–ischaemic episode is repeated); (5) the nature and rapidity of postnatal treatment.

With the exception of selective neuronal necrosis, most entities may be recognized with ultrasound especially in the late neonatal period. Focal arterial and venous infarcts are discussed elsewhere. The prevalence of echographic changes appears to be somewhat higher in deep grey matter than in white matter. In general we are confronted with mixed injury (white as well as grey matter) because asphyxia of the newborn infant often starts as prolonged hypoxia, superimposed in the end by total asphyxia due to cardiovascular collapse, extreme bradycardia or asystole. We believe sonography is superior to CT for description of late neonatal changes in the asphyxiated term infant; its strength in the first days of life is less clear and still a matter of debate. Probably diffusion-weighted MRI will become the

240

most accurate early descriptive tool, if it reaches the bedside. CT may still help for location and timing of haemorrhagic lesions.

Brain swelling starts within minutes of the insult due to cytotoxic oedema. It then subsides, returning after 6–48 hours because of delayed excitotoxic injury with both cytotoxic and vasogenic oedema. Sulci may be compressed by swollen parenchyma and become less visible with ultrasound. The ventricular cavities become slits. White matter may have diffusely increased echogenicity, and in combination with a loss of sulcal landmarks one ends up with a 'fuzzy brain' (Fig. VI.b). In the worst cases one even has problems identifying the interhemispheric and insular fissures. This stage is also characterized by relative hypoechogenicity of the caudate heads, a phenomenon which may show up as early as two hours after birth. The latter aspect is set aside for moderate or severe asphyxia with grade 2 or 3 encephalopathy in the Sarnat classification. Brain swelling must be present if one wants to use the term acute intrapartum asphyxia in a term infant. In the second half of the first week the cavities reopen. When necrosis occurs around the ventricles and/or in the basal ganglia, early ventriculomegaly *ex vacuo* may be found, sometimes with discrepant dilatation of the third ventricle when the brunt of the damage is found in deep grey matter.

In the healthy term infant the ventricular cavities may also be reduced to slits in the first hours of life; as a rule the phenomenon persists for no longer than 36 hours, whereas in the asphyxiated brain swelling may last for 3–17 days. Primary brain oedema is discussed below.

Asphyxia may generate early IVH (within hours of birth). In the term neonate this mostly starts in the choroid plexus. A special variant is due to thrombosis and venous infarction in the irrigation area of the great vein of Galen or the basal vein. The latter is typically accompanied by thalamic or striatal haemorrhage. In the first moments following ischaemia, reactive hyperaemia may give rise to primary haemorrhage in deep grey matter or internal capsule (Fig. VI.b). On the other hand tissue reaction with invasion by newly formed microvessels may occur after some days. This may in turn be accompanied by petechial haemorrhage. It is called secondary haemorrhagic conversion (Figs. VI.l–n). It may be difficult to differentiate between *haemorrhage* and infarct by ultrasound: CT or MR imaging will be necessary.

Leukomalacia has been described in section V.2. Following asphyxia, subcortical, periventricular and mixed forms of leukomalacia may be registered. Exceptionally we may observe densities in white matter that will not lead to permanent damage, probably zones where ischaemia has not caused necrosis and partial or even total recovery remains possible.

Hyperechogenicity of white matter may contrast with hypodensity of the cortex: the echogram will characteristically show a kind of 'railroad track' phenomenon (Fig. VI.c). This may be clearly seen in parasagittal sections around the cingulate sulcus. Although leukomalacia is one of the mechanisms that can explain an increase in gyral core echogenicity, we may also be confronted with venous and/or capillary congestion, and so this observation demands anatomopathological clarification. Abnormal hyperechogenicity of white matter may precede cyst formation (leukomalacia *stricto sensu*) (Fig. VI.d) or lead to ventriculomegaly without cystic intermediary (leukoencephalopathy). Severe leukomalacia is difficult to differentiate sonographically with any degree of certainty from necrosis in white matter on the one hand and brain oedema and congestion on the other in the first 48 hours following an insult.

Parasagittal cerebral (sub)cortical brain necrosis may be diagnosed given focal cystic lesions or atrophic scars at the junction between major cerebral arteries, preceded by (sub)cortical densities in the parietal lobes at a distance from the falx. Those densities are triangular, with their base towards the surface. Often the areas are only identifiable with 10 MHz scanning, under both the anterior and posterior fontanelles (Fig. VI.f). Other very focal kinds of necrosis may also be found in gyri around the upper hemispheric border, not necessarily in a border zone. Experimental analogy suggests that the lesion is perhaps sited within the area perfused by the middle cerebral artery (not in a border zone of this vessel), and that it is most prominent in perirolandic areas. We feel the entity becomes indistinguishable when associated with more extensive injury. In the literature there is no clear distinction from postasphyxial subcortical leukomalacia. We recently observed a single instance where symmetric necrosis developed in the posterior temporal lobe, showing as echogenic elliptical areas in the second part of the first week following delivery with cord prolapse. We hypothesize these infarcts may represent genuine border zone necrosis.

This 'parasagittal cerebral injury', mainly identified by technetium and PET scan, may lead to ulegyria—a band of atrophic gyri, often bilateral and along the border zones between major arteries. Any such damage will culminate in the posterior parietal areas, apparently because there is a border zone there between three major cerebral arteries. It is well known that cortex and white matter are most affected in the base of the gyrus, whereas the crown is said to be left unaffected: this results in a mushroom gyrus, due to maintenance of the gyral crown and atrophy of its stem. After disappearance of brain swelling, conventional MRI is superior to ultrasound for description of these subcortical lesions.

Ischaemia and necrosis in the diencephalon and basal ganglia have always been identified by their final anatomopathological presentation: status marmoratus. As of the second or third day of life this pattern of damage, the consequence of excitotoxicity, results in hyperechogenicity of thalamus and striatum. The lesion is by definition bilateral and symmetric. The thalamus is hyperdense (>90% of cases), with or without hyperechogenicity of the globus pallidus and putamen (about 60% of cases) (Fig. VI.g). A 'bright' thalamus may persist for months and is indicative of acute total intrapartum asphyxia. Chemical neuronal necrosis characteristically spares the internal capsule, which clearly stands out against the echodense basal ganglia as a black linear structure. On the other hand, congestion or arterial infarction may induce echogenicity in it. The posterior thalamic part, the pulvinar, is not affected and neither is the medial nucleus of the thalamus. Reservation has to be made regarding interpretation of thalamic hyperechogenicity. In children having survived undamaged, mild thalamic hyperechogenicity may temporarily show in the first two weeks after the insult. Persistence and increase of density suggest genuine necrosis.

In combination with striatal hyperechogenicity a dense thalamus acquires more prognostic potential (Fig. VI.h). It may be possible to detect hyperdensity of the dorsal part of the mesencephalon in axial sections (Fig. VI.i).

Sonographic appearances of ischaemia and haemorrhage in the basal ganglia are contrasted in Table VI.k.

TABLE VI.1
Echographic appearance of basal ganglia ischaemia *vs.* haemorrhage

Ischaemia in basal ganglia	Haemorrhage in basal ganglia
Visible from day 2–3	Visible on day 1 or after day 3–4
Soft echogenicities at first	Hard echogenicities from the start
Regular contours	Irregular contours
Symmetric	Asymmetric, often bilateral
Spared internal capsule	Internal capsule possibly affected
Without ventricular bleeding	Often with ventricular bleeding

One may suspect cortical ischaemia when finding echogenic zones around parietal or frontal sulci without the 'railroad tracks' that are so characteristic of changes in white matter. An echogenic band of variable width stretches out starting from sulcus or fissure and can be easily distinguished from less echogenic white matter (Fig. VI.e). Sulcus and cortex, with a variable border of subcortical white matter, tend to merge into one echogenic zone, consisting of minute bright dots. A similar pattern has been observed both in neonates and in older infants following apparently life-threatening events. It probably represents an extremely grave form of selective neuronal necrosis, later evolving towards (sub)cortical cystic parenchymal necrosis. This pattern of laminar echodensity is not common. The neat separation between this 'cortical' picture and gyral core hyperechogenicity deserves explanation especially in view of the similar end result: cystic necrosis under the anterior fontanelle. In a term infant with birth asphyxia following abruptio placentae we observed on day 2 a pattern of hyperechogenic white matter especially marked in the posterior parietal regions, whereas on day 10 a laminar cortical type of hyperechogenicity emerged; the brain collapsed in the late neonatal period after a transitional stage of fine cystic necrosis. Such findings emphasize the importance—if death occurs—of making every effort to correlate sequential ultrasound appearances with postmortem analysis (see Eken *et al.* 1994).

Echographic changes other than brain swelling will, as a rule, not be found after asphyxia with mild encephalopathy (Sarnat grade 1). The group for whom a diagnosis is most relevant consists of babies with moderate encephalopathy, usually hypotonic infants with clinical seizures. Typical changes in arterial flow velocity can be measured with Doppler analysis and are particularly important as far as the differentiation within this group is concerned within the first 48 hours. They are helpful in those cases where during the first days the whole picture may be falsely reassuring or hard to interpret.

Occasionally one comes across very echogenic 'fuzzy' brains, where Doppler findings are normal and where no focal change in density or ventricular dilatation occurs in the course of the second week. In such situations one may expect to have seen congestion and/or oedema without necrosis.

Detailed discussion of histopathology in the perinatal brain is beyond the scope of this book. Based on the work of Banker and Larroche (1962), Ellis *et al.* (1988) and Graham (1992), a grid of data is provided (Table VI.2) to assist in the recognition and timing of ischaemic injury. An example of its usefulness is given in Figure VI.j.

TABLE VI.2
Histopathological dating of ischaemic brain damage*

Lesion	Onset†	Duration
Astroglial swelling	30 min	
Mitochondrial swelling in neurons	2 h	
Oedema/sponginess	6–12 h	3–4 d
Axonal swelling	5–12 h	
Red cell changes	8–24 h	5–10 d
Neuronal karyorrhexis	24–36 h	± 10 d
Astroglia		
—astroglial reaction	12–24 h	Years
—gemistocytic reaction	6 d	Weeks
Microglial reaction	< 1 d	Months
Endothelial proliferation	< 1 d	Weeks
New capillaries	7 d	
Neuronal ferrugination	8–10 d	Years
Encrusted axons–capillaries	8 d	
Cavitation		
—microcavitation, liquefaction	8 d	
—macrocavitation	10–14 d	Permanent
—cystic germinolysis	7 d	Months

*The data sources (see text) do not specify fetal or postnatal ages.
†Time post-insult.

REFERENCES

Babcock, D.S., Ball, W. (1983) 'Postasphyxial encephalopathy in full-term infants: ultrasound diagnosis.' *Radiology*, **148**, 417–423.

Banker, B.Q., Larroche, J-C. (1962) 'Periventricular leukomalacia of infancy. A form of neonatal anoxic encephalopathy.' *Archives of Neurology*, **7**, 386–410.

Connolly, B., Kelehan, P., O'Brien, N., Gorman, W., Murphy, J.F., King, M., Donoghue, V. (1994) 'The echogenic thalamus in hypoxic ischaemic encephalopathy.' *Pediatric Radiology*, **24**, 268–271.

Couture, A. (1994) 'Les lésions cérébrales anoxo-ischémiques.' *In:* Couture, A., Veyrac, C., Baud, C. (Eds.) *Echographie Cérébrale du Foetus au Nouveau-né*. Montpellier: Sauramps Médical, pp. 183–248.

Cowan, F.M., Pennock, J.M., Hanrahan, J.D., Manji, K.P., Edwards, A.D. (1994) 'Early detection of cerebral infarction and hypoxic–ischemic encephalopathy in neonates using diffusion-weighted magnetic resonance imaging.' *Neuropediatrics*, **25**, 172–175.

de Vries, L.S., Eken, P., Beek, E., Groenendaal, F., Meiners, L.C. (1996) 'The posterior fontanelle: a neglected acoustic window.' *Neuropediatrics*, **27**, 101–104.

Ellis, W.G., Goetzman, B.W., Lindenberg, J.A. (1988) 'Neuropathologic documentation of prenatal brain damage.' *American Journal of Diseases of Children*, **142**, 858–866.

Eken, P., Jansen, G.H., Groenendaal, F., Rademaker, K., de Vries, L.S. (1994) 'Intracranial lesions in the full-term infant with hypoxic ischaemic encephalopathy: ultrasound and autopsy correlation.' *Neuropediatrics*, **25**, 301–307.

Graham, D.I. (1992) 'Hypoxia and vascular disorders.' *In:* Adams, J.H., Duchen, L.W. (Eds.) *Greenfield's Neuropathology, 5th Edn*. London: Edward Arnold, pp. 153–268.

Huang, C-C., Ho, M-Y., Shen, E-Y. (1987) 'Sonographic changes in a parasagittal cerebral lesion in an asphyxiated newborn.' *Journal of Clinical Ultrasound*, **15**, 68–70.

Kreusser, K.L., Schmidt, R.E., Shackelford, G.D., Volpe, J.J. (1984) 'Value of ultrasound for identification of acute hemorrhagic necrosis of thalamus and basal ganglia in an asphyxiated term infant.' *Annals of Neurology*, **16**, 361–363.

Kuenzle, C., Baenziger, O., Martin, E., Thun-Hohenstein, L., Steinlin, M., Good, M., Fanconi, S., Boltshauser,

E., Largo, R.H. (1994) 'Prognostic value of early MR imaging in term infants with severe perinatal asphyxia.' *Neuropediatrics*, **25**, 191–200.

Leech, R.W., Alvord, E.C. (1977) 'Anoxic–ischemic encephalopathy in the human neonatal period. The significance of brain stem involvement.' *Archives of Neurology*, **34**, 109–113.

Rutherford, M.A., Pennock, J.M., Schwieso, J.E., Cowan, F.M., Dubowitz, L.M.S. (1995) 'Hypoxic ischaemic encephalopathy: early magnetic resonance imaging findings and their evolution.' *Neuropediatrics*, **26**, 183–191.

Sarnat, H.B., Sarnat, M.S. (1976) 'Neonatal encephalopathy following fetal distress. A clinical and electro-encephalographic study.' *Archives of Neurology*, **33**, 696–705.

Skeffington, F.S., Pearse, R.G. (1983) 'The 'bright brain'.' *Archives of Disease in Childhood*, **58**, 509–511.

Slovis, T.L., Shankaran, S., Bedard, M.P., Poland, R.L. (1984) 'Intracranial hemorrhage in the hypoxic–ischemic infant: ultrasound demonstration of unusual complications.' *Radiology*, **151**, 163–169.

Steinlin, M., Dirr, R., Martin, E., Boesch, C., Largo, R.H., Fanconi, S., Boltshauser, E. (1991) 'MRI following severe perinatal asphyxia: preliminary experience.' *Pediatric Neurology*, **7**, 164–170.

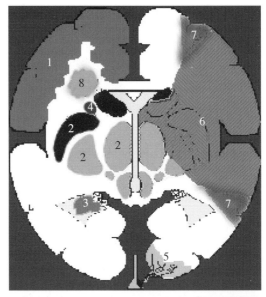

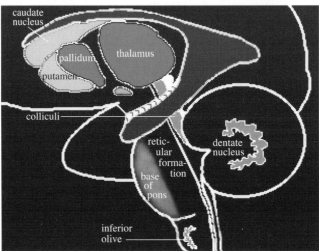

caudate nucleus

pallidum   thalamus

putamen

colliculi

retic-ular forma-tion

dentate nucleus

base of pons

inferior olive

Fig. VI.a. *(Top)* Postasphyxial perinatal brain damage is a mixture of different patterns of injury, the recognition of which is possible with careful sonography in the second part of the first week and in the second week after the insult. (Key: 1—laminar (sub)cortical necrosis; 2—deep grey matter damage; 3—congestion and plexus haemorrhage; 4—embolic infarction; 5—venous infarction and thrombosis; 6—arterial infarction; 7—interarterial infarction (border zone ischaemia); 8—subcortical and mixed leukomalacia.)

(Bottom) Vulnerable deep grey matter structures.

(Opposite) With conventional MR imaging, ischaemic change in white matter and basal ganglia is well demonstrated after disappearance of brain swelling. In particular, cortical and subcortical changes can be shown in parietal and temporal (hippocampal) areas that are hidden to the sonographer. These T_1-weighted axial images are of two different infants, both with a low Apgar score but only the *lower* one having suffered asphyxia.

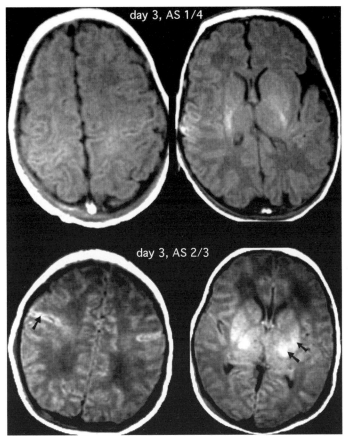

In perirolandic (sub)cortex, injury may show up due to hyperintensity in the deeper parts of the sulci and fissures *(arrow)*.

Lateral thalamus *(large arrow)* and pallidum *(small arrow)* stand out against low intensity of internal capsule.

Fig. VI.b. *Early sonographic changes following birth asphyxia (1).*

Sonographic changes in this period are quite subtle. Scans illustrating early changes and their interpretation on current knowledge are presented here (all 7.5 MHz coronal sections in four different term infants) and in Figure VI.c.

Early indicators which may be helpful in prognosis are:

1—diffuse hyperechogenicity with loss of anatomical references (sulci, fissures) and slit ventricles: the 'fuzzy brain';

2—relative hypodensity of caudate nucleus, due to increased thalamic echodensity (see section XI);

3—the appearance on day 2 of four columns in coronal section: two thalamic and two striatal ones, separated by the normally hypodense posterior limb of the internal capsule;

4—luxury perfusion: elevated diastolic flow velocity in major cerebral arteries, with lowered resistance index; or, reverse diastolic flow in major cerebral arteries (as in brain death of older children);

5—early hyperaemic haemorrhage in ischaemic areas, *e.g.* the internal capsule in the infant shown below and opposite (autopsy confirmed);

6—gyral core hyperechogenicity (Fig. VI.c).

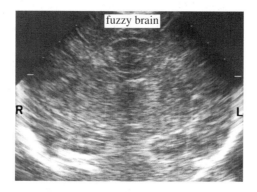

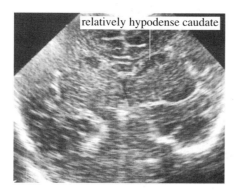

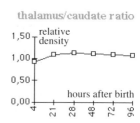

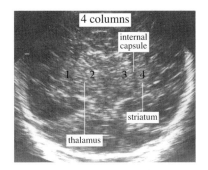

4 columns

internal capsule

1 2 3 4

striatum

thalamus

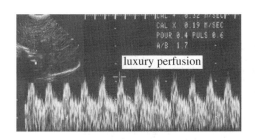

luxury perfusion

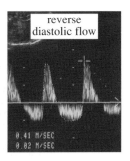

reverse diastolic flow

0.41 M/SEC
0.02 M/SEC

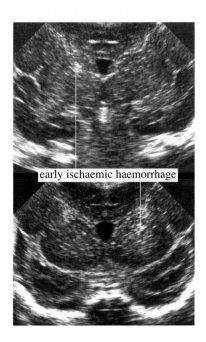

early ischaemic haemorrhage

Fig. VI.c. *Early sonographic changes following birth asphyxia (2): gyral core hyperechogenicity.*

Under normal conditions a difference in density can be observed between hypodense cortex and mildly echodense white matter. Gyral white matter core can be interpreted and compared between patients in a sagittal or coronal section through the cingulate gyrus. The best way to visualize white matter is with 7.5 MHz images (compare the three views *below left*).

It is not uncommon to observe a relative increase of echogenicity in white matter, contrasting with almost dark cortex, itself clearly separated from adjacent cortex by very bright sulcal meningovascular reflections; the triple contrast is referred to by the term 'railroad tracks'. Gyral core hyperechogenicity can be caused by venous congestion as well as white matter disease (be it an ischaemic or dystrophic process); gyral cores are not bright in periventricular leukomalacia. If in doubt, CT may help to differentiate congestion from ischaemia as the latter will show low attenuation. Serial study of gyral core echogenicity might help to differentiate ischaemia from congestion within the first post-insult days. Relative density measurements along the thick lines shown *opposite* illustrate the phenomenon.

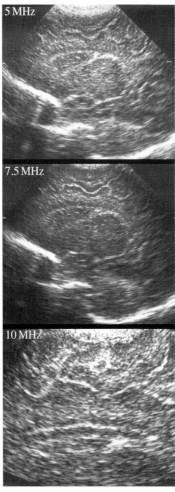

Day 1 parasagittal scans of a term infant born with difficult ventouse extraction.

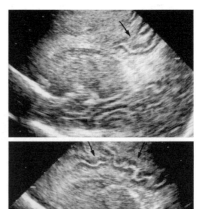

Day 2 parasagittal 7.5 MHz scans of an infant born at 39 weeks gestation following abruptio placentae: note striking gyral core to cortex contrast *(arrows)*.

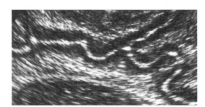

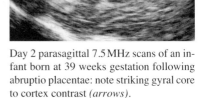

Parasagittal sonographic detail on day 2 of a term infant who had unexplained fetal distress; umbilical artery pH 6.98; meconium staining of the liquor; no neonatal seizures; and normal development at 1 year.

250

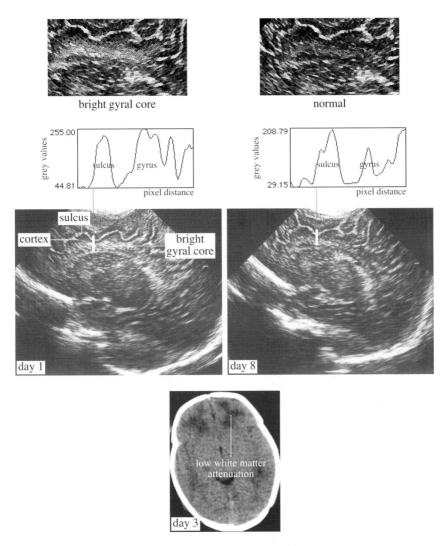

Parasagittal first day sonogram and axial third day CT scan of a term growth retarded infant who had signs of distress during labour, compared with a 'normalized' sonographic section of the same infant on day 8. No follow-up available.

Fig. VI.d. *Hyperechogenicity of white matter*, visualized with 10 MHz sonography underneath the anterior fontanelle, may precede *subcortical white matter cystic destruction*. Inevitably cortical necrosis will be also associated to a certain extent. These cysts can be seen along the mesial side of the frontal lobe, making a diagnosis of border zone infarction unlikely. The cysts are initially small but coalesce to persist for several weeks as large holes under a remnant membrane formed by the molecular layer and pial coverings. They are usually extensive and bilateral, suggesting mechanisms other than hypoperfusion. The prognosis of postasphyxial subcortical leukomalacia is gloomy, and spastic quadriplegia, severe mental retardation, microcephaly and cortical blindness may follow.

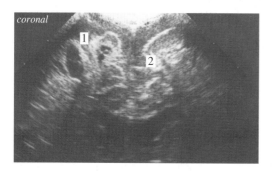

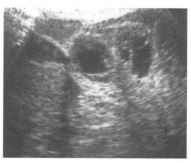

Term infant with birth asphyxia. Cystic lesions were first seen at 6 weeks of age, using a 10 MHz transducer. The child has mental retardation but did not develop cerebral palsy. Subcortical lesion spilling over from the parasagittal convexity (1) along the mesial frontal lobe cortex (2): subcortical leukomalacia or parasagittal cerebral injury?

Term infant referred for seizures on day 3: parasagittal 10 MHz section through the posterior fontanelle on day 14, showing extensive cortical and subcortical cysts. These cysts were not identified by previous sonography using the anterior fontanelle as an acoustic window. The infant developed cerebral palsy and cortical visual impairment. (Reproduced by permission from de Vries *et al.* 1996.)

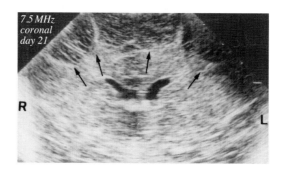

Term infant with meconium aspiration syndrome. The *arrows* point to extensive, fine cystic subcortical necrosis.

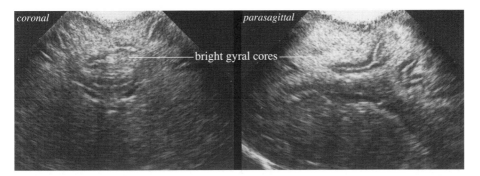

coronal   *parasagittal*

bright gyral cores

Term infant with birth asphyxia: day 5 scans. In spite of the presence of these severely echogenic areas no cysts developed over the next six weeks, and only mild ventriculomegaly was seen. The child has mental retardation but did not develop cerebral palsy.

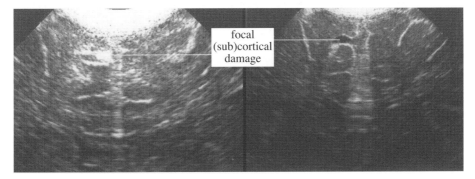

focal (sub)cortical damage

Coronal frontal 10 MHz sections on days 3 *(left)* and 22 *(right)* following birth asphyxia in a term baby. High frequency sonography may permit recognition of very subtle subcortical lesions as here in the neighbourhood of a mesial frontal sulcus to the right of the interhemispheric fissure.

Fig. VI.e. If an interest is taken in late neonatal 10 MHz sonography, a pattern other than white matter hyperechogenicity may precede (sub)cortical cyst formation in the late first and second post-insult week. *Laminar (sub)cortical hyperechogenicity* is seen as broad echodense bands that include cortex and subarcuate white matter fibres. A predilection of sulcal depths is not clearly observed. Both mesial and convexity subfontanellar cortex is affected, excluding a diagnosis of parasagittal cerebral injury. The thickness of the affected laminae may vary, thinner ones being composed of spiculae with decreasing density away from the sulcus; even thinner bands may end with extensive cystic necrosis. Ventriculomegaly is often associated even before cysts appear. This pattern may reflect extensive cortical neuronal necrosis, but not selective necrosis as glial cells also disappear in these cystic lesions. The prognosis is often as dismal as for subcortical leukomalacia (see Fig. VI.d).

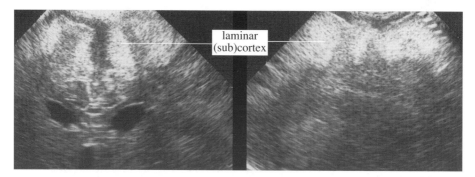

Term infant with birth asphyxia: 10 MHz scans (*left*, coronal; *right*, parasagittal).

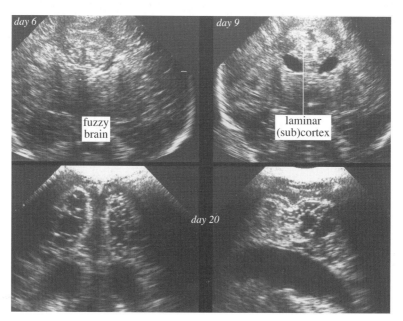

Term infant with birth asphyxia. *Top:* 7.5 MHz coronal scans. *Bottom:* 10 MHz scans (*left*, coronal; *right*, parasagittal).

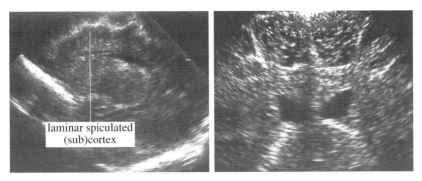

Infant born by difficult ventouse extraction following unexplained fetal distress, who subsequently had refractory seizures and subgaleal bleeding: *(left)* parasagittal scan, day 7; *(right)* coronal scan, day 21, showing extensive cysts.

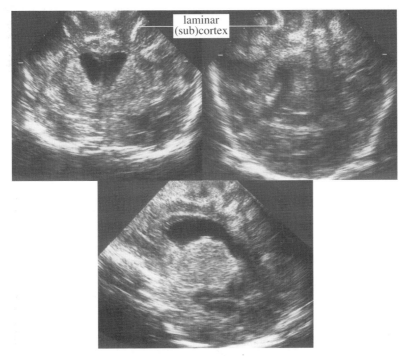

Infant with birth asphyxia (breech delivery): 7.5 MHz scans (*top*, coronal; *bottom*, parasagittal) on day 12 showing areas of increased echogenicity in cortex and subcortex.

Fig. VI.f. A common postasphyxial pattern of injury—established by postmortem reports and by technetium, PET and MR imaging, but not to our knowledge previously described sonographically—is (sub)cortical necrosis in the border zones between major cerebral arteries, especially at the parieto-occipital transition, referred to as *parasagittal cerebral injury*. In our experience one can occasionally observe a focus of hyperechogenicity at border zones, usually in between other sonographic stages between days 5 and 14. We observed bilateral, almost symmetric hyperechogenicity at the parieto-occipital transition in a few infants, and in one at the temporo-occipital transition. The foci persist for a few weeks and disappear without macroscopic cyst formation.

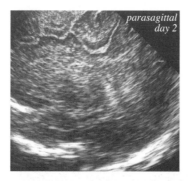

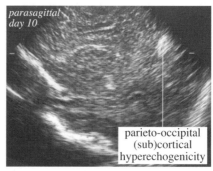

parasagittal day 2

parasagittal day 10

parieto-occipital (sub)cortical hyperechogenicity

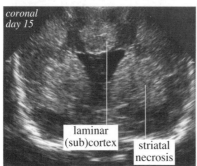

coronal day 15

Dynamic change of the ultrasound picture (all 7.5 MHz scans) in a term infant with abruptio placentae and Sarnat stage 3 encephalopathy, who survived extubation on day 3.

laminar (sub)cortex

striatal necrosis

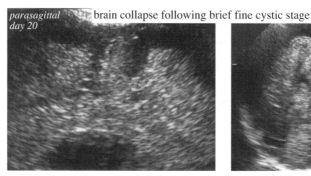

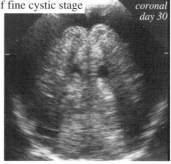

parasagittal day 20

brain collapse following brief fine cystic stage

coronal day 30

256

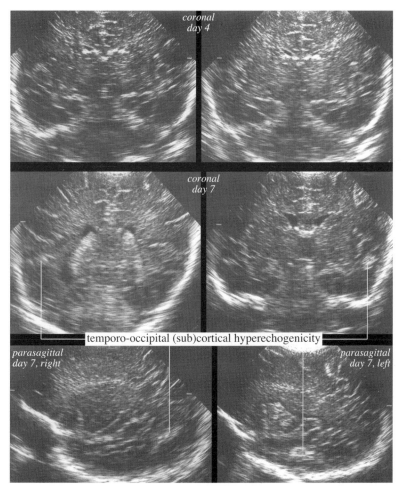

coronal
day 4

coronal
day 7

temporo-occipital (sub)cortical hyperechogenicity

parasagittal
day 7, right

parasagittal
day 7, left

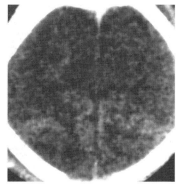

(*Above*) Term infant, second of twins, born by emergency caesarean section after cord prolapse; Sarnat stage 2 encephalopathy, seizures for 24 hours. Bilateral posterior temporal echogenic foci appeared on day 5. The outcome in this child is still unknown.

The differential density seen in some infants on uncontrasted CT at the frontoparietal transition, as shown *left* (day 2, term baby with birth asphyxia), may indicate an explanation.

257

Fig. VI.g. Thalamic ischaemia is an easily accessible sonographic marker of postasphyxial deep grey matter damage. From the second post-insult day onwards, paramedian columns of soft hyperechogenicity appear on coronal sections, with or without columns of striatal injury. If genuinely necrotic the area will remain echodense for months, its brightness increasing due to atrophic shrinkage, gliosis and neuronal ferrugination. Cysts are never seen. On parasagittal images the ventrolateral nuclei, usually most severely affected, stand out as bright areas between normally echogenic, darker internal capsule and pulvinar. If thalamic echogenicities are transient within the neonatal period, they may not carry a bad prognosis, whereas persistent densities of increasing brightness predict spastic cerebral palsy.

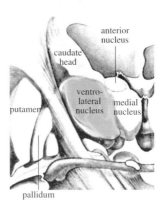

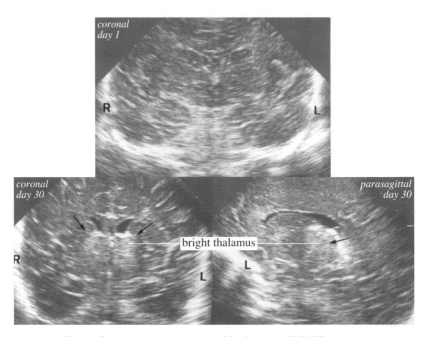

Term infant who had shown signs of fetal distress (7.5 MHz scans).

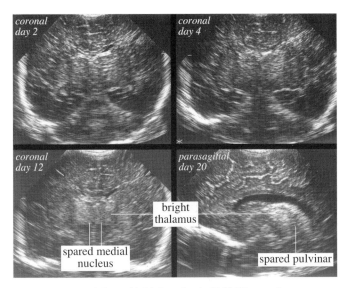

Term infant with birth asphyxia (7.5 MHz scans).

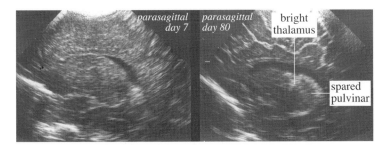

Term infant with birth asphyxia (7.5 MHz scans).

Fig. VI.h. Another way of establishing the relevance of thalamic postasphyxial brightness is by document-ing its association with *striatal injury*, whether in the putamen or pallidum. An elliptical hyperdensity, immediately in front of the posterior limb of the internal capsule on parasagittal sections, represents pallidal necrosis. If a section through the far anterior tip of the frontal horn is showing subventricular echogenicity, this will represent putaminal necrosis as well. Even without subcortical injury, the combina-tion of thalamic and striatal injury following asphyxia is never seen in normally developing infants, though it may take two years for unequivocal extrapyramidal symptoms to develop.

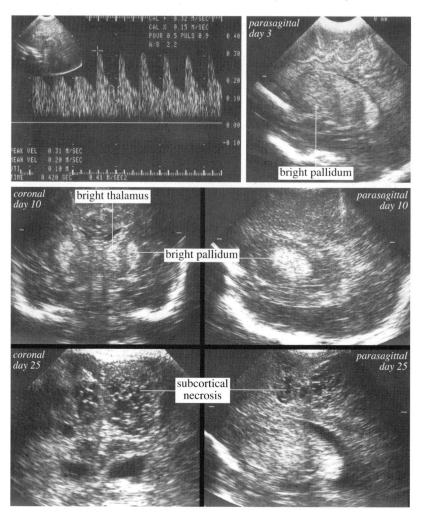

Unexplained fetal distress with later subcortical and deep grey matter necrosis. This combina-tion is not exceptional in the human infant. Striatal injury (in this case mainly pallidal) is marked. Luxury perfusion on day 4 is shown by a decrease of the resistance index below 0.55.

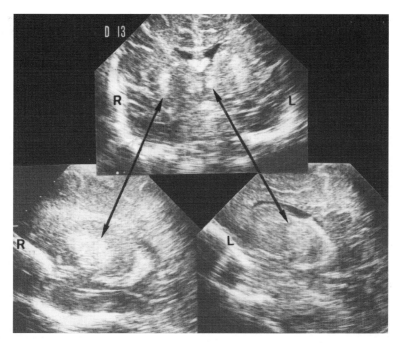

Coronal *(top)* and parasagittal *(bottom)* 7.5 MHz sections in a term infant on day 13 following birth asphyxia due to uterine rupture. The medial parasagittal section (left side) indicates thalamic injury, while the more lateral section (right side) shows striatal injury. This child developed spastic quadriplegia, microcephaly and severe mental retardation.

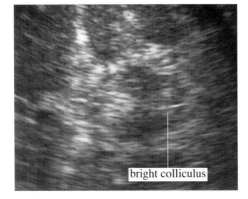

bright colliculus

Fig. VI.i. Brainstem necrosis is a common histopathological finding following severe birth asphyxia. Sometimes this is suggested on axial sonograms by hyperechogenicity of the colliculi.

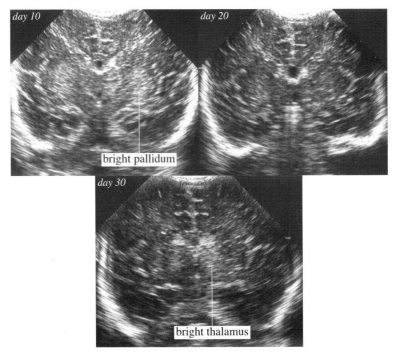

day 10

day 20

bright pallidum

day 30

bright thalamus

Fig. VI.j. Term infant with asphyxia due to abruptio placentae: coronal 7.5 MHz sections. Knowledge of the histopathological sequence of events is imperative to understand the sonographic changes observed within the neonatal period (Table VI.2):
• on day 10—the thalamus and more especially the striatum are hyperechogenic due to active neuronal and astroglial change;
• on day 20—tissue reaction has subsided to a certain extent, creating a falsely reassuring picture with no abnormal echoreflections;
• on day 30—thalamic neurons have undergone ferrugination and therefore make the area hyperechogenic again.

To make a sonographically accurate prognosis one should examine serially up to the fourth week after the insult.

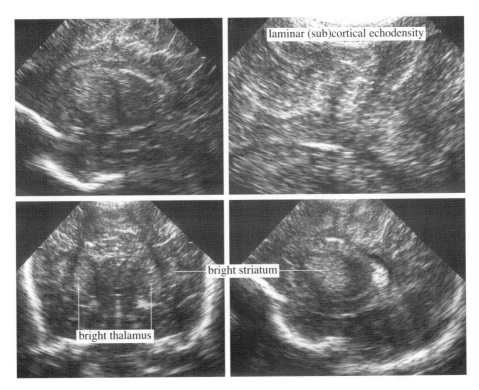

Fig. VI.k. 7.5 MHz sonograms (all parasagittal except *bottom left*, coronal) of a 2-month-old infant, 24 hours after an apparently life-threatening event, demonstrating post-asphyxial encephalopathy (Sarnat stage 3). Even at this early stage neuronal necrosis in all its severity is clearly seen: its hallmarks are thalamic and striatal hyperechogenicity, with the hypodense internal capsule in between, and laminar cortical highlighting.

Figs. VI.l–n. Three variants of *haemorrhage* exist *in association with brain necrosis*. Although bleeding will make the infarcted area even more hyperechogenic and induce irregularity into the otherwise softly echogenic zone, differentiation with certainty may still require CT scanning.

- Primary haemorrhage is confirmed by CT within 24 hours after the insult; it is probably due to early reactive hyperaemia; haemorrhage may be gross. This is a rare phenomenon.
- Secondary haemorrhagic conversion is associated with luxury perfusion and microvascular damage from the second day to the end of the first week; haemorrhage is petechial. This is the most common variant. Examples are shown in Fig. VI.l (irregular basal ganglia haemorrhage due to haemostatic defect secondary to subgaleal bleeding caused by ventouse traction) and Fig. VI.m (putaminal haemorrhagic conversion, best observed in a far anterior coronal section in front of the foramen of Monro).
- Neovascularization, peaking in the second and third week, may — if associated with enhancing circumstances like seizures or haemostatic defect — cause late haemorrhagic conversion of an infarct. An example is given in Fig. VI.n.

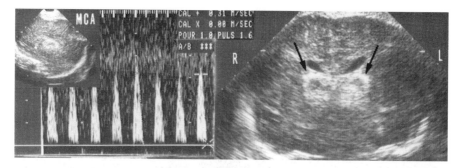

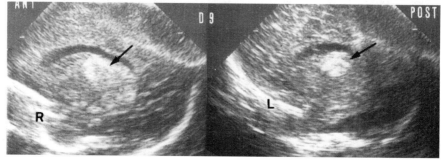

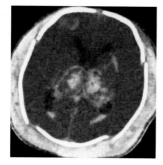

Fig. VI.l. Irregular basal ganglia haemorrhage.

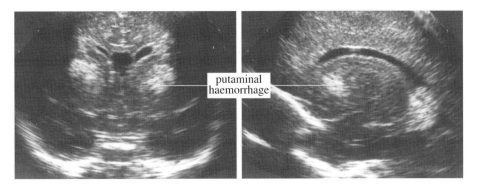

Fig. VI.m. Putaminal haemorrhagic conversion.

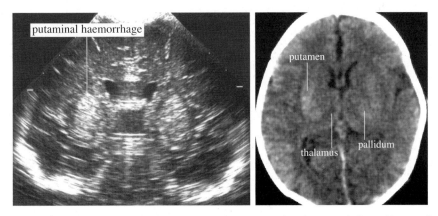

Fig. VI.n. Late haemorrhagic conversion of an infarct (asphyxiated preterm infant with putaminal necrosis that became haemorrhagic after urokinase treatment for thrombosis of the superior vena cava).

SECTION VII
PATHOLOGY: FOCAL INFARCTION

VII.1 INTRODUCTION

Classically recognized entities of focal infarction, such as complete infarction within the middle cerebral artery, may be rare, but limited foci of hyperechogenicity are more prevalent and yet scarcely studied. Entities causing bright foci in the perinatal brain include:

- middle cerebral artery infarction
- anterior cerebral artery infarction
- posterior cerebral artery infarction
- bright anterior limb of the internal capsule
- focal hyperechogenicity in the posterior limb of the internal capsule
- focal caudate hyperechogenicity
- focal pallidal echogenicity
- focal thalamic hyperechogenicity
- focal periventricular nodular hyperechogenicity
- laminar hyperechogenicity
- air embolism
- superficial venous infarction—sinus thrombosis.

Although it is difficult to define with absolute certainty every nosological entity displayed here, the attempt is based on neuropathological insight and careful sonographic and often clinical follow-up. Clearly this is an area where future study is needed.

Criteria for inclusion as an entity in this section are that the bright focus must (i) be sharply delineated, often with a linear margin, and (ii) persist as a hyperechogenic focus for at least 14 days, without cystic change in that period. The shape and evolution had to exclude abscess formation, tumour, vascular anomaly and haemorrhage. It is not always possible, however, to differentiate between arterial infarction proper and interarterial border zone ischaemia.

When a focal arterial brain infarct occurs in fetal life, the infant may ultimately be diagnosed as having Moebius syndrome, schizencephaly, focal brainstem hypoplasia, porencephaly or hydranencephaly, depending on the timing and nature of the infarct.

Infarction in the region of the posterior cerebral artery occurring with birth trauma may be associated with (i) laceration of the basilar artery, (ii) uncus herniation with arterial compression, and (iii) endoluminal occlusion via haemorrhage in the adventitia of the vertebral artery (especially in breech delivery). Two 'traumatic' mechanisms are linked with infarction of the middle cerebral artery and its branches: (i) elongation of the endothelium with thrombosis, and (ii) basal subdural haemorrhage with compression and/or vasospasm.

Arterial infarction in the term neonate will usually occur in the zone perfused by the middle cerebral artery (about 80% of cases), while the posterior and anterior arteries are responsible for 14 and 6% of cases respectively. The left middle cerebral artery is more often involved than the right. Fewer than one in four infarcts are accompanied by macroscopic haemorrhage: this may be haemorrhagic conversion after a few days or primary haematoma in the infarcted area occurring in the first hours. Between the sixth hour after its occurrence and the end of the first week, the infarcted zone is swollen, producing a mass effect. During recovery the originally necrotic zone will slowly (at least two weeks before cysts are seen) evolve towards a cortico-subcortical triangular defect that remains identifiable for years. Temporarily, from the third day until the fourth week, areas of infarcted grey matter will show up in this necrotic zone on CT and MRI. Late (after 3–6 months) atrophy of the ipsilateral thalamus, although not directly due to infarction, may be seen in complete middle cerebral artery infarction: this is based on transneuronal degeneration by disconnection from the cortex.

Although, as far as the neonatal period is concerned, little has been reported on focal infarction within any artery other than the three major ones, increased attention and fine tuning of techniques may well lead to better detection. In particular, lacunar infarcts in the divisions of the middle cerebral artery are yet to be discovered by neonatologists. Colour Doppler analysis and MR angiography will, we suspect, prove valuable in investigating focal brain infarction. MR angiography may allow noninvasive documentation of major artery occlusion. Delineation of an ischaemic area within hours after the insult can be achieved with diffusion weighted MRI. Using proton magnetic resonance spectroscopy, lactate can be found within the area of infarction, often up until a few months after the onset.

Sonography sometimes permits identification of a necrotic zone within the first hours following the insult, although it usually takes a few days before the area becomes echogenic. The affected areas are brighter due to oedema and later due to necrosis with glial reaction and new capillary formation. Tissue swelling will progressively compress regional sulci and the ipsilateral ventricle. In the early stages it is possible to register decreased flow velocities in the affected vessel as compared to the healthy side. Vascular pulsatility is reduced within the infarct and more prominent in the border zone for a few weeks. Colour Doppler analysis may demonstrate this hyperperfusion in the penumbra. In certain perilesional arteries, extremely high flow rates may be measured (>1m/s), sometimes so high that vascular malformation is suspected. The examination allows the irregular ingrowth of small arteries in the border zone to be detected after a few days. These phenomenona have been insufficiently studied.

REFERENCES

Boyce, L.H., Khandji, A.G., DeKlerk, A.M., Nordli, D.R. (1994) 'Fetomaternal hemorrhage as an etiology of neonatal stroke.' *Pediatric Neurology*, **11**, 255–257.

de Vries, L.S., Regev, R., Connell, J.A., Bydder, G.M., Dubowitz, L.M.S. (1988)' Localized cerebral infarction in the premature infant: an ultrasound diagnosis correlated with computed tomography and magnetic resonance imaging.' *Pediatrics*, **81**, 36–40.

Fischer, A.Q., Anderson, J.C., Shuman, R.M. (1988) 'The evolution of ischemic cerebral infarction in infancy: a sonographic evaluation.' *Journal of Child Neurology*, **3**, 105–109.

Giroud, M., Fayolle, H., Martin, D., Baudoin, N., André, N., Gouyon, J.B., Nivelon, J.L., Dumas, R. (1995) 'Late thalamic atrophy in infarction of the middle cerebral artery territory in neonates. A prospective clinical and radiological study in four children.' *Child's Nervous System*, **11**, 133–136.

Groenendaal, F., van der Grond, J., Witkamp, T.D., de Vries, L.S. (1995) 'Magnetic resonance spectroscopic imaging in neonatal stroke.' *Neuropediatrics*, **26**, 243–248.

Guajardo, L., Strauss, A., Amster, J. (1994) 'Idiopathic cerebral infarction and upper limb ischemia in neonates.' *American Journal of Perinatology*, **11**, 119–122.

Hernanz-Schulman, M., Cohen, W., Genieser, N.B. (1988) 'Sonography of cerebral infarction in infancy.' *American Journal of Roentgenology*, **150**, 897–902.

Hill, A., Martin, D.J., Daneman, A., Fitz, C.R. (1983) 'Focal ischemic cerebral injury in the newborn: diagnosis by ultrasound and correlation with computed tomographic scan.' *Pediatrics*, **71**, 790–793.

Mannino, F.L., Trauner, D.A. (1983) 'Stroke in neonates.' *Journal of Pediatrics*, **102**, 605–610.

Mercuri, E., Cowan, F., Rutherford, M., Acolet, D., Pennock, J., Dubowitz, L. (1995) 'Ischaemic and haemorrhagic brain lesions in newborns with seizures and normal Apgar scores.' *Archives of Disease in Childhood*, **73**, F67–F74.

Perlman, J.M., Rollins, N.K., Evans, D. (1994) 'Neonatal stroke: clinical characteristics and cerebral blood flow velocity measurements.' *Pediatric Neurology*, **11**, 281–284.

Smith, S.J., Vogelzang, R.L., Marzano, M.I., Cerullo, L.J., Gore, R.M., Neiman, H.L. (1985) 'Brain edema: ultrasound examination.' *Radiology*, **155**, 379–382.

Taylor, G.A. (1994) 'Alterations in regional cerebral blood flow in neonatal stroke: preliminary findings with color Doppler sonography.' *Pediatric Radiology*, **24**, 111–115.

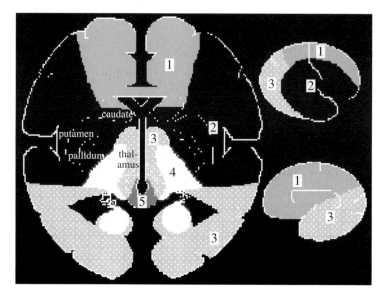

Fig. VII.1.a. Coronal view of the major arterial territories: (1) anterior cerebral artery; (2) middle cerebral artery; (3) posterior cerebral artery; (4) anterior choroidal artery; (5) posterior communicating artery.

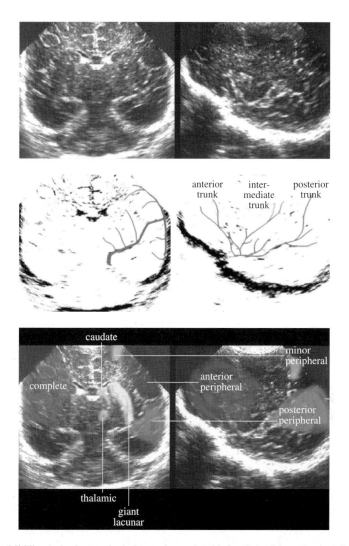

Fig. VII.1.b. Middle cerebral artery branches and associated infarction subtypes projected on 7.5 MHz coronal and parasagittal sections of a term brain. The artery arises from the internal carotid artery, its main stem coursing horizontally towards the insula; here it gives off perforators to the basal ganglia. In the insula it divides into a major anterior group of branches and a posterior group behind the insula.

TABLE VII.1
Perfusion territories of perforating arteries

Artery	Perfusion territories
Anterior cerebral artery	Rostroventral part of the head of the caudate nucleus (medial striate artery = Heubner's artery) Medial part of the anterior limb of the internal capsule Adjacent putamen
Middle cerebral artery	Lateral part of the head of the caudate nucleus Lateral pallidum Putamen Anterior thalamus (perforating thalamic branches) Lateral part of the anterior limb and genu of the internal capsule
Posterior cerebral artery	Thalamus in its lateral, inferior and paramedian parts (thalamogeniculate branches)
Anterior choroidal artery	Medial pallidum Posterior limb of the internal capsule Amygdaloid body
Posterior communicating artery	Anterior and medial thalamus (thalamotuberal branches) Hypophysis, hypothalamus Subthalamus

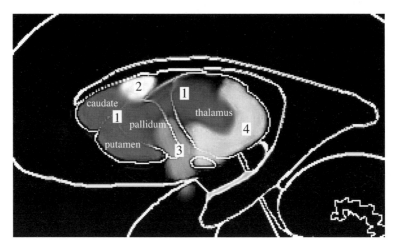

Fig. VII.1.c. Parasagittal section through the basal ganglia, showing perfusion territories of the main branches of the circle of Willis: (1) middle cerebral artery; (2) anterior cerebral artery; (3) anterior choroidal artery; (4) posterior cerebral artery.

VII.2. MIDDLE CEREBRAL ARTERY INFARCTION

Densities in the caudate nucleus or globus pallidus are the usual first indicators of complete occlusion of a middle cerebral artery (Fig. VII.2.a). Further analysis will show hyper-echogenic zones in white matter, from the ventricular border to the cortex, as early as four hours after the first hemiconvulsion. The insular region will be affected. In the first weeks one has the impression that the infarct is marginated by an echodense border due to increased vascularity in the penumbra (Figs. VII.2.a, VII.2.b). A true linear border is a diagnostic marker for arterial infarction. Ultrasound does not permit definitive diagnosis of bleeding into an infarct, although marked and clouded hyperechogenicity seems to suggest it (Fig. VII.2.b). Cystic change in the late neonatal period only confirms infarction.

We have occasionally observed focal hyperechogenicity, together with regional hypo-density on CT, without sequelae (Fig. VII.2.h). The cystic intermediary did not appear in these cases. This seems to suggest that echography allows recognition of ischaemic zones that do not necrose. This is one of the ways to explain why the diagnosis of focal arterial 'infarction' is sometimes retained without recognizing residual phenomena.

Within the irrigation area of the middle cerebral artery subtotal infarction may be recognized in an anterior portion (Figs. VII.2.c–e), a posterior parietal portion (Fig. VII.2.g) and a limited peripheral portion (Fig. VII.2.j). A giant lacunar infarct in the area of the middle cerebral artery is recognized due to its delineated echodensity in the striatum and the internal capsule: examples of capsulo-putamino-caudatal infarction in a lateral striatal artery have been observed (Figs. VII.2.i).

Abnormal findings in the first days of life may be indicative of an antenatal event, especially when they have already reached the cystic stage.

Fig. VII.2.a. Complete middle cerebral artery infarction is recognized by involvement of peripheral parenchyma (subcortex and cortex, around the insula), white matter and neostriatum as well as lateral pallidum and anterolateral thalamus. In the echogenic stage one can see a clear linear medial margin from the cranial midline to the midtemporal base. Three examples are given.

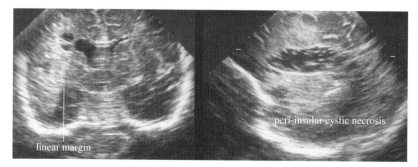

Day 30 coronal *(left)* and day 50 parasagittal *(right)* 7.5 MHz sonograms of a term infant, born with partial separation of the placenta, who aspirated blood and developed respiratory distress. The right leg turned white following placement of an arterial umbilical catheter. Subsequently complete right middle cerebral artery infarction was diagnosed.

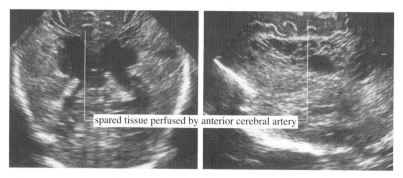

Bilateral infarction (confirmed by CT and MRI) four weeks after asphyxia and *Escherichia coli* bacteraemia: this will ultimately produce a 'basket brain'. (7.5 MHz sonograms: *left*, coronal; *right*, parasagittal.)

272

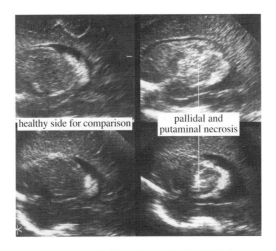

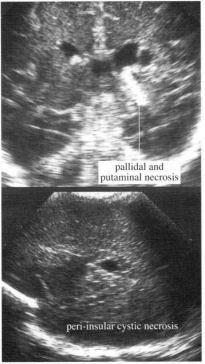

Preterm infant (35 weeks gestation) with right-sided focal seizures on day 1, brief pulmonary hypertension and early neonatal hypotension and metabolic acidosis. *Top:* 7.5 MHz parasagittal images (*upper pair*, day 13, *lower pair*, day 40). *Bottom:* 7.5 MHz images, day 40 (*upper*, coronal, *lower*, outer parasagittal).

Fig. VII.2.b. The diagnosis of middle cerebral artery infarction is made easy by recognition of (i) the spared perfusion territory of the anterior cerebral artery, (ii) involvement of putamen and caudate nucleus, and (iii) a linear mesial margin to the hyperechogenic zone.

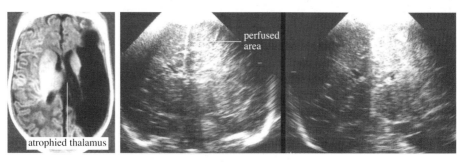

Complete middle cerebral artery infarction. Compare the end stage (MRI at 6 months) with the initial coronal sonograms of this term infant with seizures following difficult ventouse delivery. Only careful inspection allows recognition of the still perfused mesial frontal parenchyma, compressed as it is between the large swollen infarct area and the falx. The thalamus has atrophied, due to disconnection from the complexity of neuronal connections in cortex and striatum. (Reproduced by permission from Groenendaal *et al.* 1995.)

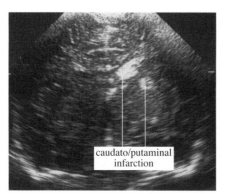

Initially, complete middle cerebral artery infarction may be difficult to detect, especially if the fontanelle is not large. In this term infant caudate and putaminal echodensities, separated by the internal capsule, were first recognized; these turned out to be haemorrhagic lesions within the large middle cerebral artery infarct (confirmed by MRI).

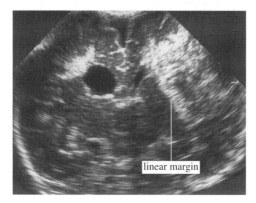

The diagnosis of middle cerebral artery infarction may not be easy if accompanied by (haemorrhagic) leukomalacia. Involvement of the basal ganglia (in this case the linear margin of a putaminal infarct) is typical of complete vessel involvement.

274

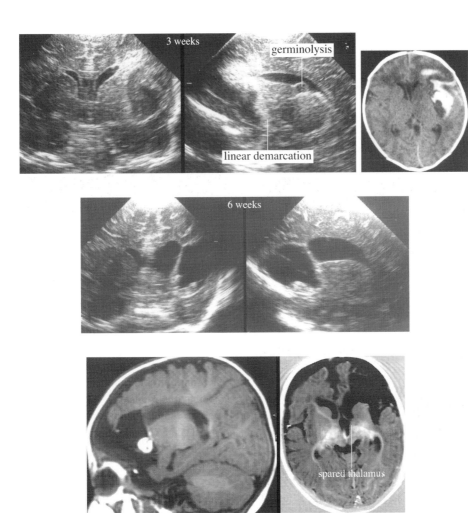

Fig. VII.2.c. *Anterior middle cerebral artery infarction*: hypoperfusion of the main insular stem artery (not shown with angiography, but probably the ascending frontal artery) before it fans out over the frontal and anterior parietal lobe. This term infant was delivered by ventouse extraction and presented with seizures on day 1. The infarct was haemorrhagic as suggested by the first week uncontrasted CT scan. Putamen and thalamus were not involved, as can be seen on follow-up MRI at 7 months. Dilatation of the ipsilateral ventricle, with a membranous remnant between it and a triangular (sub)cortical defect, is due to disconnection between basal ganglia and adjacent cortex and to extensive white matter necrosis. Germinal matrix cystic change is not easily explained, but may be due to involvement of cortical penetrating branches feeding matrix near the caudothalamic groove. Note that infarction reaches as far inward as the caudate head.

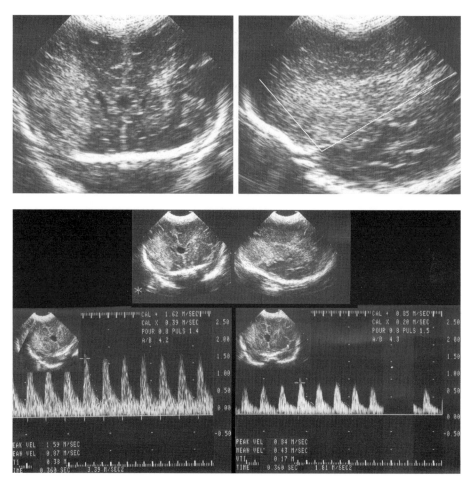

Fig. VII.2.d. *Right anterior middle cerebral artery infarction* in a growth retarded preterm infant who showed fetal distress during labour. The origin of the lesion was presumably antenatal, in or shortly before labour. *(Top)* The insular, frontal lobar and anterior parietal lobar cortex and subcortical white matter are caught in the hyperechechogenic stage on day 3 (left, coronal; right, parasagittal). *(Bottom)* Doppler flow velocities in a visibly pulsating afferent artery were lower than in the respective contralateral vessel.

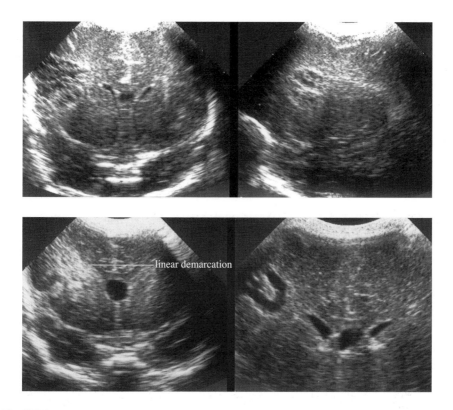

Fig. VII.2.e. *Right anterior middle cerebral artery infarction* in two different preterm infants, both presumably of antenatal origin: *(top)* 30 weeks gestation growth retarded infant, without neonatal problems (late neonatal scan); *(bottom)* 28 weeks gestation infant, one of triplets (*left*, day 1; *right*, day 10). The images clearly show two important features of arterial infarction: linear margination and extension from ventricle to pia mater.

277

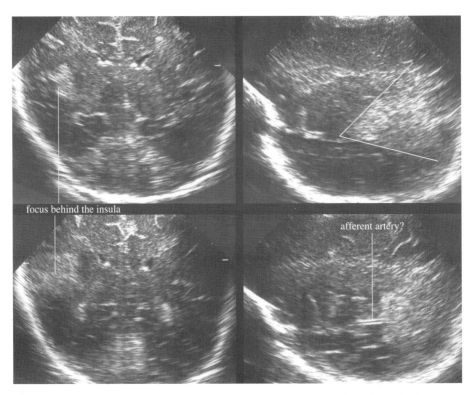

focus behind the insula

afferent artery?

Fig. VII.2.f. *Posterior middle cerebral artery infarction.* An area of hyperechogenicity with linear margins extends from the insula toward the occipitoparietal calvarium. The triangle's point is at the caudal insula, where a very pulsatile artery with brightened walls was pointing to the infarcted area; flow in this vessel exceeded 1 m/s for a few weeks. This finding was accidental in a term infant referred for a kidney mass, shown to be an adrenal cyst overlying an infarcted kidney due to thrombosis of the renal vein and involvement of the inferior vena cava. The infarct was therefore presumably embolic in origin. The vessel involved was probably the occipitotemporal artery (one of the larger vessels from the posterior trunk). The basal ganglia were spared. It took three weeks for the first sonolucent areas to become visible in the infarct. At 2 years this boy was moderately hemiplegic, with almost normal ambulation.

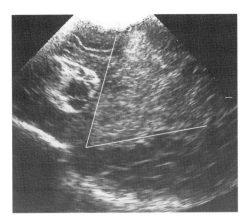

Fig. VII.2.g. Preterm infant with *Candida* endocarditis, showing a rare combination of a lobar haemorrhagic mass lesion (abscess or pure bleeding) and a *parietal middle cerebral artery infarct*, involving the insula. The involved artery may have been the intermediate trunk of the insular fan from the middle cerebral artery.

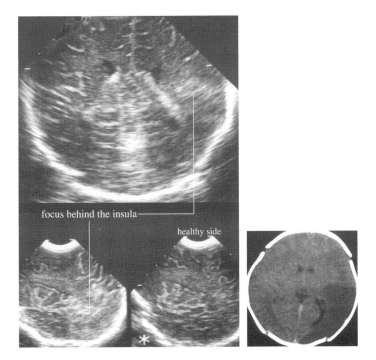

Fig. VII.2.h. An intriguing feature of sonography is its potential for recognizing *ischaemia without necrosis*. These third day sonograms and CT are from a term girl with gram-negative early onset bacteraemia and focal left EEG disturbances. At 3 years of age both the clinical examination and CT were entirely normal. The area involved is the same as in Fig. VII.2.f.

279

Fig. VII.2.i. *Giant lacunar striatal infarction* due to hypoperfusion of a lateral major perforating striatal artery from the horizontal part of the middle cerebral artery (putamino-caudate infarction). An identical triangular hyperechogenic zone, with its base against the outer lateral ventricular floor and its angle pointing to the artery involved, was found in two different infants. Part of the lateral globus pallidus may be involved as well.

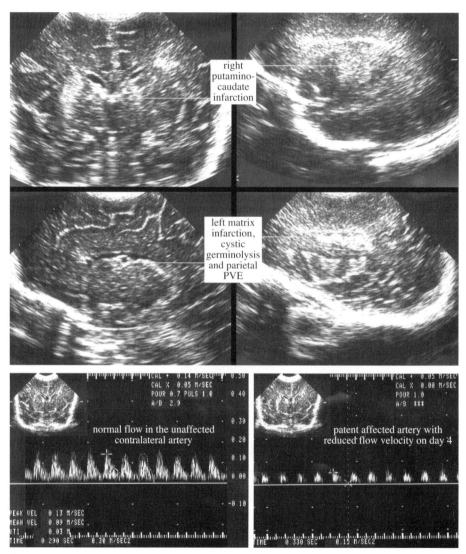

Growth retarded preterm infant with fetal distress during labour and a short period of postnatal acidosis. There is an arterial infarct on the right and a matrix haemorrhage with associated parietal periventricular echogenicity (PVE) on the left. White matter and cortex are unaffected on the right.

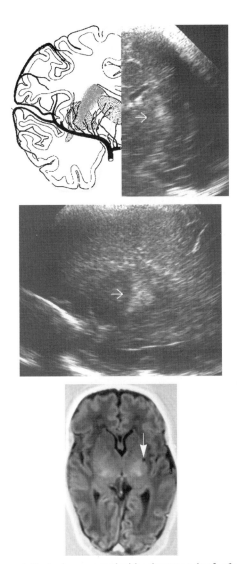

Preterm infant (31 weeks gestation) who presented with seizures on day 2, after recognition of transient hydrops due to *in utero* supraventricular tachycardia. A lacunar striatal infarct can be seen on the 7.5 MHz sonograms (*top*, coronal; *centre*, parasagittal). The MRI scan performed at term age shows a small cystic lesion in the left putamen.

Fig. VII.2.j. An infant with a *peripheral infarct of a smaller terminal branch of the middle cerebral artery* may present with focal seizures. In the early stage a very limited hyperechogenic focus in a parasagittal parietal location may be difficult to recognize. After cystic necrosis the diagnosis becomes easy, although the location may warrant differentiation from sinus thrombosis with venous subcortical infarction or from contusion.

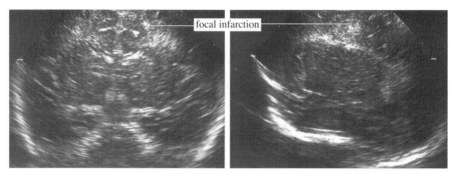

Term infant who presented with focal right-sided seizures on day 3 after an uneventful pregnancy and delivery.

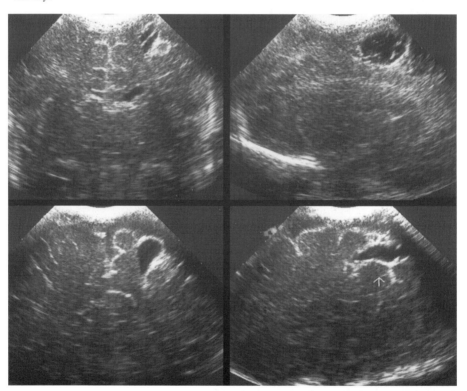

Infant born at 30 weeks gestation after death of the father. *Top row:* day 21, 7.5 MHz scans (*left*, coronal; *right*, parasagittal); *bottom row:* 10 MHz scans performed at term age (*left*, coronal; *right*, parasagittal).

VII.3. POSTERIOR AND ANTERIOR CEREBRAL ARTERY INFARCTION

Ultrasound descriptions of infarction in the area of the anterior or posterior cerebral arteries are rare.

In anterior cerebral artery infarction the hyperechogenic zone lies between the falx and the insula, is maximally frontal but stretches as far as the posterior parietal area.

In posterior cerebral artery infarction the hyperechogenic zone is mainly occipital and mesiotemporal (Figs. VII.3.a, VII.3.b).

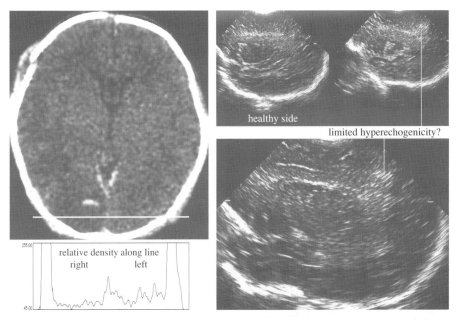

Fig. VII.3.a. Hypoperfusion and infarction in the *posterior cerebral artery* area may not be an easy diagnosis. This term infant, born after a difficult ventouse extraction, developed subgaleal bleeding and seizures; CT identified hypodensity in the right occipital lobe, with a limited parenchymal bleed in addition to subarachnoid haemorrhage. Careful sonography failed to clearly document the affected region, although minimal increase in echogenicity was suspected at the parieto-occipital transition.

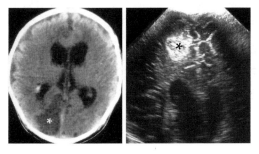

Fig. VII.3.b. Term infant treated with ECMO, with hemiconvulsions on day 16. No abnormalities were detected by sonography through the anterior fontanelle, whereas CT documented right posterior cerebral artery hypoperfusion *(asterisk)*. Subsequent (7.5 MHz) sonography through the posterior fontanelle identified an echogenic area of necrosis in the right occipital area. (Reproduced by permission from de Vries *et al.* 1996; *Neuropediatrics*, **27**, 101–104.)

VII.4 BRIGHT ANTERIOR LIMB OF THE INTERNAL CAPSULE

On parasagittal sections one can observe three echogenic areas around the head of the caudate nucleus. Just outside the caudate head physiological or pathological hyperdensity is seen in the white matter of the centrum semi-ovale. At the caudal end the hyperechogenic crossroad of the caudothalamic groove is always present. Very variable is the echogenic potential of the anterior limb of the internal capsule. In two term infants with severe anaemia at birth (one fetomaternal transfusion), soft hyperechogenic reflections were observed in and around this structure (Figs. VII.4.a, VII.4.c). The nature of the relation to anaemia is unclear. The echogenicity disappeared without ventricular dilatation or necrosis. In preterm infants the observation may be asymmetric. One clearly has to beware of not diagnosing a frontal flare on such occasions (Fig. VII.4.b). In coronal sections in front of the foramen of Monro the caudate seems surrounded by an echogenic rim. At the level of Monro's foramina the genu of the internal capsule may appear as punctiform foci. The brightness may be due to congestion, minimal bleeding or necrosis.

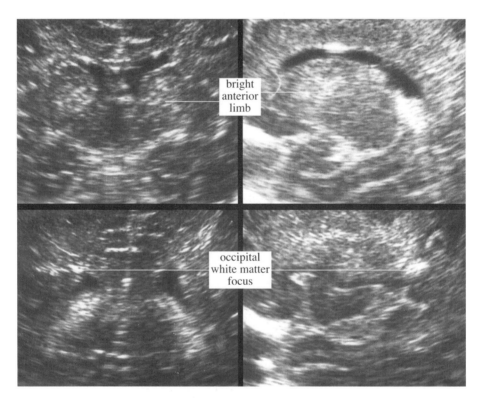

Fig. VII.4.a. Term infant with unexplained anaemia from birth and Fallot's tetralogy (7.5 MHz sections on day 2: *left*, coronal; *right*, parasagittal). Focal white matter hyperechogenicity was seen in addition to bright anterior limbs of the internal capsule.

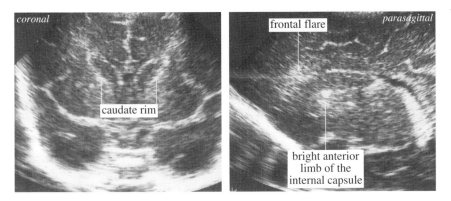

Fig. VII.4.b. Term infant with chronic fetomaternal transfusion: first day 7.5 MHz images.

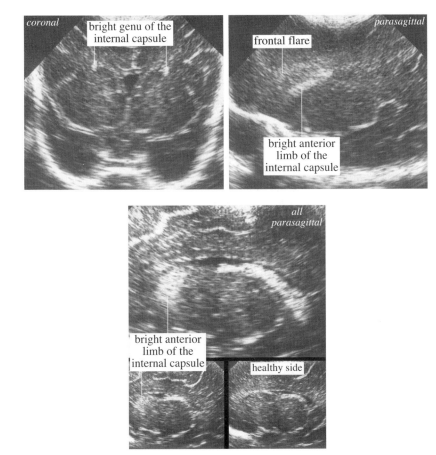

Fig. VII.4.c. Two ventilated preterm infants with respiratory distress syndrome (first week 7.5 MHz sonograms). The bright anterior crus has to be differentiated from white matter disease.

VII.5 BRIGHT FOCUS IN THALAMUS, CAUDATE HEAD OR POSTERIOR LIMB OF THE INTERNAL CAPSULE

Some fascinating lesions, the pathogenesis of which is as yet insufficiently understood, can be observed amidst the basal ganglia. These take the form of round or elliptical densities in the neostriatum, thalamus or internal capsule, or the globus pallidus (section VII.6). From a clinical context—nearly always the foci are discovered in seriously ill babies suffering from bacteraemia, pulmonary hypertension and/or asphyxia—we may suspect they are vascular insults. This is corroborated by almost obligatory unilaterality.

Should the insult be *arterial*, embolic infarction, with or without haemorrhagic conversion, may be a mechanism. These are equivalents of small lacunar infarcts in older children and adults. Even in children these lesions have only recently been recognized in life, by means of MRI. It may be useful to identify the affected vessel using angiography: penetrating branches of anterior or posterior middle cerebral arteries, of the posterior communicating artery or of the anterior choroidal artery could be involved. For thalamic infarcts at least three types exist, each with a specific clinical picture and location: thalamoperforant territory (middle cerebral artery branches entering substantia perforata anterior); thalamotuberal territory (direct branches from the posterior communicating artery); and thalamogeniculate territory (branches through the quadrigeminal plate from the posterior cerebral artery).

If *venous*, the lesion may be seen as limited deep venous thrombosis in one of the veins irrigating the internal cerebral vein or basal vein (extensive deep venous thrombosis has been described elsewhere).

If the lesion is purely thalamic or striatal, not too large and unilateral, the prognosis need not be pessimistic. However, lesions in the internal capsule, even if they are not exceptionally large (a diameter of some millimeters), may cause contralateral hemiplegia. During autopsy we have been surprised by the non-haemorrhagic character of those homogeneous densities. MRI may falsely suggest haemorrhage, due to tissue reaction with neovascularization. Sonography shows unilateral nodules in the internal capsule or thalamus. A haemorrhage may be expected to regress after a few weeks. When softening occurs, a persistence of the density is to be expected for at least three weeks.

REFERENCES

de Vries, L.S., Smet, M., Goemans, N., Wilms, G., Devlieger, H., Casaer, P. (1992) 'Unilateral thalamic haemorrhage in the pre-term and full-term newborn.' *Neuropediatrics*, **23**, 153–156.
Garg, B.P., DeMyer, W.E. (1995) 'Ischemic thalamic infarction in children : clinical presentation, etiology and outcome.' *Pediatric Neurology*, **13**, 46–49.

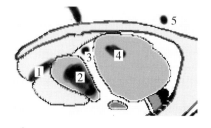

Fig. VII.5.a. Sites of bright hyperechogenic focus: (1) bright anterior limb of the internal capsule; (2) in the pallidum; (3) in the genu or posterior limb of the internal capsule; (4) in the thalamus; (5) in periventricular white matter.

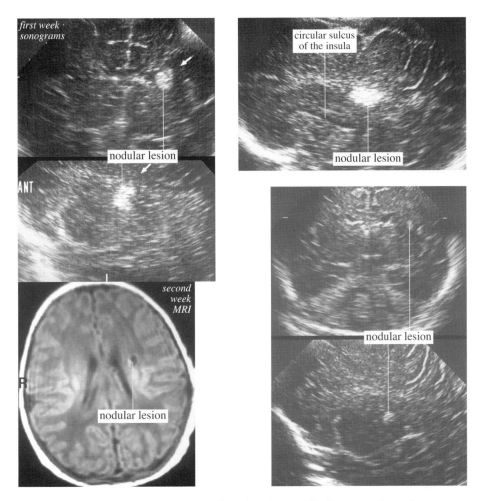

Fig. VII.5.b. Three ventilated term infants, all of whom had umbilical venous catheters inserted soon after birth. During routine sonography all were found to have a *nodular lesion in or near the left genu of the internal capsule*. The circumstances suggested embolic infarction, with or without haemorrhagic conversion, especially since two of them were ventilated for pulmonary hypertension (one after feto-maternal transfusion, the other after liver laceration during difficult breech delivery); the third had myo-tubular myopathy. The lesion is located between the circular sulcus of the insula and the head of the caudate nucleus. At least two of the infants did not develop contralteral hemiplegia, suggesting that capsular fibres were spared.

(This page and opposite, top) **Fig. VII.5.c.** A focal, lentiform density in the thalamus, anteriorly and slightly laterally, is not uncommon in sick newborn infants. The unilaterality and long persistence of the echogenicity suggest these foci are *focal arterial thalamic infarcts*. Anatomically the area involved lies anterior to the thalamogeniculate branches from the posterior cerebral artery. Thus, if the lesions are indeed true infarcts, they involve either thalamoperforating or—most likely—thalamotuberal arteries (direct branches from the posterior communicating artery). The lentiform focus is tilted with the cranial end pointing laterally. Anterior choroidal artery infarction would have to involve the posterior limb of the internal capsule and the medial pallidum (see Fig. VII.5.d)

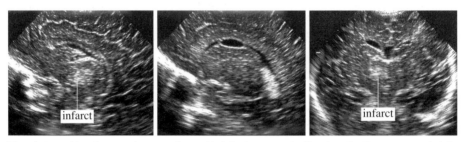

Term infant with pulmonary hypertension and brief seizures on the first day: day 7 sonograms. A right thalamic infarct was associated with a parietal white matter focus (not shown) and longstanding cystic germinolysis at the caudothalamic groove.

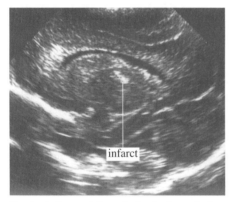

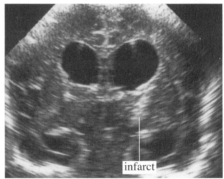

Preterm infant, recipient of a fetofetal transfusion, with hydrops and leukomalacia.

Posthaemorrhagic hydrocephalus and focal thalamic infarct following coxsackievirus myocarditis in a preterm infant (29 weeks gestation).

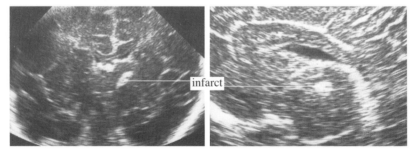

Term infant with oesophageal atresia, mediastinopleural fistula and severe acute hypoxaemia.

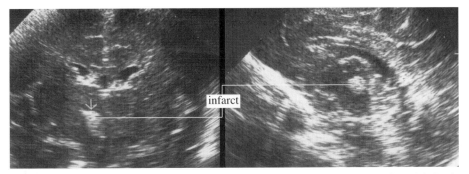

Fatal *Klebsiella* bacteraemia in a preterm infant (34 weeks gestation); autopsy confirmed thalamic infarction without haemorrhage.

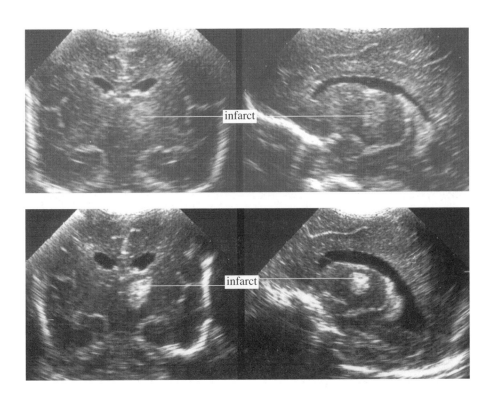

Fig. VII.5.d. Two preterm infants who presented with bacteraemia, ultrasound findings suggesting focal basal ganglia infarction. The lesions persisted for several weeks. The child in the top scans survived with mild hemiplegia, expected because of extension from the thalamus into the posterior limb of the internal capsule and medial pallidum. Although not proved, these images could fit anterior choroidal artery infarction or be analogous to the event shown in Fig. VII.5.c; they do appear larger and more rounded.

Fig. VII.5.e. Three different types of infarction in the head of the caudate nucleus. This area is perfused, in lateral and rostral parts, by the anterior cerebral artery and, in a more medial and caudal part, by branches from the middle cerebral artery. All examples were ventilated preterm infants, two with umbilical venous catheters in place in the early neonatal period. Cyst formation may occur in such cases.

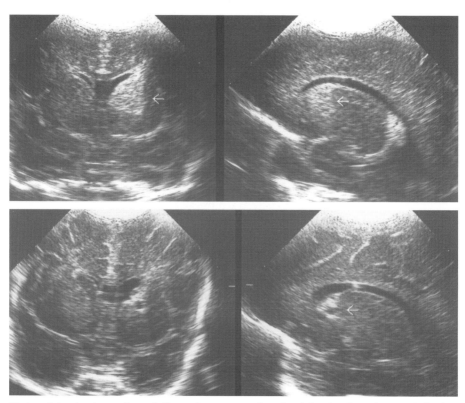

First week *(top)* and second month *(bottom)* sonograms of caudate infarction due to hypoperfusion in a striatal branch of the middle cerebral artery.

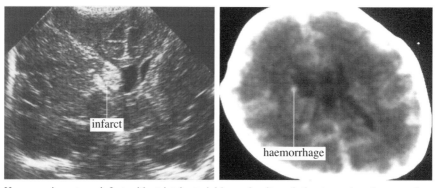

Hypoxaemic preterm infant with striatal arterial hyperdensity pointing towards a dense caudate lesion with minimal haemorrhage (see CT).

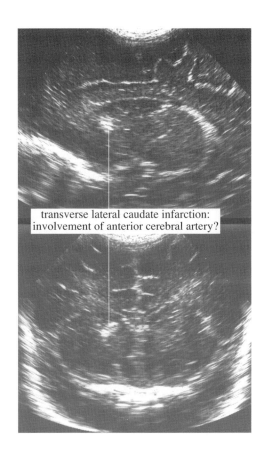

transverse lateral caudate infarction:
involvement of anterior cerebral artery?

VII.6. BRIGHT PALLIDUM

Necrosis of the globus pallidus may be seen after acute *asphyxia* (fetal or intrapartum), although, in such an instance, we also expect necrosis in the brainstem, the striatum and especially the thalamus.

With complete *infarction* in the area of the middle cerebral artery, the lateral pallidum may be very dense in the stage of coagulation necrosis preceding the cystic stage.

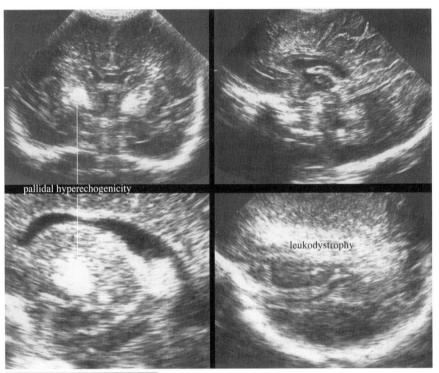

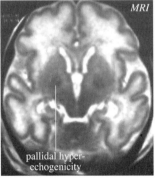

Fig. VII.6.a. Hyperechogenicity in the basal ganglia associated with an inborn error of metabolism.

(*This page* and *opposite, top*) These two infants presented with congenital lactic acidaemia, hypertrophic myocardiopathy, corneal dystrophy, extensive white matter dystrophy and pallidal hyperechogenicity; the one opposite also showed caudothalamic germinolysis.

(*Opposite, bottom*) Infant seen at 6 weeks for metabolic acidosis due to methylmalonic acidaemia. The internal capsule stood out between discretely hyperechogenic thalamus and medial pallidum.

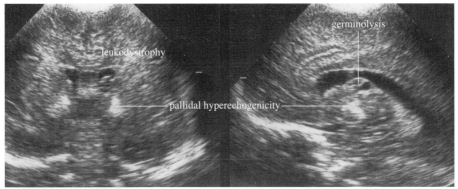

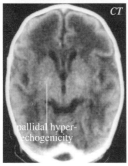

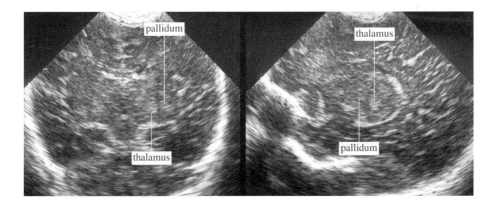

VII.7 ISOLATED PERIVENTRICULAR NODULAR ECHODENSITY

Apart from leukomalacia and periventricular damage to white matter in case of striatal vasculopathy, an echodense nodule—a small punctate unilateral lesion at the parieto-occipital transition—may occasionally be registered immediately next to the lateral ventricle. In one case we noticed that, in the weeks following the occurrence of the nodule, (sub)cortical cystic necrosis developed, compatible with infarction of the peripheral area of the middle cerebral artery (MRI excluding venous thrombosis). Context and imaging are consequently indicative of an ischaemic lesion. Focal arterial infarction in a ventriculopetal cortical branch is another possibility. (For further discussion of similar phenomena see section V.2.)

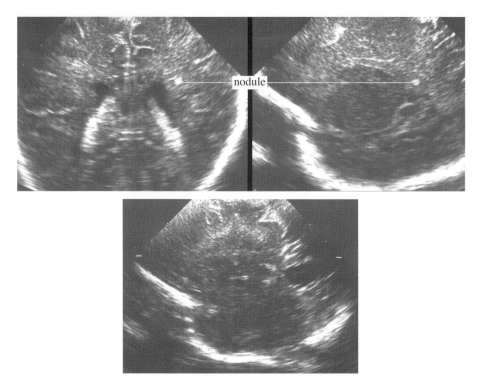

Fig. VII.7.a. Second week *(top)* and second month *(bottom)* images of a preterm infant with jugular vein thrombosis. (7.5 MHz sections: *top left*, coronal; others parasagittal.) A dense nodule preceded extensive necrosis of the entire peripheral middle cerebral artery territory.

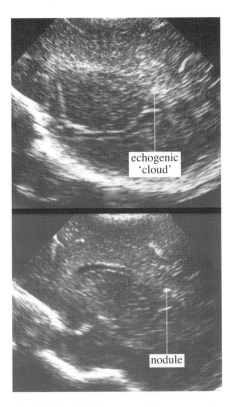

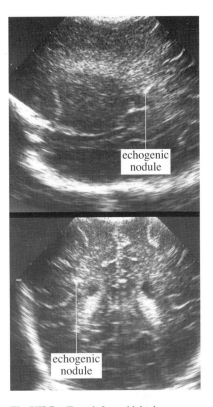

Fig. VII.7.b. 7.5 MHz parasagittal sections of a growth retarded dizygotic twin, referred on day 3 with ileal infarction (possibly of antenatal origin). The cloud of echogenicity visible on admission *(top)* had developed into a bright nodule by day 20 *(bottom)*.

Fig. VII.7.c. Term infant with hydrops, myocardial hypertrophy, pulmonary hypertension and congenital hypothyroidism: 7.5 MHz day 21 scans *(top*, parasagittal; *bottom*, coronal). No sequelae at 1 year of age.

VII.8. ECHODENSE TRAJECTORIES

Strange dense laminar trajectories have been noted in two infants during neonatal sonography, stretching from the cortex deep into brain matter.

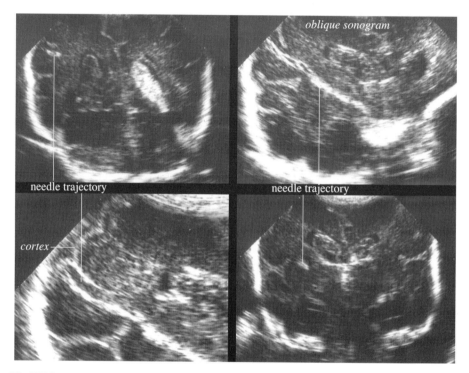

Fig. VII.8.a. This infant, born at 28 weeks gestation, presented with hydrops following fetofetal transfusion. The other twin, probably the recipient, had died *in utero*. The surviving donor died neonatally with acidosis, shock and pulmonary hypertension. Echographically a grade III intraventricular haemorrhage showed from the moment of admission (four hours after birth). Apart from that we noted on the right-hand side a dense line, with central clearing (trajectory), starting from the parietal cortex above the insula and pointing toward the third ventricle. At postmortem examination this lesion was easy to trace, with rusty brown haemorrhagic borders. On reviewing the obstetric history inadvertent fetal brain puncture during amniocentesis was considered a possible cause.

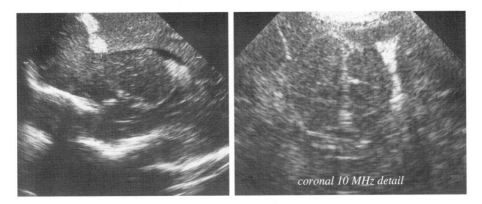

coronal 10 MHz detail

Fig. VII.8.b. This infant was referred because of preterm birth. After routine ultrasound we noted a left frontoparietal undulating laminar lesion, without central clearing, stretching from cortex to lateral ventricle. In this case no amniocentesis had been done. After six weeks the lesion remained unchanged, thus excluding haemorrhage or necrosis. MRI and colour Doppler imaging confirmed the anomaly, without getting any closer to a diagnosis. On CT the lesion was mildy hyperdense, excluding a fatty nature (possibly a hamartoma?). At 2 years of age development was within normal limits.

VII.9. AIR EMBOLISM

Air in the heart may be displaced to the brain, *e.g.* due to cardiac massage or Trendelenburg positioning. Air bubbles may be seen in the inferior vena cava, the heart or the aorta. In the brain multiple transient echogenic dots and short oblique lines are seen, aligned or in random collection in the territory of the middle cerebral artery.

REFERENCE

Sivan, Y., Nelson, M.D., Lee, S., Wood, B.P. (1990) 'Radiological case of the month: cerebral air embolism.' *American Journal of Diseases of Children*, **144**, 1351–1352.

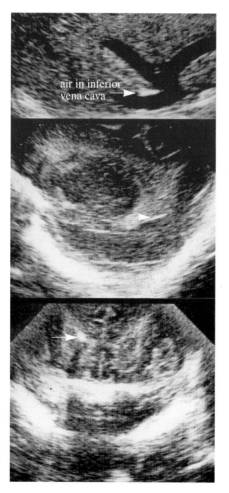

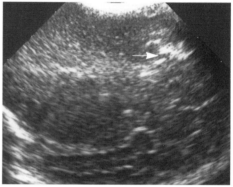

Fig. VII.9.a. Two different ventilated infants with acute deterioration due to air embolism.

(Left) Preterm infant with left pneumothorax who developed an air embolism following thoracocentesis.

(Above) Preterm infant with cardiovascular arrest following changing the pump connected to the central venous catheter. Irregular densities were noted one hour later, disappearing within 12 hours. The infant survived without adverse neurological sequelae.

VII.10 SINUS THROMBOSIS—SUPERFICIAL VENOUS INFARCTION

Venous infarction can be associated with vessel compression (as with germinal matrix haemorrhage) and with venous thrombosis. Deep venous thrombosis leads to haemorrhage in the basal ganglia and ventricles. Thrombophlebitis in smaller periventricular and cortical veins is also well known in bacterial meningitis and in fetal toxoplasmosis.

Thanks to MRI the diagnosis of perinatal cerebral sinus thrombosis has become more frequent. The seat of thrombosis is mostly the superior sagittal sinus in its parieto-occipital course. Thrombosis may propagate into anchor veins, draining a dorsal (sub)cortical part of the cerebral parenchyma. This may result in an ischaemic or (mostly) haemorrhagic 'red' infarct. Should the clot spread to the straight sinus, then the deep venous system may become involved, eventually causing a thalamoventricular haemorrhage. It has recently been shown that high frequency cranial sonography may enable identification of sinus thrombosis (Figs. VII.10.a, VII.10.b). Care should be taken not to confuse thrombus with a normal anatomic variant, such as an intraluminal septum (Fig. VII.10.c). The hypodense triangular sinusal cavity that shows on a coronal section is then filled with non-homogeneous echodense material, also showing on sagittal view. Doppler sonography will not reveal venous flow in the occluded segment. In the case of venous infarction, a subcortical zone will be hyperdense in the adjacent brain parenchyma. The peripheral location of these asymmetric hyperdense zones in white matter is indicative of a venous mechanism. A distinction needs to be made with peripheral middle cerebral artery infarction, postasphyxial parasagittal brain injury or contusion after trauma. After a few weeks cystic necrosis may be demonstrated in the affected zones. Even partial thrombosis in the superior sagittal sinus can be recognized with ultrasound (Fig. VII.10.c).

REFERENCES

Barron, T.F., Gusnard, D.A., Zimmerman, R.A., Clancy, R.R. (1992) 'Cerebral venous thrombosis in neonates and children.' *Pediatric Neurology*, **8**, 112–116.
Govaert, P., (1993) *Cranial Haemorrhage in the Term Newborn Infant. Clinics in Developmental Medicine No. 129*. London: Mac Keith Press.
— — Voet, D., Achten, E., Vanhaesebrouck, P., van Rostenberghe, H., van Gysel, D., Afschrift, M. (1992) 'Non-invasive diagnosis of superior sagittal sinus thrombosis in a neonate.' *American Journal of Perinatology*, **9**, 201–204.
Grossman, R., Novak, G., Patel, M., Maytal, J., Ferreira, J., Eviatar, L. (1993) 'MRI in neonatal dural sinus thrombosis.' *Pediatric Neurology*, **9**, 235–238.

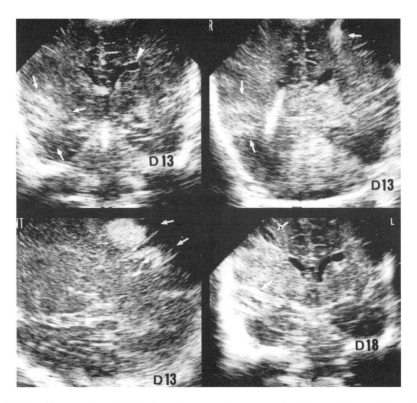

Fig. VII.10.a. Term newborn infant with nephrotic syndrome and perinatal cerebral venous thrombosis. The *arrowhead (top left)* points to a parafrontal germinolytic cyst present at birth. In the early neonatal period bilateral asymmetric subcortical echodensities appeared *(arrows)* on the right near the transverse sinus and on the left near the superior sagittal sinus. Cystic necrosis in these areas was seen by day 18. The history and the appearance of the infarcts suggested different foci of venous infarction, probably due to sinus and anchor vein thrombosis. (Reproduced by permission from Govaert 1993.)

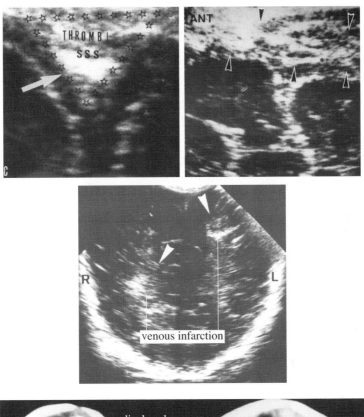

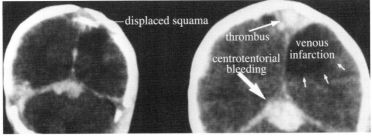

Fig. VII.10.b. Sonograms (*top*, 10 MHz; *centre*, 7.5 MHz) and coronal uncontrasted CT scans of a growth retarded term infant delivered by ventouse extraction following fetal distress. CT confirmed forward displacement of the occipital squama with subjacent thrombus formation in the superior sagittal sinus (sss). The process was also visualized with high frequency sonography: irregular bright echoes were obtained from the superior sagittal sinus, together with bilateral asymmetric subcortical occipito-parietal parenchymal echodensities *(arrowheads)*. At this stage flow was absent in the sinus. Central tentorial haemorrhage was clearly seen on CT (with dilatation of the great vein of Galen?).

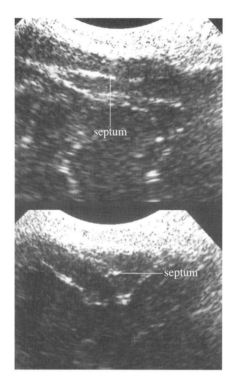 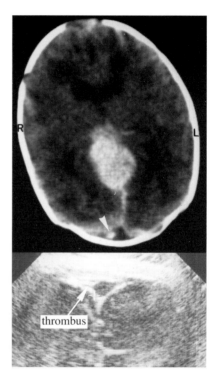

Fig. VII.10.c. With careful study, 10 MHz sonography may permit recognition of subtle intraluminal change within the superior sagittal sinus.

(Left) These scans (*top*, sagittal; *bottom*, coronal) show a normal anatomic variant, the presence of a horizontal septum from the right lateral sinus wall into the vessel cavity.

(Right) Comparison of CT and (coronal) sonographic appearance of focal thrombosis.

SECTION VIII
PATHOLOGY: MISCELLANEOUS

VIII.1 BACTERAEMIA, BACTERIAL MENINGITIS–VENTRICULITIS

During isolated bacteraemia the newborn infant may develop cerebral complications due to systemic effects. For example, an accompanying haemorrhagic diathesis may provoke a subarachnoid haematoma which is often fatal. Hypotension, hypoxia and metabolic acidosis may lead to arterial infarction and/or leukomalacia. Severely ill neonates are prone to deep venous thrombosis, which may involve the superior sagittal sinus. If meningitis–ventriculitis and/or brain abscess are also present, there may be accompanying arteritis with focal ischaemia (see arterial infarction), as brain abscess or as haemorrhagic brain necrosis.

The initial sonographic anomaly caused by meningitis and ventriculitis is brain swelling with small ventricular cavities. The sulci are wide and echogenic due to exudation in the grooves, but also due to increased echogenicity of the surrounding (sub)cortex. The latter may indicate the onset of gyral venous infarction. Foci of hyperechogenicity in white matter may occur around the ventricle and close to the cortex. After some hours the ventricles widen due to exudation and, later on, due to obstruction of CSF flow. This may occur at the level of the aqueduct, near the exit foramina of the fourth ventricle or during pericerebellar or pericerebral ascent of CSF. Hydrocephalus, both internal and external, is a potential complication. Discrepant dilatation of the fourth ventricle is possible ('isolated fourth ventricle' through occlusion above and under the ventricle).

In the second week ependymitis will show as a dense ventricular lining. Glial reaction along the ependyma or on choroid plexus creates intraventricular strands (septation) with compartmentalization (Fig. VIII.1.a). During the first few days fine intraluminal linear and nodular reflections may show, commonly called 'debris'. Mostly those reflections appear in the occipital or frontal horns. They are also associated with intraventricular haemorrhage and are consequently not diagnostic of ventriculitis, whereas septation tends to be.

The combination of infection and venous infarction (thrombophlebitis) eventually gives rise to periventricular cysts, sometimes of a porencephalic nature. The distinction between the loculated part of a ventricle and a periventricular postnecrotic cavity, infected or not, is not always easy. Later periventricular calcification may be expected.

Haemorrhagic necrosis of the brain may occur in fulminating gram-negative brain infections (*e.g.* with *Proteus* spp., *Escherichia coli* or *Pseudomonas aeruginosa*). We have observed the echographic changes in the brain parenchyma of a preterm infant suffering from a fatal *Pseudomonas* bacteraemia with meningitis (Fig. VIII.1.b). After a few days the brain substance was granularly hyperdense everywhere, as if crowded by small haemorrhages or areas of infarction. Within five days there was rapid progression toward scattered generalized microcystic necrosis with, in the ventricle, septation on top of blood clot. Even without postmortem confirmation this was compatible with meningo-encephalitis and ventriculitis.

A brain abscess usually starts as a focal infarct caused by thrombophlebitis in white matter. Extension of a subependymal or cortical micro-infarct might also lead to abscess formation. In the cortex itself no abscesses are formed. At first one sees a circular echodensity caused by inflammation and coagulation necrosis. This is followed by central dissolution, possibly with a level between fluid and necrotic debris. An abscess may eventually be identified by a thick and irregular capsule, though in the neonatal period this is less obvious (Fig. VIII.1.c). About 10 to 14 days after the onset of 'cerebritis' the mass-effect, if any, disappears. It may be difficult to differentiate from a sterile postnecrotic cavity. Focal arterial infarction or haemorrhage sometimes present with very similar echographic pictures. At a later stage one will see a residual cavity that may be integrated into the ventricle or give rise to a glial nodule with calcification.

Subdural collections of fluid, whether sterile or purulent, are comparatively rare in the neonatal period. A round or biconvex echogenic collection may be found between the bone and compressed brain cortex. Compression and not dilatation of the underlying sulci allows differentiation from a subarachnoid collection due to CSF retention. The echoreflections in the subdural collection are fine and may show strand formation. Interhemispheric location may occur. Sonography cannot differentiate between a sterile or a purulent effusion.

REFERENCES

Berman, P.H., Banker, B.Q. (1966) 'Neonatal meningitis. A clinical and pathological study of 29 cases.' *Pediatrics*, **38**, 6–24.

Enzmann, D.R., Britt, R.H., Lyons, B., Carroll, B., Wilson, D.A., Buxton, J. (1982) 'High-resolution ultrasound evaluation of experimental brain abcess evolution: comparison with computed tomography and neuropathology.' *Radiology*, **142**, 95–102.

Gallagher, P.G., Ball, W.S. (1991) 'Cerebral infarctions due to CNS infection with *Enterobacter sakazakii*.' *Pediatric Radiology*, **21**, 135–136.

Han, B.K., Babcock, D.S., McAdams, L. (1985) 'Bacterial meningitis in infants: sonographic findings.' *Radiology*, **154**, 645–650.

Hill, A., Shackelford, G.D., Volpe, J.J. (1981) 'Ventriculitis with neonatal bacterial meningitis: identification by real-time ultrasound.' *Journal of Pediatrics*, **99**, 133–136.

Hung, K-L. (1986) 'Cranial ultrasound in the detection of post-meningitic complications in the neonates.' *Brain and Development*, **8**, 31–36.

Lorber, J., Pickering, D. (1966)' Incidence and treatment of post-meningitic hydrocephalus in the newborn.' *Archives of Disease in Childhood*, **41**, 44–50.

Reeder, J.D., Sanders, R.C. (1983) 'Ventriculitis in the neonate: recognition by sonography.' *American Journal of Neuroradiology*, **4**, 37–41.

Ries, M., Deeg, K-H., Heininger, U., Stehr, K. (1993) 'Brain abscesses in neonates—report of three cases.' *European Journal of Pediatrics*, **152**, 745–746.

Schellinger, D., Grant, E.G., Manz, H.J., Patronas, N.J., Uscinski, R.H. (1986) 'Ventricular septa in the neonatal age group: diagnosis and considerations of etiology.' *American Journal of Neuroradiology*, **7**, 1065–1071.

Veyrac, C., Couture, A., Baud, C. (1994) 'La pathologie infectieuse.' *In:* Couture, A., Veyrac, C., Baud, C. (Eds.) *Echographie Cérébrale du Foetus au Nouveau-né.* Montpellier: Sauramps Médical, pp. 371–382.

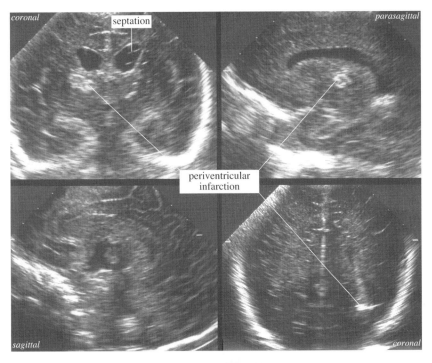

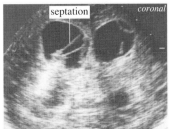

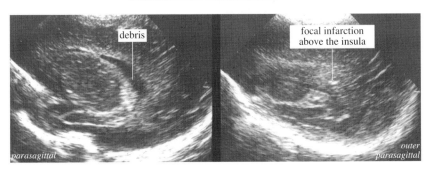

Fig. VIII.1.a. The consequences of meningitis and ventriculitis are shown by virtue of three different infants with neonatal *E. coli* meningitis; the top infant was scanned in the second week (with moderate ventriculomegaly), the middle one 1 month after onset of sickness (with hydrocephalus) and the bottom one at the end of the first week of life. (All 7.5 MHz scans, except *middle*, 5 MHz.)

305

Fig. VIII.1.b. *Haemorrhagic necrosis of the brain.* Initially, scattered small hyperechogenic foci (pellets) are seen; in the course of a few days these coalesce to form large plaques of necrosis. The end result is a fuzzy brain where anatomic landmarks, except for the ventricles, have disappeared. Two examples are given; in both cases the basal ganglia are spared.

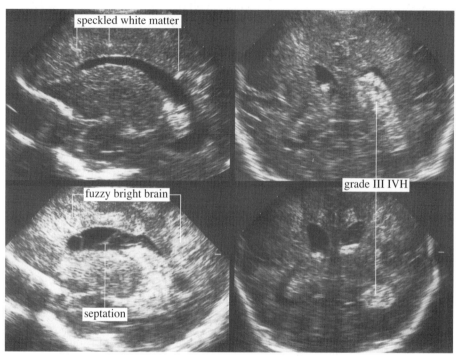

Preterm infant, two days *(top)* and six days *(bottom)* after onset of *Pseudomonas aeruginosa* bacteraemia. A grade III intraventricular haemorrhage is also apparent. (7.5 MHz scans: *left*, parasagittal; *right*, coronal.)

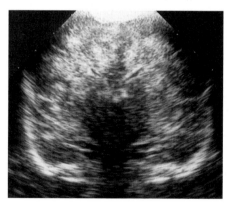

Preterm infant with *E. coli* infection: 7.5 MHz scan showing fuzzy bright brain with clouds of necrosis and haemorrhage.

Fig. VIII.1.c. An *abscess* in the brain can be caused by a variety of organisms. On ultrasound a level can be seen between fluid and necrotic debris, or debris fills the whole cavity. The capsule is finely echogenic; location in the internal capsule may explain contralateral motor impairment.

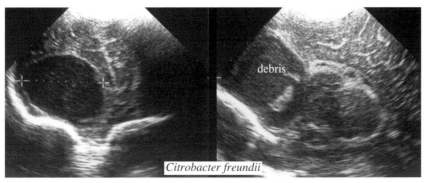

Preterm infant (26 weeks gestation), scanned at 2 weeks of life. The abscess was drained and there were no adverse sequelae at follow-up.

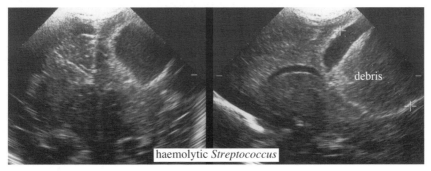

Term infant who became ill at 2 weeks of age; she died soon after admission.

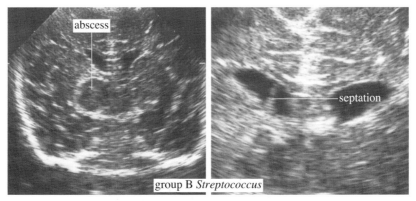

Term infant presenting with seizures and bacteraemia, and a right adrenal haemorrhage. Severe contralateral hemiplegia had developed by the age of 3 years.

307

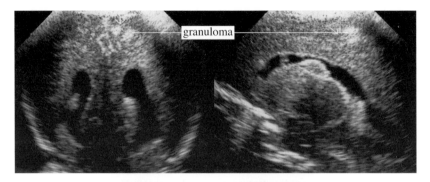

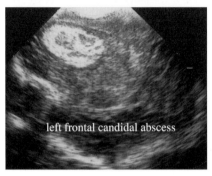

Fig. VIII.1.d. Brain infection with *Candida albicans* takes the form of meningitis but also of perivascular *granuloma* formation. The granulomas are subcortical in location and asymmetrically dispersed. Early abscess formation is presumed where a bigger focus is visible. The examples above were both preterm infants; neither survived.

VIII.2 NEONATAL BRAIN TUMOUR

The most frequent clinical sign of brain tumour is abnormally increasing head circumference with a tense fontanelle. Papilloedema is extremely rare. Cranial sonography has a clear but limited place in diagnosis. Due to its non-invasive simplicity it is an excellent exploratory tool; MRI will provide essential detail.

Ultrasound offers recognition and crude localization of the mass. Displacement of the sylvian sulcus from the midline to one or other side will suggest hemispheric localization. Deformation and displacement of the third ventricle suggests a midline supratentorial lesion. Displacement of the fourth ventricle with hydrocephalus suggests an intraventricular or posterior fossa lesion. It is possible to distinguish a well-defined mass from an infiltrating space-occupying process, the latter suggesting malignancy. Surrounding oedema or recent haemorrhage into the lesion may cause tumour size to be exaggerated.

The internal structure can be heterogeneous with cysts and calcification (teratoma) or extremely homogeneous and dense (plexus papilloma). The tumour is, almost by definition, echogenic in the middle of normal parenchyma. Astrocytomas of the posterior fossa are often cystic and behave benignly, unless they are located in the brainstem. Plexus papilloma often has a frontal vessel pedicle with intense venous blood flow; it is rarely malignant and may be multilocular. Hydrocephalus with papilloma results from CSF overproduction, mechanical obstruction of foramina or channels and occlusion pathways with tumorous debris.

During follow-up of a solid tumour treated with chemotherapy, a positive effect, *i.e.* necrosis in the mass, may sometimes show echographically: a previously homogeneous structure now shows denser foci of necrosis.

Tumoural processes show up in the differential diagnosis of hydrocephalus, unexplained parenchymal haemorrhage, intraventricular haemorrhage at term, thalamoventricular haemorrhage, and brain abscess.

Congenital hamartoma may look like a tumour. An 'accessory' brain structure has been described as a neuroglial tumour between diencephalon and telencephalon. This structure contained an abortive ventricle with ependyma and plexus.

REFERENCES

Body, G., Darnis, E., Pourcelot, D., Santini, J.J., Gold, F., Soutol, J.H. (1990) 'Choroid plexus tumors: antenatal diagnosis and follow-up.' *Journal of Clinical Ultrasound*, **18**, 575–578.

Buetow, P.S., Smirniotopoulos, J.G., Done, S. (1990) 'Congenital brain tumors: a review of 45 cases.' *American Journal of Roentgenology*, **155**, 587–593.

Cappe, I.P., Lam, A.H. (1985) 'Ultrasound in the diagnosis of choroid plexus papilloma.' *Journal of Clinical Ultrasound*, **13**, 121–123.

Chow, P.P., Horgan, J.G., Burns, P.N., Weltin, G., Taylor, K.J.W. (1986) 'Choroid plexus papilloma: detection by real-time and Doppler sonography.' *American Journal of Neuroradiology*, **7**, 168–170.

Han, B.K., Babcock, D.S., Oestreich, A.E. (1984) 'Sonography of brain tumors in infants.' *American Journal of Neuroradiology*, **5**, 253–258.

Harris, C.P., Townsend, J.J., Klatt, E.C. (1994) 'Accessory brains (extracerebral heterotopias): unusual prenatal intracranial mass lesions.' *Journal of Child Neurology*, **9**, 386–389.

Lipman, S.P., Pretorius, D.H., Rumack, C.M., Manco-Johnson, M.L. (1985) 'Fetal intracranial teratoma: US diagnosis of three cases and a review of the literature.' *Radiology*, **157**, 491–494.

Osborn, R.A., McGahan, J.P., Dublin, A.B. (1984) 'Sonographic appearance of congenital malignant astrocytoma.' *American Journal of Neuroradiology*, **5**, 814–815.

Radkowski, M.A., Naidich, T.P., Tomita, T., Byrd, S.E., McLone, D.G. (1988) 'Neonatal brain tumors: CT and MR findings.' *Journal of Computer Assisted Tomography*, **12**, 10–20.

Sauerbrei, E.E., Cooperberg, P.L. (1983) 'Cystic tumors of the fetal and neonatal cerebrum: ultrasound and computed tomographic evaluation.' *Radiology*, **147**, 689–692.

Schellhas, K.P., Siebert, R.C., Heithoff, K.B., Franciosi, R.A. (1988) 'Congenital choroid plexus papilloma of the third ventricle: diagnosis with real-time sonography and MR imaging.' *American Journal of Neuro-radiology*, **9**, 797–798.

Shawker, T.H., Schwartz, R.M. (1983) 'Ultrasound appearance of a malignant fetal brain tumor.' *Journal of Clinical Ultrasound*, **11**, 35–36.

Strassburg, H.M., Sauer, M., Weber, S., Gilsbach, J. (1984) 'Ultrasonographic diagnosis of brain tumors in infancy.' *Pediatric Radiology*, **14**, 284–287.

Winkler, P., Helmke, K. (1985) 'Ultrasonic diagnosis and follow-up of malignant brain tumors in childhood. A report of 4 cases and a review of the literature.' *Pediatric Radiology*, **15**, 215–219.

TABLE VIII.1
Neonatal intracranial tumours

Tumour	Location	Sonographic aspects
Astrocytoma/glioma	Suprachiasmatic	Homogeneous and softly echogenic
	Lateral supratentorial	Heterogeneous
	Cerebellar	Often cystic
	Brainstem	Homogeneous, infiltrating
Plexus papilloma	Lateral ventricle	Homogeneous, very echogenic, lobulated; fixed
	Fourth ventricle floor	to plexus with a small frontal or temporal
	Third ventricle roof	pedicle; if cystic, malignancy more likely
Ependymoma	Around a ventricle	With a broad basis in a ventricular wall; infiltrating more towards parenchyma than to ventricular lumen; homo- or heterogeneous
Medulloblastoma	In the midline on vermis; grows into cerebellar hemisphere and through tentorial incisura	Round, homogeneous and echogenic; often metastasizes into spinal canal and up along supratentorial ventricles, *e.g.* over caudate head
Teratoma	Pineal	Less mass-effect than expected; soft
	Third ventricle floor	hyperechogenic stroma with cysts and
	Posterior fossa	calcification or teeth
Lipoma	Corpus callosum	Very echogenic; possibly with marginal
	Choroid plexus	calcification; often associated with spina bifida,
	Hypothalamus	cephalocele, agenesis of corpus callosum

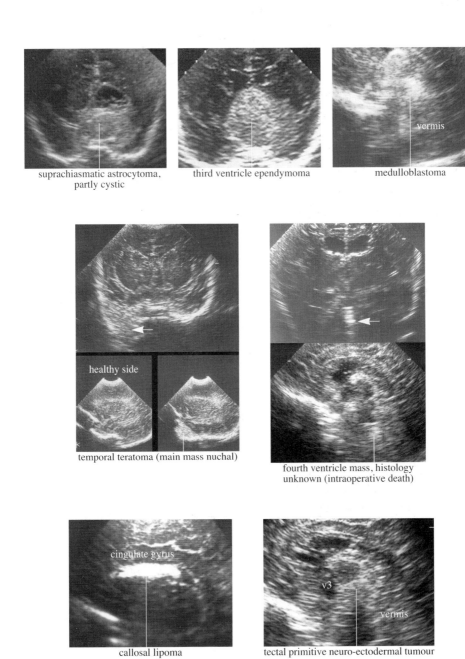

suprachiasmatic astrocytoma,
partly cystic

third ventricle ependymoma

medulloblastoma

vermis

healthy side

temporal teratoma (main mass nuchal)

fourth ventricle mass, histology
unknown (intraoperative death)

cingulate gyrus

callosal lipoma

v3

vermis

tectal primitive neuro-ectodermal tumour

Fig. VIII.2.a. Ultrasound appearance of different types of intracranial tumours.

VIII.3 CRANIOCEREBRAL EROSION

Weeks or even months following traumatic interruption of the dural membrane, as with rupture of the fontanelle or a bone fracture, cystic erosion of the fracture margins may occur. Any such growing fracture, better known as craniocerebral erosion, has the tendency to invade the underlying brain parenchyma, aiming at the ipsilateral ventricle. It is accepted that pulsatile arachnoid vessels and cells erode surrounding tissue by displacement. A similar observation has been made in extremely preterm infants, with bilateral, parietal, progressive haemorrhagic necrosis stretching from cortex to ventricle (see section IV.8).

REFERENCE

Voet, D., Govaert, P., Caemaert, J., de Lille, L., D'Herde, K., Afschrift, M. (1992) 'Leptomeningeal cyst: early diagnosis by color Doppler imaging.' *Pediatric Radiology*, **22**, 417-418.

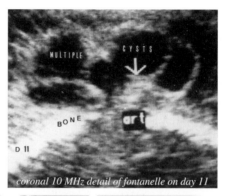

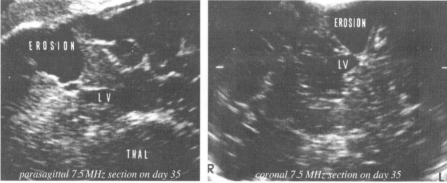

Fig. VIII.3.a. Term infant delivered by very difficult ventouse extraction, presenting with subgaleal haemorrhage; subsequent craniocerebral erosion occurred through the anterior fontanelle immediately near the superior sagittal sinus. A multilocular cyst invaded the subgaleal space together with cerebrofugal vessels in the margin of the defect. (The *arrow* indicates a cerebrofugal artery leaving the brain to enter the subgaleal space; LV = lateral ventricle.)The arterial character of those vessels was demonstrated with colour Doppler imaging. In spite of resection of the extracranial tumour with closure of the dural membrane on day 29, active erosion of the parietal parenchyma occurred in the direction of the ipsilateral ventricle. This unilocular erosion formed a cone with its base against the fontanelle. Contralateral hemiparesis was not observed on follow-up.

VIII.4. PHAKOMATOSIS

Tuberous sclerosis (Fig. VIII.4.a)

As early as the second trimester, this autosomal dominant neuroectodermal disorder may present with cerebral anomalies in a number of cases. Traditionally we encounter three lesions: subependymal nodules, giant cell astrocytomas and hamartomas. Megalencephaly may be part of the neonatal presentation (see below).

Subependymal nodules, consisting of immature neuroglial cells, are spread against the ependyma of the lateral and possibly third or fourth ventricles, like fat dripping off a candle. Those nodules may allow a provisional diagnosis in preterm infants presenting with cardiac failure due to an associated rhabdomyoma or, much less commonly, with large renal cysts. Especially in parasagittal sonographic sections they show up as small round echodensities in the floor or lateral wall of the body of the lateral ventricle. They are typically found in the caudothalamic groove.

Around the foramen of Monro a *giant cell astrocytoma* may be found, possibly causing unilateral hydrocephalus through compression. Discrete hyperdensity of periventricular white matter may show. Similar masses may give rise to aqueductal stenosis.

In the third trimester (sub)cortical foci of hamartomatosis may be found in the form of a solid *tuber*, replacing normal local structures. Particularly affected are the frontal lobes, and also occasionally the cerebellum. From the outside a tuber resembles a wart. Between these tubers and the ventricle a trace of heterotopic and dysplastic immature nerve cells may be found. In some cases calcification may occur in the neonatal period in both periventricular and peripheral hamartomas. All these lesions are echogenic, but may be iso- or hypodense on CT, unless calcified.

REFERENCES

Barth, P.G., Stam, F.C., van der Harten, J.J. (1978) 'Tuberous sclerosis and dysplasia of the corpus callosum. Case report of their occurrence in a newborn.' *Acta Neuropathologica*, **42**, 63–64.

Frank, L.M., Chaves-Carballo, E., Earley, L.M. (1984) 'Early diagnosis of tuberous sclerosis by cranial ultrasonography.' *Archives of Neurology*, **41**, 1302–1303.

Lago, P., Boniver, C., Casara, G.L., Laverda, A.M., Fiore, A., Salvadori, S., Carollo, C., Saia, O.S. (1994) 'Neonatal tuberous sclerosis presenting with intractable seizures.' *Brain and Development*, **16**, 257–259.

Legge, M., Sauerbrei, E., Macdonald, A. (1984) 'Intracranial tuberous sclerosis in infancy.' *Radiology*, **153**, 667–668.

Östör, A.G., Fortune, D.W. (1978) 'Tuberous sclerosis initially seen as hydrops fetalis. Report of a case and review of the literature.' *Archives of Pathology and Laboratory Medicine*, **102**, 34–39.

Fig. VIII.4.a. Sonographic presentation of tuberous sclerosis in three cases, two with CT confirmation.

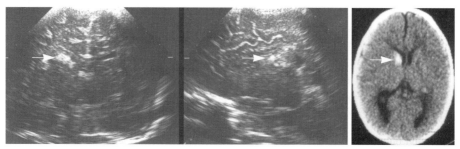

Neonatal seizures: right subependymal nodule.

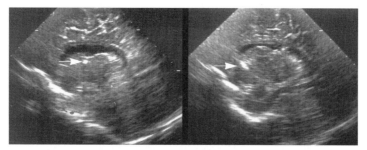

Infantile seizures and polycystic kidney disease: subependymal nodules.

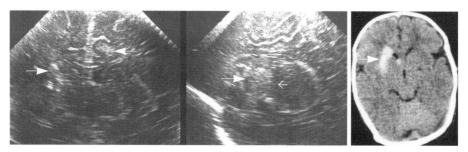

Neonatal seizures (the mother had seizures at age 16 years): hamartoma.

Neurofibromatosis type I (NF1)

Reports of the documentation by ultrasound of neonatal presentation of NF1 are lacking.

Sturge–Weber disease (Fig. VIII.4.b)

This disease presents in the neonatal and early infantile period with pial venous angioma over frontal and/or occipital lobes. After some evolution ipsilateral choroid plexus hypertrophies and dilated deep venous collaterals develop around the lateral ventricle. The underlying parenchyma may necrose, with intralesional calcification that may show already in the neonatal period. Cortex and subcortical white matter are irregularly and focally hyperechogenic. The gyri are readily identified due to increased reflections from the sulci.

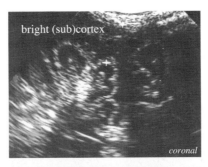

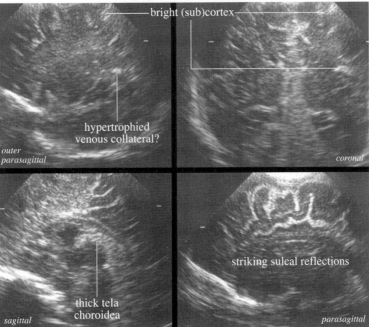

Fig. VIII.4.b. Infant with seizures and facial angioma (later operated on): *(top)* 10 MHz section; *(bottom)* 7.5 MHz sections.

Epidermal naevus syndrome (linear naevus sebaceus) (Fig. VIII.4.c)

This neuro-ectodermosis is often associated with hemimegalencephaly ('hemipachygyria with colpocephaly'). Exceptionally hamartomas, arachnoid cysts or arterial aneurysms are observed. An association with subtotal cerebellar agenesis has been described. Branches of the ipsilateral middle cerebral artery may be exceptionally large.

REFERENCES

El-Shanti, H., Bell, W.E., Waziri, M.H. (1992) 'Epidermal nevus syndrome: subgroup with neuronal migration defects.' *Journal of Child Neurology*, **7**, 29–34.
Wang, P.J., Maeda, Y., Izumi, T., Yasjima, K., Hara, M., Kobayashi, N., Fukuyama, Y. (1983) 'An association of subtotal cerebellar agenesis with organoid nevus. A possible new variety of neurocutaneous syndrome.' *Brain and Development*, **5**, 503–508.

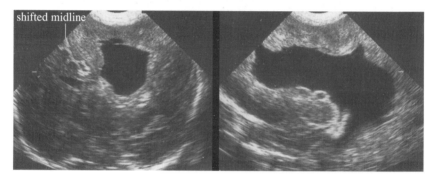

Fig. VIII.4.c. Preterm infant (32 weeks gestation) with seizures and typical linear naevus sebaceus of Jadassohn. There was left-sided megalencephaly with displacement of the midline and ipsilateral ventricular dilatation. In this dysplastic hemisphere glial hyperplasia and hypertrophy, together with altered neuroblast migration, give the ventricle roof an irregular appearance.

Hypomelanosis of Ito

This phakomatosis is important because it can trigger encephaloclastic brain lesions. Focal or global brain atrophy may occur together with porencephaly. Involvement of white matter may, with hypodensity on CT, imitate a leukodystrophic process. Neuronal heterotopia and pachygyria are well known.

REFERENCES

Glover, M.T., Brett, E.M., Atherton, D.J. (1989) 'Hypomelanosis of Ito: spectrum of the disease.' *Journal of Pediatrics*, **115**, 75–80.
Gordon, N. (1994) 'Hypomelanosis of Ito (incontinentia pigmenti achromians).' *Developmental Medicine and Child Neurology*, **36**, 271–274.
Rosemberg, S., Arita, F.N., Campos, C., Alonso, F. (1984) 'Hypomelanosis of Ito. Case report with involvement of the central nervous system and review of the literature.' *Neuropediatrics*, **15**, 52–55.

Incontinentia pigmenti (Fig. VIII.4.d)

This disease may be categorized along with disorders of perinatal white matter (see also Fig. VI.c, p. 216). A destructive encephalopathy is rare but can occur in the neonatal period.

REFERENCES

Chatkupt, S., Gozo, A.O., Wolansky, L.J., Sun, S. (1993) 'Characteristic MR findings in a neonate with incontinentia pigmenti.' *American Journal of Radiology*, **160**, 372–374.
Shuper, A., Bryan, R.N., Singer, H.S. (1990) 'Destructive encephalopathy in incontinentia pigmenti: a primary disorder?' *Pediatric Neurology*, **6**, 137–140.

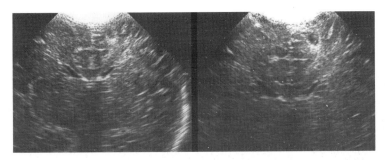

Fig. VIII.4.d. Term infant presenting with seizures: coronal 7.5 MHz sections. The scan made on admission *(left,* day 4*)* shows an area of increased echogenicity in the subcortical white matter. Following the development of the localized subcortical cysts *(right,* day 20), a vesicular skin eruption appeared and the diagnosis of incontinentia pigmenti was made.

Megalencephaly due to phakomatosis

By definition we are dealing with macrocrania without ventriculomegaly and without widening of the subarachnoid spaces. Macrocephaly need not be fetal in onset.

Cerebral gliomatosis, in its diffuse form without tumour formation, may present in the neonatal period with convulsions. The affected zones may initially be asymmetric, giving rise to hemimegalencephaly without ventriculomegaly.

REFERENCES

Gooskens, R.H.J.M., Willemse, J., Bijlsma, J.B., Hanlo, P.W. (1988) 'Megalencephaly: definition and classification.' *Brain and Development*, **10**, 1–7.
Jennings, M.T., Frenchman, M., Shehab, T., Johnson, M.D., Creasy, J., LaPorte, K., Dettbarn, W.D. (1995) 'Gliomatosis cerebri presenting as intractable epilepsy during early childhood.' *Journal of Child Neurology*, **10**, 37–45.

Naevoid basal cell carcinoma syndrome (Gorlin syndrome)

This entity may present at birth with macrocephaly, retinal tumour, myocardial tumour, bifid ribs and/or hemivertebrae. Mild hydrocephalus of the communicating type may be present. Other markers may be cysts in the choroid plexus and ependymal nodules spilling over into a ventricle. Rarely this syndrome will be associated with agenesis of the corpus callosum and medulloblastoma.

REFERENCE

Cramer, H., Niederdellmann, H. (1983) 'Cerebral gigantism associated with jaw cyst basal cell naevoid syndrome in two families.' *Archiv für Psychiatrie und Nervenkrankheiten*, **233**, 111–124.

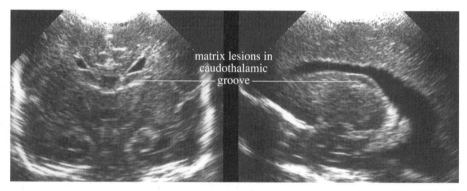

Fig. VIII.4.e. Preterm infant (29 weeks gestation), whose mother was known to have Gorlin syndrome. These day 1 scans show the typical matrix lesions associated with the syndrome.

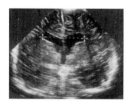

Fig. VIII.4.e. Communicating hydrocephalus in a term infant with cardiac tumour, macrocephaly and odontogenic cysts.

VIII.5 CALCIFICATION

Cerebral or cerebellar calcification usually indicates that there has been preceding necrosis. Dense and sizeable calcifications throw off an acoustic shadow. Sound waves are strongly absorbed by and reflect upon a calcified fleck, preventing deeper substance from throwing echoreflections. Calcification may follow intrauterine and neonatal infection, global antenatal brain ischaemia, severe birth asphyxia, and venous thrombosis with infarction; it also occurs in certain neuroectodermal disorders (Sturge–Weber syndrome, tuberous sclerosis), tumours (*e.g.* teratoma, lipoma, astrocytoma), vascular anomalies (*e.g.* aneurysm of the great vein of Galen), and in a group of rare syndromes (see references).

Size, location and shape of the calcifications may give some hint of the underlying disorder. Thus periventricular calcification may follow fetal infection with such organisms as cytomegalovirus, *Toxoplasma gondii*, herpes simplex virus, rubella virus and others. Superficial perisulcal calcification and calcium deposits in the hypothalamic region follow leptomeningeal thrombophlebitis and microarteritis which occur with these infections; such peripheral calcification is often present for example in congenital toxoplasmosis. If CMV infection occurs early in the second trimester, fine subcortical calcification may be present. Inflammation of the striatal arteries occurs in many fetal infections, and their walls may be calcified. Calcification in basal grey matter and in frontal and temporal lobes may follow neonatal HSV infection.

Dead neurons, particularly those in the thalamus, accumulate calcium, phosphorus and iron, remaining recognizable as fossilized cells. Soft symmetric hyperdensity due to calcification of the lateral thalamic nuclei can subsequently be evident on ultrasound two weeks after global antenatal brain ischaemia, though not evident on conventional skull X-rays.

However, there can be uncertainty about the calcific nature of lesions seen on ultrasound, and a small calcification may not be identified by MRI. CT scanning can still be important in doubtful situations.

REFERENCES

Aicardi, J., Goutières, F. (1984) 'A progressive familial encephalopathy in infancy with calcifications of the basal ganglia and chronic cerebrospinal fluid lymphocytosis.' *Annals of Neurology*, **15**, 49–54.

Ambler, M., O'Neill, W. (1975) 'Symmetrical infantile thalamic degeneration with focal cytoplasmic calcification.' *Acta Neuropathologica*, **33**, 1–8.

Ansari, M.Q., Chincanchan, C.A., Armstrong, D.L. (1990) 'Brain calcification in hypoxic–ischemic lesions: an autopsy review.' *Pediatric Neurology*, **6**, 94–101.

Billard, C., Dulac, O., Boulouche, J., Echenne, B., Lebon, P., Motte, J., Robain, O., Santini, J.J. (1989) 'Encephalopathy with calcifications of the basal ganglia in children. A reappraisal of Fahr's syndrome with respect to 14 new cases.' *Neuropediatrics*, **20**, 12–19.

Boltshauser, E., Steinlin, M., Boesch, C., Martin, E., Schubiger, G. (1991) 'Magnetic resonance imaging in infantile encephalopathy with cerebral calcification and leukodystrophy.' *Neuropediatrics*, **22**, 33–35.

Bönneman, C.G., Meinecke, P. (1992) 'Encephalopathy of infancy with intracerebral calcification and chronic spinal fluid lymphocytosis—another case of the Aicardi–Goutières syndrome.' *Neuropediatrics*, **23**, 157–161.

Burn, J., Wickramasinghe, H.T., Harding, B., Baraitser, M. (1986) 'A syndrome with intracranial calcification and microcephaly in two sibs, resembling intrauterine infection.' *Clinical Genetics*, **30**, 112–116.

Eicke, M., Briner, J., Willi, U., Uehlinger, J., Boltshauser, E. (1992) 'Symmetrical thalamic lesions in infants.' *Archives of Disease in Childhood*, **67**, 15–19.

Fasanelli, S., Perrotta, F., Fruhwirth, R. (1989) 'Computed tomography of the "near miss syndrome" with basal ganglion calcification.' *Pediatric Radiology*, **19**, 435.

Fujimoto, S., Yokochi, K., Togari, H., Nishimura, Y., Inukai, K., Futamura, M., Sobajima, H., Suzuki, S., Wada, Y. (1992) 'Neonatal cerebral infarction: symptoms, CT findings and prognosis.' *Brain and Development*, **14**, 48–52.

Grant, E.G., Williams, A.L., Schellinger, D., Slovis, T.L. (1985) 'Intracranial calcification in the infant and neonate: evaluation by sonography and CT.' *Radiology*, **157**, 63–68.

Habibi, P., Strobel, S., Smith, I., Hyland, K., Howells, D.W., Holzel, H., Brett, E.M., Wilson, J., Morgan, G., Levinsky, R.J. (1989) 'Neurodevelopmental delay and focal seizures as presenting symptoms of human immunodeficiency virus I infection.' *European Journal of Pediatrics*, **148**, 315–317.

Illum, N., Reske-Nielsen, E., Skovby, F., Askjaer, S.A., Bernsen, A. (1988) 'Lethal autosomal recessive arthrogryposis multiplex congenita with whistling face and calcifications of the nervous system.' *Neuropediatrics*, **19**, 186–192.

Magliocco, A.M., Demetrick, D.J., Sarnat, H.B., Hwang, W.S. (1992) 'Varicella embryopathy.' *Archives of Pathology*, **116**, 181–186.

Parnes, S., Hunter, A.G.W., Jimenez, C., Carpenter, B.F., MacDonald, I. (1990) 'Apparent Smith–Lemli–Opitz syndrome in a child with a previously undescribed form of mucolipidosis not involving the neurons.' *American Journal of Medical Genetics*, **35**, 397–405.

Patel, P.J. (1987) 'Some rare causes of intracranial calcification in childhood: computed tomographic findings.' *European Journal of Pediatrics*, **146**, 177–180.

Pérez Fontán, J.J., Herrera, M., Fina, A., Peguero, G. (1982) 'Periventricular calcifications in a newborn associated with aneurysm of the great vein of Galen.' *Pediatric Radiology*, **12**, 249–251.

Razavi-Encha, F., Larroche, J.C., Gaillard, D. (1988) 'Infantile familial encephalopathy with cerebral calcifications and leukodystrophy.' Neuropediatrics, 19, 72–79.

Sabatino, G., Domizio, S., Verrotti, A., Ramenghi, L.A., Pelliccia, P., Morgese, G. (1994) 'Fetal encephalopathy with cerebral calcifications: a case report.' *Child's Nervous System*, **10**, 195–197.

Samsom, J.F., Barth, P.G., de Vries, J.I.P., Menko, F.H., Ruitenbeek, W., van Oost, B.A., Jakobs, C. (1994) 'Familial mitochondrial encephalopathy with fetal ultrasonographic ventriculomegaly and intracerebral calcifications.' *European Journal of Pediatrics*, **153**, 510–516.

Schiffmann, J.H., Wessel, A., Brück, W., Speer, C.P. (1992) 'Idiopathische infantile Arterienverkalkung. Eine seltene kardiovaskulärer Erkrankung unklarer Ätiologie—Falbericht und Literaturübersicht.' *Monatsschrift für Kinderheilkunde*, **140**, 27–33.

Takahashi, H., Sato, Y., Urata, S., Kaneko, K. (1990) 'A case of neonatal herpes simplex virus encephalitis with calcifications of thalamus and basal ganglia.' *No To Hattatsu*, **22**, 179–183. *(In Japanese.)*

Takashima, S., Becker, L.E. (1985) 'Basal ganglia calcification in Down's syndrome.' *Journal of Neurology, Neurosurgery, and Psychiatry*, **48**, 61–64.

Troost, D., van Rossum, A., Veiga Pires, J., Willemse, J. (1984) 'Cerebral calcifications and cerebellar hypoplasia in two children: clinical, radiologic and neuropathological studies—a separate neurodevelopmental entity.' *Neuropediatrics*, **15**, 102–109.

Venkatesh, S., Coulter, D.L., Kemper, T.D. (1994) 'Neuroaxonal dystrophy at birth with hypertonicity and basal ganglia mineralization.' *Journal of Child Neurology*, **9**, 74–76.

Voit, T., Lemburg, P., Neuen, E., Lumenta, C., Stork, W. (1987) 'Damage of thalamus and basal ganglia in asphyxiated full-term neonates.' *Neuropediatrics*, **18**, 176–181.

Fig. VIII.5.a. Unexplained brain disorders with striking calcification, illustrating three important features of neonatal brain calcium deposition: association with necrosis; association with antenatal infection (sometimes unspecified); and lack of acoustic shadow due to minute size of the flecks of calcium, so that CT confirmation is often necessary.

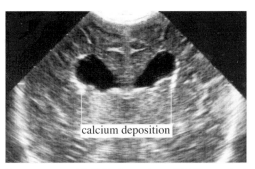

Term neonate with Fallot's tetralogy, falciform retinal dysplasia and an elevated serum IgM of 1.58 g/L.

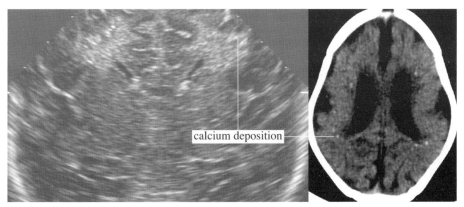

Term baby with hypotonia, refractory seizures and elevated serum IgM (1.5 g/L): coronal first week 7.5 MHz sonogram and follow-up CT at 6 months. Echogenic white matter shows bright foci near the cortex, later evident as focal calcium deposits.

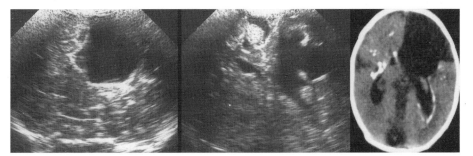

In this case cerebellar hypoplasia was detected at 20 weeks of gestation; return for follow-up only at 33 weeks, with loss of fetal movement, negative umbilical arterial diastolic flow and fetal heart decelerations. The scans (7.5 MHz coronal sonograms, day 1; CT, day 14) reveal a severe encephaloclastic process with calcification from ventricle to cortex and left frontal expansive porencephaly; cause uncertain.

321

SECTION IX
ULTRASOUND OF THE LOWER SPINAL CANAL

Frederik J.A. Beek

Sonographic examination of the contents of the lower spinal canal is readily accomplished in young babies. The posterior parts of the vertebral arches are still cartilaginous and transmit ultrasound waves. If an abnormality is detected, additional MR scanning will generally be performed. It provides a good overview, allows some degree of tissue characterization, and produces a record for possible comparison at an older age when sonographic examination is no longer possible.

Indications
Ultrasound is suitable as a screening tool for examination of the lower spinal canal in infants with cutaneous abnormalities that can be associated with intraspinal abnormalities, in those with congenital abnormalities of other organ systems that may be present with intraspinal abnormalities, and in those in whom a spinal origin of a back mass needs to be confirmed or excluded quickly. The value of ultrasound lies in the demonstration of a normal intraspinal anatomy, obviating the need for further imaging.

Technique
The patient can be examined in a prone or lateral decubitus position. In a lateral decubitus position the examination is easy to perform. In a prone position it can be more troublesome to limit the baby's movements. In this position the infant can hyperextend the back which hampers sonographic access.

The examination is preferably done with a 5–10 MHz linear array transducer. On sagittal views the location of the medullary cone can be related to the lumbar vertebral bodies. If a plain X-ray is available the ossified lumbosacral vertebral bodies can be counted. With this number in mind during the sonographic examination, the ossified vertebral bodies can be counted from the distal sacrum upwards. If plain X-rays are not at hand the lumbosacral junction can be used as a landmark. Transverse views are useful to detect slight hydromyelia or a thickened filum terminale.

Normal anatomy
The normal anatomy is depicted in Figures IX.a–f. At birth the medullary cone of term infants is located between the twelfth thoracic and the third lumbar vertebral bodies. In preterm infants it may be lower.

On sagittal views the spinal cord is visible as a long hypoechogenic structure with an echogenic central stripe. The cord widens at the medullary cone. The cauda equina consists of a collection of echogenic strands. Both spinal cord and cauda equina can show rhythmic movements which are related to respiration and heart beat. The coccyx is seen as a hypoechogenic to anechogenic concave structure.

On transverse views the cord and medullary cone are visible as hypoechogenic oval structures with a central echogenicity. The left-to-right diameter is larger than the anteroposterior diameter. The cauda equina is visualized as an assemblage of echogenic round structures, often arranged in four groups. The ossified parts of the vertebrae are echogenic, the cartilaginous parts hypoechogenic.

Pathology

Congenital abnormalities of the lower spinal canal can be classified according to Byrd *et al.* (1991). Three main groups can be distinguished:

1 — Spinal dysraphism with a mass that is not skin-covered: myelomeningocele; myelocele.
2 — Spinal dysraphism with a skin-covered mass: lipomyelomeningocele; myelocystocele; posterior meningocele.
3 — Occult spinal dysraphism: diastematomyelia; dorsal dermal sinus; intradural lipoma; tight filum terminale; anterior sacral meningocele; hydromyelia; caudal regression syndrome.

Byrd *et al.* also mention the split notochord syndrome and the lateral thoracic meningocele. These abnormalities are very rare and will not be discussed.

Ultrasound is not indicated in patients with a group 1 abnormality (Fig. IX.g) because it has little impact on treatment planning. After surgical closure of the defect the spinal cord can easily be detected during the first years of life. It has a stretched appearance, is abnormally thin, and is fixed at the site of surgical repair. The margins of the spinal cord are more echogenic than normal.

The abnormalities of group 2 are often apparent clinically (Fig. IV.1.h). Ultrasound can quickly confirm the clinical diagnosis and MRI can be performed at a later date. The anomalies are often extensive, exceeding the sonographic field of view. In lipomyelomeningocele the lipomatous component is echogenic. In posterior meningocele a normal spinal cord is present. The meningocele can contain some roots.

From a sonographic point of view the group 3 abnormalities are the most interesting (Figs. IX.i–n). In infants with cutaneous lumbar abnormalities and in those with an anorectal malformation combined with vertebral deformities, a tight filum terminale can be found, sometimes associated with an intradural lipoma or hydromyelia. A normal filum terminale is hardly or not visible. According to the literature a filum thickness exceeding 2 mm is abnormal. It often contains some fat and is visible as an echogenic strand on sagittal views or as an echogenic round to oval structure on transverse views.

Diastematomyelia is a duplication of the spinal cord in which both cords have an incomplete set of sensory and/or motor nerve roots. In diplomyelia both cords have a complete set of nerve roots. Diastematomyelia is easily recognized by the two cords, often of unequal size. At the caudal site of the duplication a bony or fibrous spur can be discerned just above the point of reunion.

If the spinal cord terminates above the first lumbar vertebral body in babies with a caudal regression syndrome with partial or complete sacral agenesis, a wedge-shaped cord terminus is present. It is a malformed medullary cone of which the dorsal portion extends further caudally than the ventral portion. MRI shows this abnormality more clearly than ultrasound.

Ultrasound can be of value in infections and tumours in and around the spinal canal. However, the sonographic overview is limited, and MRI can often demonstrate these processes to better advantage. Ultrasound can also be used in the examination of sacrococcygeal teratomas. Presacral extension can be shown. In the postoperative patient remnants or recurrences can be diagnosed, but masses must be distinguished from fibrosis and postoperative fluid collections. The use of ultrasound in the examination of spinal birth injuries is described in the literature.

ACKNOWLEDGMENT

The author wishes to thank Jan de Groot for his photographic assistance and Rodger Laplam for the corrections in style and grammar.

REFERENCES

Albright, A.L., Gartner, J.C., Wiener, E.S. (1989) 'Lumbar cutaneous hemangiomas as indicators of tethered spinal cords.' *Pediatrics*, **83**, 977–980.

Barkovich, A.J., Raghavan, N., Chuang, S., Peck, W.W. (1989) 'The wedge-shaped cord terminus: a radiographic sign of caudal regression.' *American Journal of Neuroradiology*, **10**, 1223–1231.

Beek, F.J.A., Van Leeuwen, M.S., Bax N.M.A., Dillon, E.H., Witkamp, T.D., Van Gils, A.P.G. (1994) 'A method for sonographic counting of the lower vertebral bodies in newborns and infants.' *American Journal of Neuroradiology*, **15**, 445–449.

Byrd, S.E., Darling, C.F., McLone, D.G. (1991) 'Developmental disorders of the pediatric spine.' *Radiologic Clinics of North America*, **29**, 711–752.

Fotter, R., Sorantin, E., Schneider, U., Ranner, G., Fast, C., Schober, P. (1994) 'Ultrasound diagnosis of birth-related spinal cord trauma: neonatal diagnosis and follow-up and correlation with MRI.' *Pediatric Radiology*, **24**, 241–244.

Gryspeerdt, G.L. (1963) 'Myelographic assessment of occult forms of spinal dysraphism.' *Acta Radiologica*, **1**, 702–717.

Nelson, M.D., Sedler, J.A., Gilles, F.H. (1989) 'Spinal cord central echo complex: histoanatomic correlation.' *Radiology*, **170**, 479–481.

Robbin, M.L., Filly, R.A., Goldstein, R.B. (1994) 'The normal location of the fetal conus medullaris.' *Journal of Ultrasound in Medicine*, **13**, 541–546.

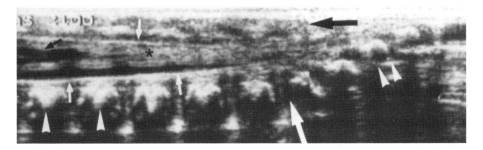

Fig. IX.a. Sagittal view of the lower spinal canal with a split screen, dual image function (*large black arrow* indicates transition between the two images). The ossified parts of the vertebral bodies appear as echogenic, rather square structures *(single white arrowheads)*. The spinal cord and medullary cone are seen as a hypoechogenic tapering structure with a central echogenic line *(small black arrow)*. The spinal nerve roots that form the cauda equina are visible as a collection of mildly echogenic strands *(asterisk)* surrounded by anechogenic CSF. The dura mater *(small white arrows)* is represented by a ventral and dorsal echogenic line along and between the vertebral bodies and arches. The lumbosacral junction shows as a lordotic transition *(large white arrow)* between the lumbar vertebral bodies, whose dorsal surfaces form an almost straight line, and the concave sacrum *(double white arrowheads)*.

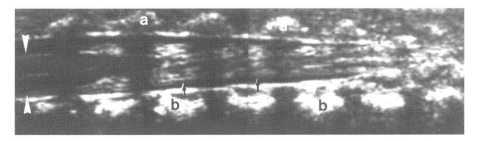

Fig. IX.b. Composite sonogram, sagittal view of the thoracolumbar spinal canal. The cord is seen as a hypoechogenic structure *(arrowheads)* with a central echogenic line. The dural sac curves dorsally and tapers; it contains the spinal nerve roots of the cauda equina *(arrows)*. The ossification centres of the vertebral bodies (b) are echogenic; those of the vertebral arches (a) cast dorsoventral drop-out shadows.

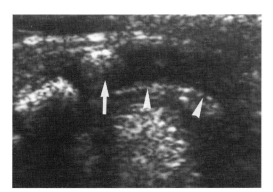

Fig. IX.c. Sagittal view of the sacrococcygeal spinal column (same infant as Fig. IX.b): the kyphosis of the sacrococcyx is well seen; the fifth sacral vertebral body shows by its ossification centre *(arrow)*; the cartilaginous coccyx is hypoechogenic *(arrowheads)*; no differentiation can be made between different coccygeal elements.

325

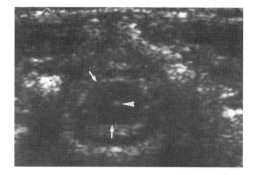

Fig. IX.d. Transverse view of the medullary cone *(arrows)*. The cord has an oval shape, the transverse being larger than the sagittal diameter. These diameters are greater then those of the spinal cord at low thoracic level but correspond to the diameters of the lumbar intumescence. The central echo complex is still visible *(arrowhead)*.

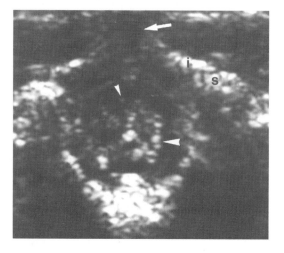

Fig. IX.e. Transverse view through the cauda equina at the level of the third lumbar vertebra. The nerve roots are seen as a collection of echogenic dots *(large arrowhead)*. Some arachnoid strands *(small arrowhead)* are visible in the subarachnoid space. The superior (s) and inferior (i) articular processes of an intervertebral joint are shown. The posterior part of the vertebral arch is still cartilaginous and thus hypoechogenic *(arrow)*.

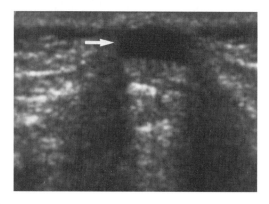

Fig. IX.f. Transverse view of the coccyx, seen as an ovoid hypoechogenic structure *(arrow)* with enhanced acoustic transmission. This almost anechoic structure should not be mistaken for an abscess or tumour; sagittal views will demonstrate the typical shape of a coccyx.

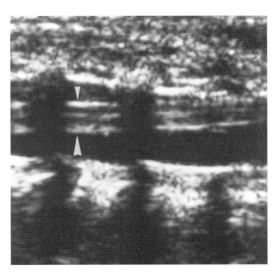

Fig. IX.g. 1-month-old boy after closure of a myelomeningocele: sagittal view cranial to the site of repair. The rims of the spinal cord *(arrowheads)* are highly echogenic and the central echogenicity complex is prominent. The cord runs in a dorsal direction and blends into the dorsal tissues at the site of repair.

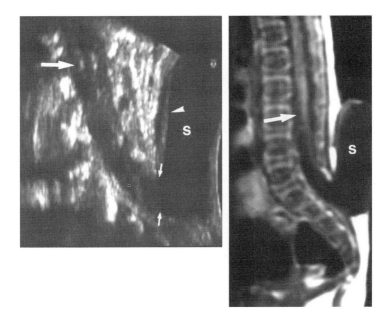

Fig. IX.h. Posterior meningocele in a 1-week-old boy with a skin-covered sac in the lower lumbar region. The sagittal ultrasound picture and sagittal T_1-weighted MRI depict the medullary cone *(large arrows)* cranial to the neck *(small arrows)* of the herniating sac(s). The thickened filum terminale *(arrowhead)* travels towards the roof of the sac.

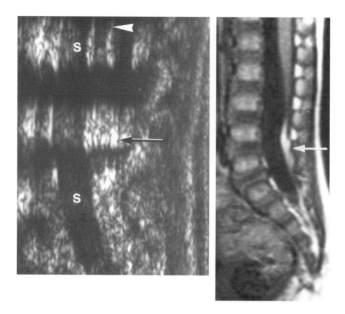

Fig. IX.i. Tight filum terminale syndrome: 2-month-old boy with a lumbosacral dimple. The sagittal sonogram shows a medullary cone at L3 *(arrowhead)*. A thick, moderately echogenic filum terminale is seen distal to the conus; one part of it is more echogenic *(arrow)*, compatible with fat (s = subarachnoid space). T_1-weighted sagittal MRI obtained at the age of 7 months demonstrates the fatty infiltrated filum terminale *(arrow)*.

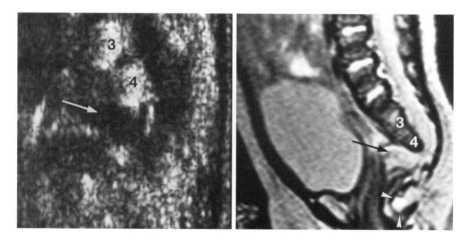

Fig. IX.j. 1-month-old girl with rectal stenosis. During bladder sonography an anechogenic mass was found behind the bladder; a pelvic X-ray demonstrated partial agenesis of the right sacrum and absence of the fifth sacral vertebra. The sagittal sonogram and T_2-weighted MRI shown here demonstrate a dural sac running too far caudally and curving forward into the pelvis below the right sacral remnant, forming a meningocele *(arrow)*. An associated teratoma *(arrowheads)* was not recognized with ultrasound. (3, 4 = third and fourth sacral vertebrae.)

328

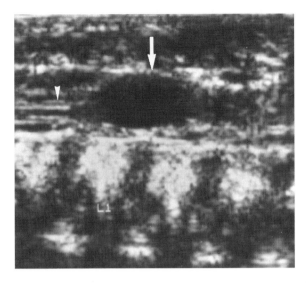

Fig. IX.k. 2-month-old boy after repair of a low lumbar myelomeningocele at birth. Syringohydromyelia is seen at the L1/L2 level *(arrow)* proximal to the site of repair. The central canal is slightly dilated *(arrowhead)*. During examination the anechogenic collection moved simultaneously with the spinal cord in a craniocaudal direction.

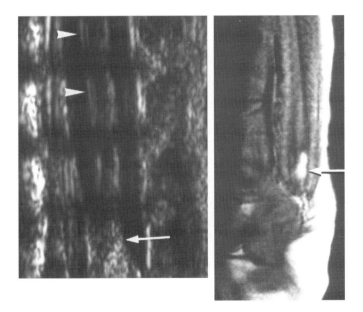

Fig. IX.l. 6-day-old girl with caudal regression syndrome. Three vertebrae of a lumbar type were present and one hypoplastic vertebra of sacral type. The distal sacrum was absent. Axial sonogram and T_1-weighted MRI show a fatty mass distal to the medullary cone *(arrow)*. The sonographic image shows a slight hydromyelia *(arrowheads)*. Note almost complete absence of the sacrum on MRI.

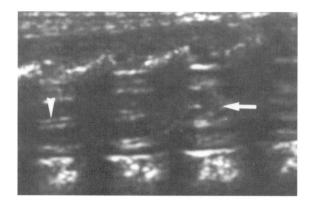

Fig. IX.m. Newborn infant with an anorectal malformation and agenesis of the distal coccyx. A blunt cord terminus *(arrow)* with slight hydromyelia *(arrowhead)* is visible. This image is probably equivalent to the wedge-shaped cord terminus observed with MRI in patients with caudal regression (MRI failed in this patient due to motion artefact).

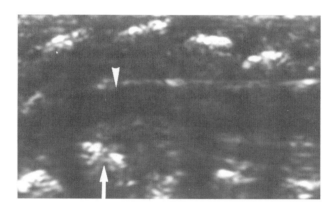

Fig. IX.n. Sagittal view of the midthoracic vertebral column in a newborn infant with spondylodiscitis. A kyphotic curve is seen with compression of the spinal canal *(arrowhead)*; the cord is not well seen. A vertebral body is destroyed by inflammation *(arrow)*. MRI showed paravertebral extension of infection, overlooked by sonography.

SECTION X
THREE-DIMENSIONAL BRAIN
SONOGRAPHY

Recent advances in volumetric sonography have proved useful in obstetrics and urology. It is thought that recognition of fetal dysmorphism and skeletal anomalies will become easier. The principle change with this method is that, instead of sweeping the scanhead through a volume of tissue in a series of consecutive planes, the steady scanhead itself contains a fast sweeping or rotating sector plane. Images generated in a plane are stored for an entire brain volume within 5–10 seconds. Afterwards any orthogonal plane in the stored volume can be inspected in the absence of the patient. For teaching purposes this may become very useful. Measurement of a lesion in an unorthodox plane presents few problems. Thresholding at the upper and lower end of the grey scale permits volume and surface rendering. The images presented here were generated on the Combison 530 apparatus (courtesy of Kretztechnik, Belgium). Some first impressions indicate possibilities for further study.

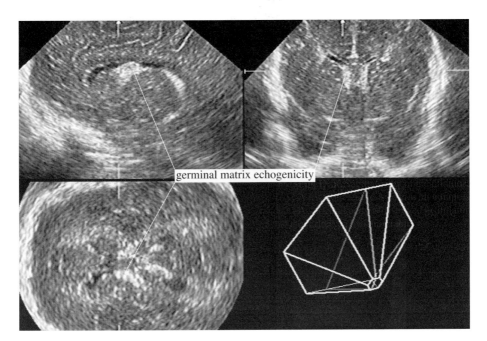

germinal matrix echogenicity

Fig. X.a. Coronal, parasagittal and reconstructed axial views as seen on the ultrasound machine's display, together with a diagram showing the volume captured *(bright lines)* and the plane of section represented on the screen *(grey lines)*. The images are from a 6-day-old infant with chronic lung disease under steroid treatment. Germinal matrix in such infants may become very echogenic in the late neonatal period, after which cystic germinolysis precedes regression of matrix in the caudothalamic groove.

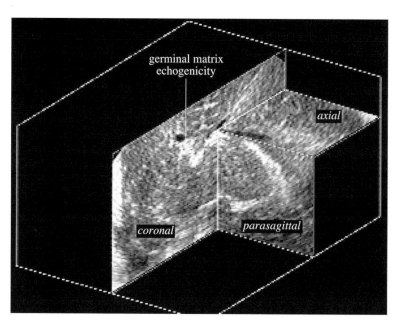

Fig. X.b. The technique permits inspection in three dimensions at the same time and in the same image. Here, the same patient as in Fig. X.a. is represented by sections in three planes through the left caudothalamic groove.

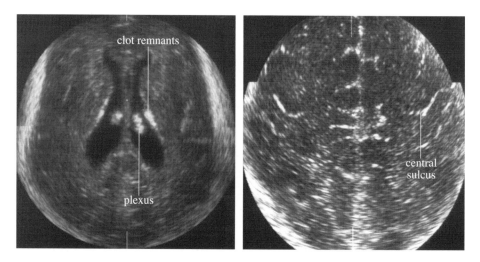

Fig. X.c. Three-dimensional sonography will permit observations in planes that are otherwise inaccessible to classic ultrasound technique. Two examples are shown of axial reconstructed images in a captured brain volume. *(Left)* Preterm infant with minimal ventricular dilatation following grade II intraventricular haemorrhage: remnant clot is seen lateral to sectioned plexus tissue. *(Right)* Term infant without neurological problems: superficial gyri can be inspected to a certain extent.

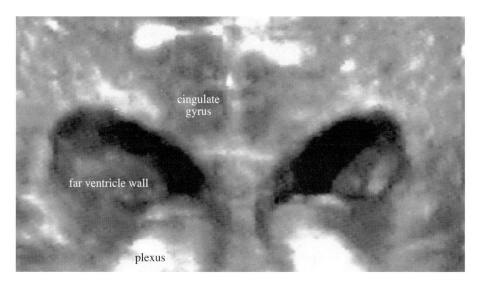

Fig. X.d. Upper and lower thresholding (elimination of grey scales above and/or below certain limits) in a volume of captured reflections can render 'depth' and 'volume' to brain spaces. (Example is a preterm infant with posthaemorrhagic ventricular dilatation, sectioned in a coronal plane.)

SECTION XI
MEASUREMENT OF ECHODENSITY
AND COLOUR SONOGRAPHY

XI.1 ECHODENSITY

Preliminary observations suggest potential benefits from the measurement of echodensity. The impetus for such research comes from obvious difficulties in the interpretation of hyperechogenic change in white matter or basal ganglia following leukomalacia or asphyxia. This limitation of sonography tends to make it unpopular and gives rise to differences of interpretation between clinicians and radiologists. Further, technicians may be left to undertake the examination, leaving records for later viewing. We think sonography should be carried out by those looking after the baby, preferably a neonatologist versed in the likely neuropathology of this age period, who can consider the possibilities as the scan moves through brain tissue. Exceptions to this rule will be radiologists or sonologists with a clinical interest out of the ordinary.

Our current method of measuring relative echodensity of brain structures is based on digitization of the video signal from the ultrasound machine, in our case an ATL Ultramark 4 (Fig. XI.1.a). The detected signal s(r) in the ultrasound machine is first demodulated (*i.e.* rectified, filtered and amplified); the resultant signal v(r) is then amplified, producing $v_a(r)$, the video signal. The amplification factor depends on user-selectable gain and time gain compensation (tgc); we have obtained good results for tgc settings when the total gain is kept close to 100%. The video signal is digitized and then displayed as p(r) with an analogue-to-digital convertor (ADC). All linear video signals are finally digitized using a frame grabber and then compensated for the machine's settings. Measurements are made using NIH Image software (Wayne Rasband for National Institutes of Health, USA, version 1.55), designed to assess grey values in medical imaging. This setting usually permits good image quality in 7.5 MHz scanning mode. The video signal is converted to an image file comprising a 256 value grey-scale. The highest value (256) is attached to white, the lowest (0) to black. In the uncompensated setting, bone density averages around 240, plexus density around 210, and CSF around 20 (Fig. XI.1.b). Healthy thalamus and white matter range between 50 and 150, while ischaemic thalamus varies between 150 and 200, ischaemic white matter between 150 and 240. After compensation for tgc and depth, these values are considerably lower.

With the method described above only *relative* echodensity can be measured with accuracy. Absolute values of the potential to reflect sound waves depend on too many variables to be controlled by this approach.

Possible approaches include measurement of grey values ascribed to pixels along a line, with subsequent estimation of an area under the curve, and measurement of mean echodensity and range of grey values in a random or standardized area of tissue, as exemplified in Figure XI.1.c.

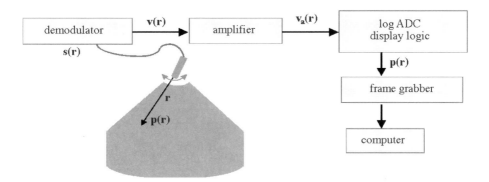

Fig. XI.1.a. Conversion of analogue ultrasound signals for computerized measurement of relative echodensity.

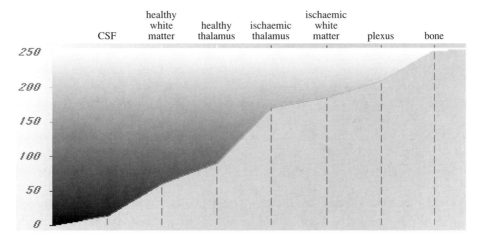

Fig. XI.1.b. Relative echodensities within the brain as measured on a 256 value grey scale.

In a limited number of neurologically healthy infants admitted to the neonatal unit of Gent Children's Hospital we measured echodensity in a standard square area in five different structures on a parasagittal section (Fig. XI.1.d). Ratios of densities can be measured, and for two items the results were plotted against gestational age (Fig. XI.e). Given calibration or compensation as described above, the values measured were different from the NIH Image values (plexus with a grey value around 210 now measures around 50). For the ratio of occipital white matter to thalamus the value varied around parity, starting above 1 at 28 weeks and ending below 1 at term. For this slope, regression analysis yielded an R-value of 0.47. Although such observations need confirmation, they suggest that occipital white matter loses echogenicity relative to the thalamus, with maturation in the third trimester.

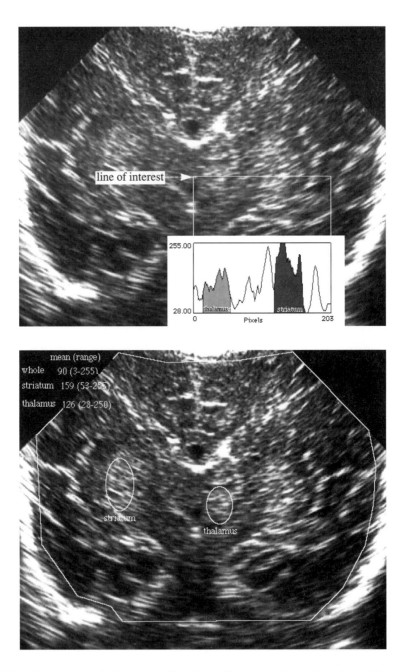

Fig. XI.1.c. Measurement of echodensity values along a line *(top)* and in a selected area of brain tissue *(bottom)*. The 7.5 MHz images shown here are from a 10-day-old infant delivered at term with birth asphyxia and necrosis in the thalamus and striatum.

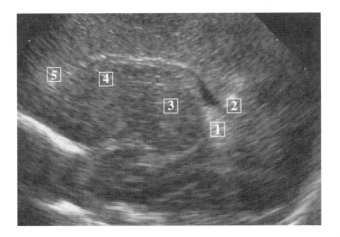

Fig. XI.1.d. Standard square areas measured in brain tissue comparative echodensity study: (1) choroid glomus, (2) occipital white matter, (3) thalamus, (4) caudate nucleus head, (5) frontal white matter.

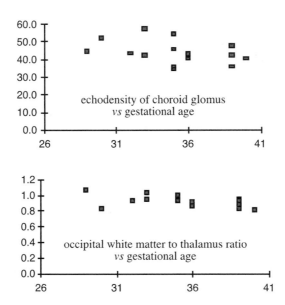

Fig. XI.1.e. Variation in echodensity (grey-scale values) with gestational age (in weeks) as measured in a small sample of neurologically healthy infants (see text for details).

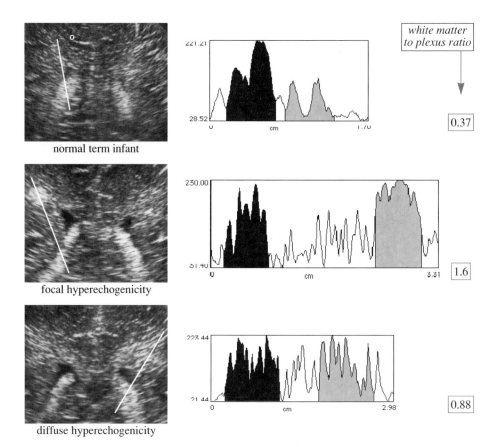

Fig. XI.1.f. White matter to plexus ratio measured in a normal term infant and in two infants with, respectively, focal and diffuse hyperechogenicity. Echodensity is measured along a line and its profile plotted. The area under the curve is measured for that part of the line traversing plexus *(black shading)* and a region of white matter *(grey shading)*.

The entities of white matter hyperechogenicity or flaring are still awaiting accurate definition, as explained in the sections on leukomalacia (V.2) and asphyxia (VI). Figure XI.1.f illustrates an attempt to objectively define two different types of ischaemic white matter injury, one focal and the other more diffuse, both belonging to the heterogeneous group of leukomalacias. One would hope that subtle relative changes in echogenicity may help to predict the outcome of minimal white matter injury.

Other examples of the potential use of objective echodensity are shown in Figure VI.b (early caudate hypoechogenicity relative to thalamus, p. 248), Figure VI.c (gyral core hyperechogenicity, p. 250), and Figure VII.3.a (posterior cerebral artery infarction, p. 283).

A major problem in this context will be to show superiority of objective measurement over subjective visual interpretation. In the study of ischaemic brain disease we also need

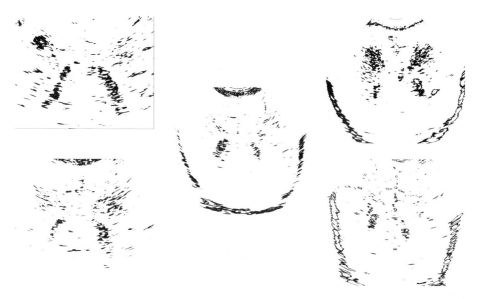

Fig. XI.1.g. Binary images (*i.e.* black and white, with grey values digitally removed) for five different coronal sections in NIH Image. The central image is from a healthy term baby, the others represent white matter injury with hyperechogenic clouds within flares. Although further sonography did not show cystic changes in white matter, the infant developed mild spastic diplegia. Compare white matter reflections with those from the choroid glomus.

a reproducible and easy method to define mild ventriculomegaly with great accuracy. High quality neurological follow-up is a prerequisite as it will take years for some mild changes to translate into clinical problems.

XI.2. COLOUR SONOGRAPHY

Given the fact that the human visual system is limited in its ability to differentiate grey values (up to around 128), it would be logical to attempt brain sonography in colour scales. Higher resolution analysis with a colour scale for the interesting areas (*e.g.* ischaemic white matter) may prove useful. Processing of the captured video signal with commercial 'photo-shop' software or density slicing in NIH Image are available rudimentary examples for the time being. To avoid drowning in colour chaos, research will have to focus on the ideal resolu-tion of the digitized sound signal, the kind of colours to be used and the range across which they should be employed. An example of the different effects that can be produced in colour enhancement of white matter hyperechogenicity is given in Figure XI.2.a. It seems impera-tive when attempting colour presentation to indicate both the grey values and their corre-sponding colour codes.

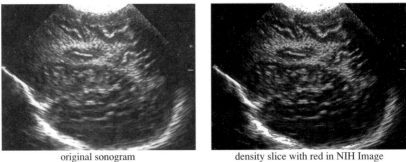

original sonogram   density slice with red in NIH Image

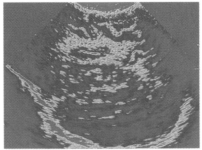

change to 'spectrum' colours

Fig. XI.2.a. Parasagittal 7.5 MHz sonogram: effect of colour enhancement on delineation of white matter hyperechogenicity (unknown cause; subject is the term infant of a diabetic mother).

SECTION XII
CEREBRAL BLOOD FLOW VELOCITY
WAVEFORM CHARACTERISTICS
(DOPPLER ULTRASOUND)

Frank van Bel

Since 1979, the year in which Henrietta Bada and her co-workers introduced the use of Doppler-derived cerebral (arterial) blood flow velocity (CBFV) to assess changes in neonatal cerebral blood flow, the development of this noninvasive technique in neonatology has been tremendous. This section summarizes the use of (colour) Doppler ultrasonography to assess changes in neonatal vascular cerebral resistance and cerebral perfusion, including its limitations and pitfalls. It further describes how to identify, insonate and determine reliable blood velocity waveforms from cerebral arteries and veins. Finally, the role of perinatal cerebral Doppler studies as a tool in both research and clinical settings is briefly discussed.

Technical aspects and quantification of cerebral blood flow velocity
The Doppler principle: calculation of blood flow velocity and actual blood flow
Measurement of the velocity of blood in a vessel depends on the Doppler principle, first described by C.J. Doppler in 1843. When an ultrasound beam is placed over a blood vessel, blood passes through the beam and reflection of ultrasound occurs by moving particles in the blood, predominantly red blood cells. The frequency shift (the difference between emitted and reflected frequency) is proportional to the velocity of these red blood cells (Fig. XII.a). When the angle of insonation (*i.e.* the angle between the emitted ultrasound beam and the vessel under investigation) is known, and the frequency shift is measured, the velocity of the blood can be calculated using the formula: $V = (c \times \Delta f)/(2 \times f_o \times \cos@)$, where c = velocity of sound waves in brain tissue (1540 m/s), Δf = change of frequency of emitted ultrasound, f_o = emitted frequency, @ = angle between emitted ultrasound beam and vessel under investigation. At small angles of insonation ($<15°$) the potential inaccuracy of CBFV determination is small because the cosine varies little between 0 and 15°, but with larger angles precise quantification of this angle is essential for reliable determination (Eldridge *et al.* 1983). For instance, a one degree error in determination of the angle of insonation near 70° introduces a 6% error in the velocity measured.

Theoretically, the flow Q (mL/min) can be measured if the cross-sectional area (A) of the vessel is known, since: $Q = V \times A \times 60$; A equals πr^2, where r represents the internal radius of the vessel under investigation. However, one should realize that reliable measurement of internal diameter in any human neonatal artery is not achievable because clear depiction with grey-scale duplex ultrasound is impossible (see also below) due to their

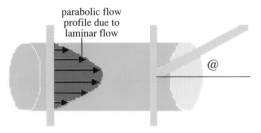

parabolic flow
profile due to
laminar flow

@

Fig. XII.a. Sonographic imaging of cerebral blood flow (see text for explanation).

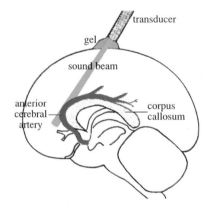

transducer

gel

sound beam

anterior
cerebral
artery

corpus
callosum

Fig. XII.b. Insonation of the anterior cerebral artery.

small size (1 to 2 mm), whereas depiction of the vessel with colour Doppler flow imaging is much too crude for accurate measurement of its diameter (van Bel *et al.* 1990).

The Doppler systems used
The early studies using Doppler ultrasound to investigate neonatal cerebral perfusion were performed with continuous wave Doppler instruments. These devices were inexpensive, portable and user friendly. The continuous wave transducers emit and receive ultrasound in an uninterrupted fashion because one crystal emits the ultrasound waves and a second crystal in the same transducer receives the reflected signals. The penetration capacity of the emitted ultrasound waves is determined by the emission frequency: the lower the frequency the greater the penetration. All moving structures which lie in the ultrasonic beam will produce frequency shifts. Doppler ultrasound studies of the neonatal cerebral circulation with this method have used almost exclusively the anterior cerebral artery (ACA) or its pericallosal branch because of their favourable course in the midline, just beneath the anterior fontanelle which can be used as an acoustic window (Bada *et al.* 1979). Insonation was performed mostly blind, but audible signals and the visual display helped the investigator to adjust the transducer position in order to obtain the optimum velocity waveform of the ACA (Fig. XII.b).

When the combined pulsed Doppler two dimensional (2D) ultrasound devices (duplex sonography) became available, it was possible to identify other important intracerebral arteries and even veins to determine velocity within these vessels with much more precision. The *pulsed Doppler* system, which uses the same crystal to emit bursts of ultrasound at a regular rate to tissue (pulse repetition frequency or PRF) and to receive the reflected signals, is an alternative device. It has the advantage that it is able to selectively detect blood flow velocity in a single vessel of the neonatal brain (Doppler sample volume), at specific distance from the transducer, but the disadvantage that the maximum detectable frequency shift is limited to one-half the PRF.

If the frequency shift exceeds this limit, aliasing occurs: the high frequency portion of the waveform is cut off and reinserted as a negatively shifted component (Eldridge *et al.* 1983). Pronounced aliasing may mimic a disturbed turbulent flow velocity waveform. Practically, however, aliasing is not a problem when dealing with the neonatal cerebral circulation, because flow velocities are relatively low in the cerebral vascular bed. In combination with 2D ultrasound systems, which can identify the vascular anatomy, the vessel of choice can be insonated under an angle of insonation as small as possible and the optimum velocity waveform of the blood can then be determined. With grey scale Duplex sonography, neonatal cerebral arteries are identified mainly by their pulsatile action; it is usually not possible to depict their entire course, prohibiting accurate measurement of the angle of insonation (Raju and Zikos 1987, Wladimiroff and van Bel 1987).

In contrast to grey scale Duplex sonography, colour Doppler flow imaging (CDFI) of the neonatal brain enables rapid and accurate identification of the cerebral vascular anatomy and full-field blood flow information, which is colour coded. The direction of motion of the blood (red cells) is encoded in red (mostly used to depict blood moving toward the transducer) or blue (mostly used to depict blood moving away from the transducer), while frequency shifts, related to the velocity of the blood, are reflected in the degree of colour saturation, less colour indicating higher velocities (Mitchell *et al.* 1988, van Bel *et al.* 1993). The most important advantages of CDFI in noninvasive investigation of neonatal brain perfusion, as compared to grey scale imaging, are: (i) the possibility to choose the optimum position for the Doppler sample volume in larger cerebral arteries, including arteries normally not detectable with grey scale ultrasound, to obtain reliable and virtually absolute measurements of blood velocities (see also below); (ii) the possibility of identifying the deep and superficial veins; and (iii) the possibility of identifying smaller arteries in regions of the (preterm) neonatal brain which are particularly vulnerable to ischaemic and/or haemorrhagic damage, such as the basal ganglia, periventricular white matter and subcortex (Mitchell *et al.* 1988, Wigglesworth 1989, van Bel *et al.* 1993). With regard to this last possibility, success depends largely upon the sensitivity and characteristics of the colour Doppler imaging system used. Finally, it has shown its clinical usefulness in the determination of cerebral vascular malformations (Tessler *et al.* 1989, van Bel *et al.* 1993).

Determination of cerebral vascular resistance and CBFV and its relation to actual cerebral blood flow
Changes in blood flow velocity in major intracranial arteries are often—but not always—

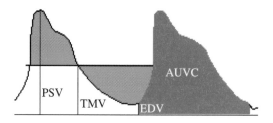

Fig. XII.c. Cerebral blood velocity curve: PSV = peak systolic velocity; TMV = temporal mean velocity; EDV = end-diastolic velocity; AUVC = area under the velocity curve.

indicative of changes in actual cerebral blood flow. Experimental as well as clinical studies in newborn animals and human (preterm) neonates show acceptable correlations between several CBFV waveform indices and actual cerebral blood flow. The equilibration of blood flow velocity with actual blood flow through a large cerebral artery is based on the assumption that large arteries are conduit vessels, without important changes in internal vascular diameter, whereas changes in resistance of the vascular bed, served by this artery, are exclusively caused by the arterioles and the precapillary bed, which are situated far distally to the artery under investigation. It becomes more and more clear, however, that large arteries do have the ability to contribute substantially to the total resistance in the vascular bed under investigation by changing their internal diameter (Brant *et al.* 1987, Faraci and Heistad 1990, Belik 1994). It is important to take this into account when interpreting CBFV indices from cerebral arteries.

Because it was not possible to quantify blood flow velocity in cerebral arteries (*i.e.* the ACA) using the continuous wave Doppler device with blind insonation of the vessel (angle of insonation unknown), Bada instead used a measure of cerebral vascular resistance, the resistance index (RI), which was originally introduced by Pourcelot in 1975. The RI is derived by dividing the difference between peak systolic blood velocity (PSV) and end-diastolic blood velocity (EDV) by the PSV (PSV–EDV/PSV) (Fig. XII.c). Because it is a ratio, the RI is independent of the angle of insonation. The RI is in common use in neonatology. Other Doppler ratios reported in the literature are the pulsatility index (PI: PSV–EDV/TMV) and the PSV/EDV ratio (TMV = temporal mean velocity, AUVC = area under the velocity curve—see below). These ratios are mainly used in obstetrics (maternally as well as fetally). A high RI correlates with increased cerebral vascular resistance and a decreased blood velocity, and a low RI with a decreased resistance and increased blood velocity. The above statements are true only if resistance-related changes in blood velocity are mainly related to EDV, because this waveform variable has been thought to be influenced in particular by the peripheral vascular resistance, whereas PSVs reflect not only changes in cerebrovascular resistance but also changes in pump function of the heart (van Bel *et al.* 1992*b*) and in compliance of the cerebral vascular bed (van Bel *et al.* 1988*a*).

Moreover, the interpretation that the RI of large intracranially situated arteries is directly related to cerebral vascular resistance (also accounting for vascular beds of other organ systems) is not correct from a fluid dynamics viewpoint: the concept of vascular resistance

TABLE XII.1
Correlation coefficients (*r*) in the various studies which investigated the relation between actual
cerebral blood flow and the Doppler ultrasound derived variables of the neonatal CBFV
waveform(see text for abbreviations)

	PSV vs CBF	TMV/AUVC vs CBF	EDV vs CBF	RI vs CBF
Experimental studies*	0.49 to 0.76	0.51 to 0.90	0.49 to 0.72	–0.41 to 0.20
Clinical studies**	0.21	0.75 to 0.77	0.65 to 0.82	–0.56 to –0.67

*Batton *et al.* (1983), Hansen *et al.* (1983), Rosenberg *et al.* (1985), Sonesson and Herin (1988), Martin *et al.* (1990).
**Risberg and Smith (1980, in adults), Greisen *et al.* (1984), Perlman *et al.* (1985*b*).

is defined by the relation R (resistance) = P (arteriovenous pressure difference)/Q (flow rate), which shows that determination of resistance requires both pressure and flow data. Several studies report on the relationship between RI and actual blood flow—experimental studies in newborn animals (Batton *et al.* 1983, Hansen *et al.* 1983, Rosenberg *et al.* 1985, Martin *et al.* 1990) as well as clinical studies in human (preterm) babies (Greisen *et al.* 1984, Perlman *et al.* 1985*b*) and adults (Risberg and Smith 1980). A summary of the results is shown in Table XII.1: it is obvious from these data that the relation between RI and actual cerebral blood flow is not strong.

Duplex ultrasonography and especially CDFI offer the possibility to place the sample volume of the Doppler transducer in the vessel of choice with a minimal angle of insonation (<15°). It has become increasingly common to estimate changes in blood velocity by angle of insonation dependent velocity waveform indices. Figure XII.c gives a graphical representation of these indices, which are mentioned below. The CBFV waveform variable most frequently investigated as a measure of changes in actual cerebral blood flow is the mean blood velocity. This can be obtained by a time-averaged electronic integration of the waveform (time-averaged or temporal mean velocity: TMV) or can be represented by the maximum spectral velocity (the area under the velocity curve: AUVC). These measurements show a very close interrelationship (Batton *et al.* 1983). Other angle of insonation dependent indices are the EDV and the PSV. The latter is, as already stated, also dependent on myocardial contractility and compliance of the vascular bed under investigation.

It is important to stress that the cross-sectional blood flow velocity profile, and the location and size of the sample volume of the transducer, have, at least theoretically, a substantial impact on the PSV, TMV and EDV: the red cells in the cerebral vessels have the highest velocity in the centre of the vessel as compared to those streaming near the vascular wall (parabolic flow profile, Fig. XII.a), implying that the magnitude of the blood velocity depends on the position (and size) of the sample volume. Practically, in the newborn baby, the internal diameter of even the largest cerebral arteries will mostly not exceed the sample volume size. Hence, almost always the whole vessel under investigation will be insonated. It remains important, especially when dealing with grey scale duplex sonography in which the intracerebral arteries are identified only by their pulsatile action, to use audible signals and the visual display in order to obtain the optimum velocity waveform (highest velocities). In this respect the use of CDFI is preferable for proper placement of the sample volume of the pulsed Doppler system in order to obtain absolute values of blood velocities in cerebral arteries and veins. Indeed, we found when using CDFI in healthy preterm and term neonates that velocities in the major cerebral arteries were substantially higher than those reported in comparable neonates, using continuous wave devices or grey scale duplex ultrasound systems. These findings strongly suggest that (i) the measurement of the angle of insonation was more accurately determined, and (ii) placement of sample volume was optimal when using CDFI.

Effects of Doppler ultrasound on developing brain tissue
Three potential hazards leading to tissue damage are important in relation to ultrasound: (1) heat, (2) cavitational effects, and (3) damage to chromosomes.

When ultrasound energy is absorbed by tissue a heating effect occurs. Although brain tissue does not have a high acoustic absorption coefficient, it remains important to reckon with the possibility of generation of heat, which is highest when using pulsed Doppler systems in developing brain tissue (Ter Haar *et al.* 1989). The American Institute of Ultrasound in Medicine (AIUM) proposed safe threshold values for ultrasound devices and clinical use (O'Brien *et al.* 1979, AIUM Bioeffects Committee 1988): they stated that total duration of ultrasound exposure should be as short as possible (*i.e.* it should not exceed 1 minute towards a particular point), whereas the output intensity should remain below $100\,mW/cm^2$.

It must be stated that cavitation (formation of small gaseous cavities) is merely hypothetical when dealing with the clinical situation, or at least it has never been detected in such a context. Nonetheless, experimental studies on the larva of the fruit fly have revealed this possibility (Sirry *et al.* 1995).

Identification and insonation of intracerebral vessels
Major cerebral arteries
ANTERIOR CEREBRAL ARTERY (ACA)
The ACA can easily and reliably be detected and insonated in the (para)sagittal plane using the anterior fontanelle as an acoustic window. CDFI mostly depicts the entire course of this artery (Fig. XII.d). The correct site for insonation and placement of the sample volume of the ACA is anterior to the genu of the callosal body, commonly just proximal to the origin of the pericallosal artery, or in the proximal portion of the ACA before it curves around the callosal body.

INTERNAL CAROTID ARTERY (ICA)
In the parasagittal plane when using CDFI, almost the entire intracranial course of the ICA, including its course through the carotid canal, can be depicted and the vertical part of this artery can easily be insonated (Fig. XII.d). Alternatively, the coronal plane through the anterior fontanelle and dorsum sellae can be used. Where the ICA leaves the carotid canal just lateral to the dorsum sellae, the vertical orientation of the artery always permits its proper insonation.

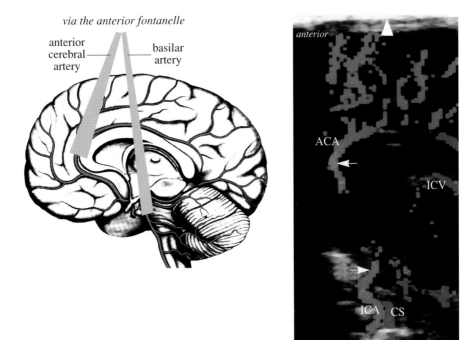

Fig. XII.d. *(Left)* Optimum sites for Doppler insonation of the anterior cerebral artery (ACA) and internal carotid artery (ICA). *(Right)* Parasagittal image through the anterior fontanelle, showing the distal course of the ACA, and the ICA coursing through the carotid canal. (ICV = internal cerebral vein, CS = cavernous sinus.) The *arrowhead* points at the anterior fontanelle. (Adapted from van Bel *et al.* 1993.)

BASILAR ARTERY (BA)

The BA can be insonated in the midsagittal plane through the anterior fontanelle during its course just anterior to the pons, or in the coronal (frontal) plane using the anterior fontanelle as an acoustic window (Figs. XII.d, XII.e). The optimum plane is situated only a few millimetres posterior to the plane through the dorsum sellae, used to insonate the ICA. The BA is then situated in the midline. When using CDFI it is often possible in this coronal plane, depending on the CDFI device used, to depict the intracranially situated distal parts of both vertebral arteries where they merge to form the BA.

MIDDLE CEREBRAL ARTERY (MCA)

The axial plane through the squamous temporal bone, just above and in front of the ear, at the level of the cerebral peduncles is the plane of choice to insonate the proximal course of the MCA in the lateral (sylvian) sulcus. The MCA is the largest branch of the ICA and in fact its continuation. When using CDFI, it is often possible to depict the entire circle of Willis, including the MCA, the posterior communicating arteries, the posterior cerebral arteries and the proximal (A1 segments) parts of both ACAs. Figure XII.f shows the circle

347

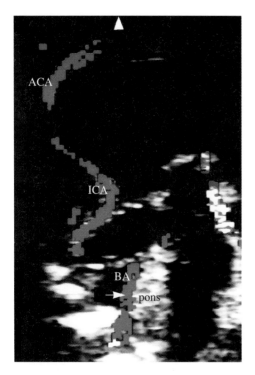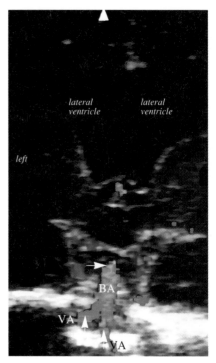

Fig. XII.e. Insonation of the basilar artery (BA): *(left)* image through the midsagittal plane depicting the BA where it courses anterior to the pons (ACA = anterior cerebral artery, ICA = internal carotid artery); *(right)* image through a coronal plane just behind the dorsum sellae, depicting the BA and distal parts of both vertebral arteries (VA)—the lateral ventricles are moderately enlarged. *Arrows* indicate optimal sites for Doppler insonation. (Adapted from van Bel *et al.* 1993.)

of Willis and the optimum site for placement of the Doppler sample volume to insonate the MCA (anatomical relationships are depicted in section I.9).

Identification/insonation of important regional arteries

STRIATE ARTERIES (SA)

The medial and lateral SAs, which are proximal branches from the MCA and important for the blood supply to the ependyma, basal ganglia and periventricular white matter, can be depicted with CDFI and reliably insonated using the parasagittal and/or coronal planes. Figure XII.g shows CDFI images and a characteristic blood flow velocity waveform of these arteries.

Identification/insonation of the cerebral veins

Although it is possible to insonate important venous vessels within the neonatal brain using grey scale duplex ultrasound (Winkler and Helmke 1989), CDFI greatly facilitates identification and insonation of these vessels.

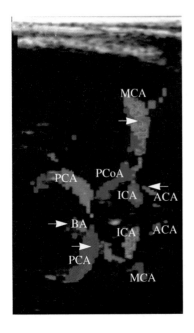

Fig. XII.f. CDFI representation of the circle of Willis, using an axial plane at the level of the cerebral peduncles (MCA, ACA, PCA = middle, anterior and posterior cerebral arteries; PCoA = posterior communicating artery). *Arrows* indicate the optimum site for insonation of the various arteries. (Adapted from van Bel *et al.* 1993.)

INTERNAL CEREBRAL VEINS

These veins can be insonated in the parasagittal plane close to the midline using the anterior fontanelle. The junction of the internal cerebral veins to form the great vein of Galen can be imaged in the coronal plane through the anterior fontanelle and trigones of the lateral ventricles (Fig. XII.h). The superior sagittal sinus can be imaged in the near field of the sagittal plane, but the angle of insonation is less favourable then (Fig. XII.g).

Neonatal cerebral blood velocity waveform patterns

Physiological variables and the (arterial) CBFV waveform

Normal values of blood velocity during the neonatal period in the most important (regional) cerebral arteries and the great vein of Galen, obtained by CDFI, are summarized in Table XII.2. A number of physiological variables influence the neonatal CBFV waveform.

DEVELOPMENTAL VARIABLES

The most important variables are gestational age, body weight and postnatal age (Bode 1988, Deeg and Rupprecht 1988, Horgan *et al.* 1989, Fenton *et al.* 1990, van Bel *et al.* 1993). PSV, TMV and EDV of all major cerebral and striate arteries and the TMV of large intracranial veins are positively related to gestational age and body weight, but the RI of these arteries is largely independent of these variables (Table XII.2). Several investigators report that PSV, TMV, EDV and RI of the intracranial arteries show a sustained increase (PSV, TMV, EDV) or decrease (RI) respectively during the neonatal period, but the largest change occurs during the first day of life (Bode 1988, Deeg and Rupprecht 1988, Meerman *et al.* 1990) (Table XII.3).

349

TABLE XII.2

Normal values (mean ± SD) and correlations (*r*) with birthweight (BW) and gestational age (GA) of blood flow velocities (PSV, TMV, EDV and resistance index of Pourcelot (RI) of the anterior cerebral artery (ACA), internal carotid artery (ICA), middle cerebral artery (MCA), basilar artery (BA) and lateral striate arteries (LSA), and of the great vein of Galen (GVG)

Doppler variables	ACA	ICA	MCA	BA	LSA	GVG*
PSV (cm/s)						
mean ± SD	38.1 ± 12.3	40.2 ± 7.4	48.0 ± 11.9	40.7 ± 7.9	10.1 ± 2.2	—
r (BW)	0.58, $p<0.05$	0.89, $p<0.01$	0.65, $p<0.01$	0.74, $p<0.01$	0.59, $p<0.05$	
r (GA)	0.49, $p<0.05$	0.86, $p<0.01$	0.43, $p<0.05$	0.69, $p<0.01$	0.70, $p<0.01$	
TMV (cm/s)						
mean ± SD	18.9 ± 8.3	20.7 ± 5.9	20.3 ± 5.2	21.0 ± 2.2	7.2 ± 1.9	7.6 ± 1.7
r (BW)	0.54, $p<0.05$	0.71, $p<0.01$	0.61, $p<0.05$	0.63, $p<0.05$	0.72, $p<0.05$	0.64, $p<0.01$
r (GA)	0.47, $p<0.05$	0.62, $p<0.05$	0.50, $p<0.05$	0.56, $p<0.05$	0.61, $p<0.05$	0.57, $p<0.05$
EDV (cm/s)						
mean ± SD	8.9 ± 3.9	10.7 ± 4.6	8.3 ± 2.5	11.0 ± 2.7	4.3 ± 1.4	—
r (BW)	0.63, $p<0.05$	0.41, *ns*	0.64, $p<0.01$	0.41, *ns*	0.59, $p<0.05$	
r (GA)	0.53, $p<0.05$	0.19, *ns*	0.55, $p<0.05$	0.26, *ns*	0.49, *ns*	
RI						
mean ± SD	0.77 ± 0.03	0.74 ± 0.07	0.82 ± 0.03	0.80 ± 0.03	0.58 ± 0.08	—
r (BW)	-0.50, $p<0.05$	0.02, *ns*	-0.12, *ns*	-0.02, *ns*	-0.61, $p<0.05$	
r (GA)	-0.37, *ns*	0.03, *ns*	-0.23, *ns*	0.05, *ns*	0.11, *ns*	

Data derived from a cohort of 24 stable newborn infants (van Bel *et al.* 1993). (See text for abbreviations.)
*Cohort of 15 infants.

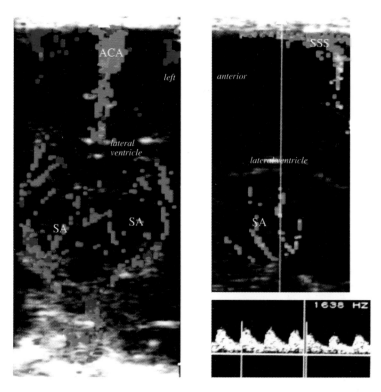

Fig. XII.g. Coronal *(left)* and parasagittal *(right)* sections through the anterior fontanelle, depicting medial and lateral striate arteries (SA). The trace at *bottom right* shows a characteristic flow velocity waveform of a striate artery. (SSS = superior sagittal sinus.). (Adapted from van Bel *et al.* 1993.)

TABLE XII.3
PSV, TMV, EDV and RI of the middle cerebral artery (mean ± SD) at 6, 12, 24 and 48 hours of life in 22 healthy term newborn infants†

Postnatal age	6 h	12 h	24 h	48 h
PSV (cm/s)	27 ± 12	31 ± 14	35 ± 12*	34 ± 12*
TMV (cm/s)	13 ± 5	18 ± 9*	20 ± 7*	19 ± 6*
EDV (cm/s)	7 ± 2	11 ± 6*	12 ± 4*	11 ± 4*
RI	0.70 ± 0.12	0.63 ± 0.06	0.64 ± 0.10	0.66 ± 0.07

†Data from Meerman *et al.* (1990).
*$p < 0.05$ *vs* 6 h postnatal age.

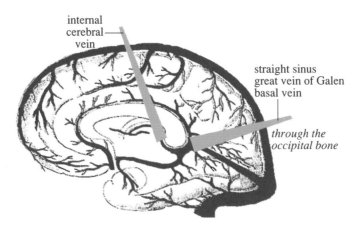

internal
cerebral
vein

straight sinus
great vein of Galen
basal vein

*through the
occipital bone*

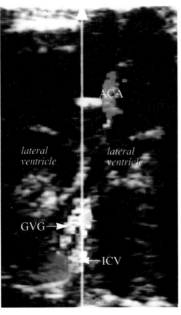

ACA

lateral
ventricle

lateral
ventricle

GVG→

←ICV

Fig. XII.h. *(Above)* Insonation sites for viewing the internal cerebral vein, straight sinus, great vein of Galen and basal vein. *(Left)* CDFI image in a coronal plane through the atria of the lateral ventricles. Note the internal cerebral veins (ICV) as they course toward the great vein of Galen (Adapted from van Bel *et al.* 1993.)

VARIABILITY IN THE CBFV WAVEFORM

Beat-to-beat variability of the CBFV waveform is a well known phenomenon and was first described by Perlman and co-workers (1983, 1985*a*). These fluctuations are thought to be caused mainly by respiration-induced cardiovascular variability (Bignall *et al.* 1988) and are especially reported in artificially ventilated preterm babies with cardiovascular instability (Perlman *et al.* 1983, 1985*a*; Cowan and Thoresen 1987; Bignall *et al.* 1988; Rennie 1989), though they can also occur in the term neonate during spontaneous respiration (Deeg and Rupprecht 1988). Synchronization of the respirator, muscle paralysis and cardiovascular support have all been found to significantly reduce beat-to-beat variability (Perlman *et al.* 1983, Rennie 1989).

Recently, a much slower cyclic variation of the CBFV waveform has been established in healthy preterm and term babies with up to 5 cycles per minute, independent of gestational or postnatal age (Anthony *et al.* 1991). Finally, behavioural state dependent variations in CBFV waveform are reported in healthy term infants (Ramaekers *et al.* 1989, Winkler and Helmke 1990): greater variability of CBFV was described during active sleep (REM sleep) as compared to non-REM sleep or during active wakefulness.

CHANGES IN ARTERIAL CARBON DIOXIDE TENSION (P_aCO_2), ARTERIAL OXYGEN TENSION (P_aO_2) AND HAEMATOCRIT

Changes in P_aCO_2 are known to influence cerebral vascular resistance. Several experimental and clinical studies using Doppler ultrasound established a relationship between PSV, TMV, EDV and RI of the intracranial arteries and P_aCO_2 (Daven *et al.* 1983, Archer *et al.* 1986a, Sonesson and Herin 1988, van Bel *et al.* 1988b, Pryds *et al.* 1989). Changes in EDV and RI in particular are related to changes in P_aCO_2 (van Bel *et al.* 1988b). Preterm babies, especially during the first hours of life, often show a blunted or even an absent reactivity of the CBFV waveform to changes in P_aCO_2 (Levene *et al.* 1988). Furthermore, conditions such as asphyxia, intracranial haemorrhage and changes in haematocrit are known to influence P_aCO_2 reactivity (van Bel *et al.* 1987b, Raju 1991, Raju and Kim 1991). Although less obvious, changes in P_aO_2 are also related to changes in the CBFV waveform (Niijima *et al.* 1988, van Bel *et al.* 1988b). Haematocrit has been known to influence CBFV: a low haematocrit causes an increase in blood velocity, and the occurrence of turbulence (Rosenkrantz and Oh 1982), polycythaemia and hyperviscosity cause decreased blood velocities and increased RI values (Rosenkrantz and Oh 1982, Bada *et al.* 1986, Maertzdorf *et al.* 1993).

CHANGES IN MYOCARDIAL CONTRACTILITY

Changes in (neonatal) myocardial contractility are reported to influence the CBFV waveform. Experimental studies in dogs (van Bel *et al.* 1992b) and newborn lambs (van Bel *et al.* 1991) showed a relationship between myocardial contractility and the PSV and acceleration time of the CBFV waveform (time from onset of ejection to PSV; Fig. XII.i). These studies further revealed that TMV and EDV of the CBFV waveform were not influenced by the pump function of the heart. A clinical study in preterm and term neonates confirmed the results obtained from these experimental studies (Molicki *et al.* 1995). These studies indicate that when using the PSV of arteries supplying the brain or indices which combine PSV with TMV or EDV, such as the RI, to assess changes in actual cerebral blood flow one must be sure that myocardial contractility remains stable. On the other hand, acceleration time of cerebral arteries may be used in the assessment of changes in neonatal cardiac function (van Bel *et al.* 1991): a decrease in acceleration time of the blood velocity in cerebral arteries indicates an increase in myocardial contractility (Fig. XII.i).

The (arterial) CBFV waveform and perinatal complications
A number of abnormal fetal and neonatal conditions in preterm as well as in term neonates carry haemodynamic consequences for the cerebral circulation, often inducing a characteristic

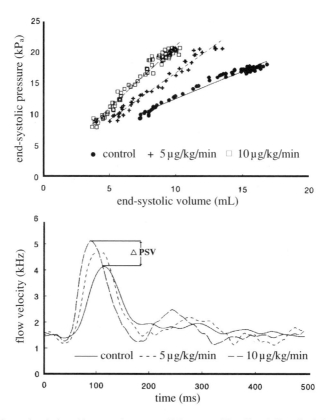

Fig. XII.i. Dobutamine-induced increase in myocardial contractility (5 and 10 µg/kg/min) as indicated by a change in the end-systolic pressure volume relationship (steeper curve shifted to the left); this was associated with an increase of the peak systolic blood flow velocity (PSV) in the vertebral artery as showed in the lower plot. Temporal and end-diastolic flow velocities (TMV, EDV) did not change significantly (van Bel *et al.* 1992*b*).

arterial (and sometimes venous) CBFV waveform during early neonatal life. Knowledge of these waveform characteristics may therefore be helpful to identify pathological conditions and to assess the success of established therapy. The following summary briefly discusses those conditions which are linked to abnormal changes in the CBFV waveform.

NEONATAL CBFV AND IMPAIRED FETAL GROWTH

Intrauterine hypoxia due to reduced uteroplacental blood flow induces preferential perfusion of vital organs such as the brain, myocardial tissue and the adrenals, to meet the metabolic requirements of these important organ systems (Wladimiroff *et al.* 1988). We found lower RI values and higher EDV values of the anterior cerebral artery during the first five days of life in growth retarded newborn infants, indicating a continuation of preferential cerebral blood perfusion during the early neonatal period (van Bel *et al.* 1986).

354

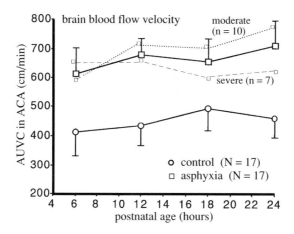

Fig. XII.j. AUVC (mean ± SD) of the anterior cerebral artery (ACA) in 17 asphyxiated infants and 17 matched controls on the first day of life. AUVC was significantly higher in the asphyxiated infants (*p*<0.01), suggesting an increase of actual cerebral blood flow.

NEONATAL CBFV, PERINATAL HYPOXIC–ISCHAEMIC EVENTS AND NEURODEVELOPMENTAL OUTCOME

In a longitudinal study in which serial measurements were performed of the blood velocity waveform of the anterior cerebral artery in 17 severely asphyxiated and 17 healthy mature newborn infants, matched for gestational age and birthweight, we found lower RI values and higher AUVC values in the asphyxiated neonates from 6 hours after birth up to 4 days of life (Fig. XII.j) (van Bel *et al.* 1987*c*). Other studies reported similar results (van Bel *et al.* 1984, van Bel and van de Bor 1985, Levene *et al.* 1989). A study by Archer *et al.* (1986*b*) established a relationship between abnormally low RI values of the anterior cerebral artery and adverse neurodevelopmental outcome. It was suggested that this phenomenon was re-lated to postasphyxial oedema (van Bel *et al.* 1984, 1987*b*; van Bel and van de Bor 1985), although Archer *et al.* attributed these low RI values to a decreased or even absent P_aCO_2 reactivity of the cerebral vascular bed, which is vasodilated and paralysed, leading to hyper-perfusion of the neonatal brain. Bada *et al.* (1979) reported low RI values in the anterior cerebral artery of preterm babies suffering perinatal asphyxia, although these were less pronounced than in the more mature neonate. Van Bel *et al.* (1987*b*) found that an abnor-mally fluctuating CBFV waveform in the anterior cerebral artery preceded the onset of periventricular–intraventricular haemorrhage and that both this fluctuating pattern and an increased AUVC in that artery preceded its extension. They also found that, contrary to find-ings in the more mature infant, consistently higher RI values (mainly due to elevated PSV values) in the first week of life in preterm babies born before the 34th gestational week were related to a neurodevelopmental delay at 2 years of age (van Bel *et al.* 1989*a*). In summary, serial CBFV waveform determinations can be used as an additional tool to assess the prob-ability of adverse neurodevelopmental outcome and the onset and extension of intracranial bleeding in preterm infants.

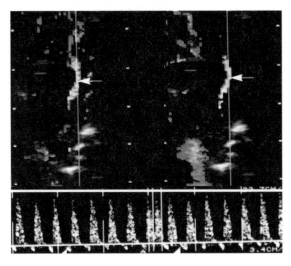

Fig. XII.k. Sequential CDFI images of the ACA during one cardiac cycle in a preterm baby with PDA (*arrows* = insonation points). Note the conversion from red (indicating anterograde flow) during the end-systolic phase *(left)* to blue (indicating retrograde flow) during the end-diastolic phase *(right)*: this illustrates reversal of cerebral blood flow towards the heart in diastole, as also shown in the waveform with retrograde flow.

CBFV AND A HAEMODYNAMICALLY IMPORTANT DUCTUS ARTERIOSUS (PDA)

A significant left-to-right shunt through the ductus arteriosus has profound influence on cerebral haemodynamics and thus CBFV waveform (Perlman *et al.* 1981, Lipman *et al.* 1982, Martin *et al.* 1982). There is a decreased EDV in all cerebral arteries, with sometimes even a retrograde flow during diastole (Perlman *et al.* 1981, Lipman *et al.* 1982, Martin *et al.* 1982, Ellison *et al.* 1983) (Fig. XII.k). Van Bel *et al.* (1995) also reported an increase in PSV with abnormally high RI of the cerebral arteries in preterm babies during PDA, with normalization of PSV values after ductal closure, probably indicating an increment of compliance of the cerebral vascular bed to compensate for ductal steal during PDA. Some studies report a decrease in CBFV during PDA (Lipman *et al.* 1982, Martin *et al.* 1982), but other investigators found no significant difference between TMV values of cerebral arteries during PDA and TMV values after ductal closure (van Bel *et al.* 1995). The RI has been used as a semiquantitative measure of the severity of the left-to-right shunt due to PDA. A positive relationship between the RI of the anterior cerebral artery and the severity of PDA has been established (van Bel *et al.* 1987*a*). Kupferschmid *et al.* (1988) reported that an absent or even retrograde diastolic flow velocity in the anterior cerebral artery predicted PDA with a high sensitivity and specificity. Although CBFV waveform changes can be used as a simple additional means to diagnose PDA, especially in situations in which cardiac echographic evaluation is not desirable or possible, it is important to realize that similar changes can be caused by complications other than PDA alone such as hydrocephalus, cardiac malformations with a large left-to-right shunt or profound hypotension (see below).

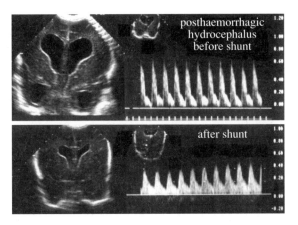

Fig. XII.l. Typical CBFV waveform changes during posthaemorrhagic hydrocephalus in a preterm infant (basilar artery flow velocity): abnormally high PSV and low EDV, with normalization after shunting.

CBFV AND HYDROCEPHALUS

In infants with (posthaemorrhagic) hydrocephalus the RI of cerebral arteries appears to be increased, whereas after placement of a shunt normalization of the CBFV waveform takes place (Hill and Volpe 1982, Saliba *et al.* 1985). More recent studies of the anterior cerebral and internal carotid arteries (Alvisi 1985, van Bel *et al.* 1988*a*) showed that an initial increase and a moderate decrease occurs in the PSV and EDV respectively (Fig. XII.l). In this situation MFV was not altered, suggesting preservation of blood flow in these vessels. When hydrocephalus was progressive and/or long-standing, the RI increased further and the EDV became absent or negative indicating reverse flow. A recent study in infants with progressive hydrocephalus, in which cerebral haemodynamics were monitored using transcranial Doppler ultrasound, concluded that the current Doppler indices obtained from the CBFV waveform (PSV, TMV, EDV, PI and RI) were inadequate to assess the complex intracranial haemodynamic responses in patients with raised intracranial pressure (Hanlo *et al.* 1996).

(COLOUR)DOPPLER ULTRASOUND DERIVED IDENTIFICATION OF VASCULAR ABNORMALITIES

Full-field real time flow information using colour Doppler imaging provides instantaneous information about vascular malformations. Moreover, the flow velocity pattern in malformations and in vessels feeding these malformations gives useful functional information (Fig. XII.m). With serial measurements it is possible to monitor the haemodynamic situation (Tessler *et al.* 1989, van Bel *et al.* 1993).

Research applications of (colour) Doppler ultrasound
Neonatal CBFV and drugs frequently used in neonatal care
Doppler ultrasound investigations of the neonatal cerebral circulation have produced a substantial amount of information concerning the haemodynamic activity of drugs often used in (preterm) babies.

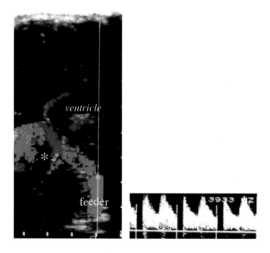

Fig. XII.m. Sagittal CDFI image of an arteriovenous malformation (great vein of Galen) and a blood flow velocity waveform of a feeding artery. The black area *(asterisk)* indicates a clot within the aneurysm. (Adapted from van Bel *et al.* 1993.)

SURFACTANT

Several studies using Doppler ultrasound have investigated the effect of exogeneous surfactant on neonatal brain perfusion, reporting heterogeneous results. Transient increases as well as decreases in CBFV are reported after endotracheal instillation of artificial or natural surfactant (Jorch *et al.* 1989, Cowan *et al.* 1991, van de Bor *et al.* 1991, van Bel *et al.* 1992*a*). During surfactant treatment CBFV was found to be extremely low, while in the same study a transient increase in RI of the anterior cerebral artery occurred, compatible with a surfactant-induced left-to-right shunt through the ductus arteriosus (van Bel *et al.* 1992*a*).

INDOMETHACIN

Indomethacin, used for noninvasive closure of PDA, is another important drug with a very profound and prolonged effect on the neonatal (cerebral) circulation (Cowan 1986). Depending on the infusion rate, a rapid (bolus) injection (van Bel *et al.* 1989*c*) or more protracted (10–30 min) injection (Colditz *et al.* 1989) decreases in PSV, TMV and EDV in the important cerebral arteries have been documented, indicating a constrictive effect of this drug on resistance vessels. This results in a decrease in brain perfusion of up to 40% as compared to pre-indomethacin values. This perfusion reducing effect may last for up to one or two hours after administration (van Bel *et al.* 1989*c*). A very recent study in preterm babies revealed that a very slow continuous infusion prevented any haemodynamic perturbation of the cerebral circulation as indicated by unchanged CBFV waveforms (Hammerman *et al.* 1995). This is an important finding because of the possible beneficial effect of indomethacin on the incidence of severe periventricular–intraventricular haemorrhage in extremely preterm babies (Ment *et al.* 1994).

Corticosteroids are being increasingly used to prevent or mitigate chronic lung disease in the extremely preterm baby. Preliminary studies using Doppler ultrasound (Ohlsson *et al.* 1994, Pellicer *et al.* 1995) showed a corticosteroid-induced change of CBFV, although these reports gave conflicting results. Further research is needed to elucidate the effects of corticosteroids on brain perfusion.

MATERNAL COCAINE USE

Cocaine use by the mother appears to cause high blood flow velocity in the anterior cerebral artery during the first day of life in (preterm) babies. A dopamine-related effect has been suggested (van de Bor *et al.* 1990).

CAFFEINE AND THEOPHYLLINE

Several studies of the newborn infant using Doppler ultrasound investigated the possible effect on cerebral haemodynamics of these drugs (Rosenkrantz and Oh 1984, Mathew and Wilson 1985, Ghai *et al.* 1989, Saliba *et al.* 1989, van Bel *et al.* 1989*b*). Although the results were divergent, some studies claimed a reduction of CBFV. It appeared that these changes are probably related to drug-induced decreases in P_aCO_2 tensions and not directly to the drug itself.

Clinical suitability of (colour)Doppler ultrasound examination of the newborn brain

Doppler ultrasound investigation of the neonatal brain has contributed significantly to a better understanding of normal and abnormal changes in brain perfusion of the (preterm) baby in the peri- and neonatal period and appears to be a powerful clinical research tool. Although its clinical applications are at present rather limited, characteristic changes in the CBFV waveform are used in our neonatal intensive care unit as an additional tool to support the diagnosis of PDA and to estimate the severity of its left-to-right shunt, and to assess the optimum timing for drainage of (posthaemorrhagic) hydrocephalus. With the ongoing improvement of Doppler technology it seems reasonable to suppose that this noninvasive technique will be increasingly used as a diagnostic and perhaps prognostic tool. In particular, colour Doppler imaging may play an important role in the description of arteriovenous malformations, not only to provide anatomical information but also to identify feeding vessels and functional data concerning turbulence and the magnitude of the shunt. It therefore may delay or decrease the need for more invasive diagnostic methods.

Finally one has to mention Colour Doppler Energy or CDE, a new imaging technique which calculates the energy of the returning Doppler signal, rather than velocity, and translates these signals into colour (Tessler and Rifkin 1994). The advantage of CDE is its independency of the angle of insonation. It has, therefore, the potency to investigate areas of the newborn brain that have a very low blood flow (velocity). This technique may enable us to monitor the microcirculation in important regions of the (preterm) neonatal brain such as the basal ganglia and (periventricular) white matter. These areas are related to periventricular–intraventricular haemorrhage and periventricular leukomalacia in the extremely preterm baby and asphyxia-related hypoxic–ischaemic damage in the more mature newborn baby.

REFERENCES

Alvisi, C., Cerisoli, M., Guilioni, M., Monari, P., Salvioli, G.P., Sandri, F., Lippi, C., Bovicelli, L., Pilu, G. (1985) 'Evaluation of cerebral blood flow changes by transfontanelle Doppler ultrasound in infantile hydrocephalus.' *Child's Nervous System*, **1**, 244–247.

American Institute of Ultrasound in Medicine Bioeffects Committee (1988) 'Bioeffects considerations for the safety of diagnostic ultrasound.' *Journal of Ultrasound Medicine*, **7** (Suppl.), S1–S38.

Anthony, M.Y., Evans, D.H., Levene, M.I. (1991) 'Cyclical variations in cerebral blood velocity.' *Archives of Disease in Childhood*, **66**, 12–16.

Archer, L.N.J., Evans, D.H., Paton, J.Y., Levene, M.I. (1986a) 'Controlled hypercapnia and neonatal cerebral artery Doppler ultrasound waveforms.' *Pediatric Research*, **20**, 218–221.

—— Levene, M.I., Evans, D.H. (1986b) 'Cerebral artery Doppler ultrasonography for prediction of outcome after perinatal asphyxia.' *Lancet*, **2**, 1116–1118.

Bada, H.S., Hajjar, W., Chua, C., Sumner, D.S. (1979) 'Noninvasive diagnosis of neonatal asphyxia and intraventricular hemorrhage by Doppler ultrasound.' *Journal of Pediatrics*, **95**, 775–779.

—— Korones, S.B., Kolni, H.W., Fitch, C.W., Ford, D.L., Magill, H.L., Anderson, G.D., Wong, S.P. (1986) 'Partial plasma exchange transfusion improves cerebral hemodynamics in symptomatic neonatal polycythemia.' *American Journal of the Medical Sciences*, **291**, 157–163.

Batton, D.G., Hellmann, J., Hernandez, M.J., Maisels, M.J. (1983) 'Regional cerebral blood flow, cerebral blood velocity, and pulsatility index in newborn dogs.' *Pediatric Research*, **17**, 908–912.

Belik, J. (1994) 'Myogenic response in large pulmonary arteries and its ontogenesis.' *Pediatric Research*, **36**, 34–40.

Bignall, S., Bailey, P.C., Rivers, R.P.A., Lissauer, T.J. (1988) 'Quantification of cardiovascular instability in premature infants using spectral analysis of waveforms.' *Pediatric Research*, **23**, 398–401.

Bode, H. (1988) 'Results.' *In:* Bode, H. (Ed.) *Pediatric Applications of Transcranial Doppler Sonography.* New York: Springer-Verlag, pp. 25–27.

Brant, A.M., Teodori, M.F., Kormos, R.L., Borovetz, H.S. (1987) 'Effect of variations in pressure and flow on the geometry of isolated canine carotid arteries.' *Biomechanics*, **20**, 831–838.

Colditz, P., Murphy, D., Rolfe, P., Wilkinson, A.R. (1989) 'Effect of infusion rate of indomethacin on cerebrovascular responses in preterm neonates.' *Archives of Diseases of Children*, **64**, 8–12.

Cowan, F. (1986) 'Indomethacin, patent ductus arteriosus, and cerebral blood flow.' *Journal of Pediatrics*, **109**, 341–344.

—— Thoresen, M. (1987) 'The effects of intermittent positive pressure ventilation on cerebral arterial and venous blood velocities in the newborn infant.' *Acta Paediatrica Scandinavica*, **76**, 239–247.

—— Whitelaw, A., Wertheim, D., Silverman, M. (1991) 'Cerebral blood flow velocity changes after rapid administration of surfactant.' *Archives of Disease in Childhood*, **66**, 1105–1109.

Daven, J.R., Milstein, J.M., Guthrie, R.D. (1983) 'Cerebral vascular resistance in premature infants.' *American Journal of Diseases of Children*, **137**, 328–331.

Deeg, K.H., Rupprecht, T.H. (1988) 'Dopplersonographische Messung der Normalwerten der Flußgeschwindigkeiten in der Arteria carotis interna bei Frühgeborenen, Neugeborenen und Säuglingen.' *Monatsschrift für Kinderheilkunde*, **136**, 193–199.

Doppler, J.C. (1843) 'Uber das farbige Licht der Dopplersterne und einiger anderer Gestirne des Himmels.' *Abhandlungen der Königlichen Böhmischen Gesellschaft der Wissenschaften*, **2**, 465–482.

Eldridge, M.W., Alverson, D.C., Howard, E.A., Berman, W. (1983) 'Pulsed Doppler ultrasound: principles and instrumentation.' *In:* Berman W (Ed.) *Pulsed Doppler Ultrasound in Clinical Pediatrics.* New York: Futura, pp. 5–40.

Ellison, P., Eichorst, D., Rouse, M., Heimler, R., Denny, J. (1983) 'Changes in cerebral hemodynamics in preterm infants with and without patent ductus arteriosus.' *Acta Paediatrica Scandinavica*, Suppl. 311, 23–27.

Faraci, F.M., Heistad, D.D. (1990) 'Regulation of large cerebral arteries and cerebral microvascular pressure.' *Circulation Research*, **66**, 8–17.

Fenton, A.C., Shortland, D.B., Papathoma, E., Evans, D.H., Levene, M.I. (1990) 'Normal range for blood flow velocity in cerebral arteries of newly born term infants.' *Early Human Development*, **22**, 73–79.

Ghai, V., Raju, T.N.K., Kim, S.Y., McCulloch, K.M. (1989) 'Regional cerebral blood flow velocity after aminophylline therapy in premature newborn infants.' *Journal of Pediatrics*, **114**, 870–873.

Greisen, G., Johansen, K., Ellison, P.H., Fredriksen, P.S., Mali, J., Friis-Hansen, B. (1984) 'Cerebral blood flow in the newborn infant: comparison of Doppler ultrasound and [133]xenon clearance.' *Journal of Pediatrics*, **104**, 411–418.

Hammerman, C., Glaser, J., Schimmel, M.S., Ferber, B., Kaplan, M., Eidelman, A.I. (1995) 'Continuous versus multiple rapid infusions of indomethacin: effects on cerebral blood flow velocity.' *Pediatrics*, **95**, 244–248.

Hanlo, P.W., Gooskens, R.H.J.M., Nijhuis, I.J.M., Faber, J.A.J., Peters, R.J.A., Van Huffelen, A.C., Tulleken, C.A.F., Willemse, J. (1996) 'The value of transcranial Doppler indices in predicting raised intracranial pressure in children with hydrocephalus.' *Child's Nervous System*, **11**, 595–603.

Hansen, N.B., Stonestreet, B.S., Rosenkrantz, T.S., Oh, W. (1983) 'Validity of Doppler measurements of anterior cerebral artery blood flow velocity: correlation with brain blood flow in piglets.' *Pediatrics*, **72**, 526–531.

Hill, A., Volpe, J.J. (1982) 'Decrease in pulsatile flow in the anterior cerebral arteries in infantile hydrocephalus.' *Pediatrics*, **69**, 4–7.

Horgan, J.G., Rumack, C.M., Hay, T., Manco-Johnson, M.L., Merenstein, G.B., Esola, C. (1989) 'Absolute intracranial blood-flow velocities evaluated by duplex Doppler sonography in asymptomatic preterm and term neonates.' *American Journal of Roentgenology*, **152**, 1059–1064.

Jorch, G., Rabe, M., Michel, E., Gortner, L. (1989) 'Acute and protracted effects of intratracheal surfactant application on internal carotid blood flow velocity, blood pressure and carbon dioxide tension in very low birth weight infants.' *European Journal of Pediatrics*, **148**, 770–773.

Kupferschmid, C., Lang, D., Pohlandt, F. (1988) 'Sensitivity, specificity and predictive value of clinical findings, m-mode echocardiography and continuous-wave Doppler sonography in the diagnosis of symptomatic patent ductus arteriosus in preterm infants.' *European Journal of Pediatrics*, **147**, 279–282.

Levene, M.I., Shortland, D., Gibson, N., Evans, D.H. (1988) 'Carbon dioxide reactivity of the cerebral circulation in extremely premature infants: effects of postnatal age and indomethacin.' *Pediatric Research*, **24**, 175–179.

—— Fenton, A.C., Evans, D.H., Archer, L.N.J., Shortland, D.B., Gibson, N.A. (1989) 'Severe birth asphyxia and abnormal cerebral blood-flow velocity.' *Developmental Medicine and Child Neurology*, **131**, 427–434.

Lipman, B., Serwer, G.A., Brazy, J.E. (1982) 'Abnormal cerebral hemodynamics in preterm infants with patent ductus arteriosus.' *Pediatrics*, **69**, 778–781.

Maertzdorf, W.J., Tangelder, G.J., Slaaf, D.W., Blanco, C.E. (1993) 'Effects of partial plasma exchange transfusion on blood flow velocity in large arteries of arm and leg, and in cerebral arteries in polycythaemic newborn infants.' *Acta Paediatrica*, **82**, 12–18.

Martin, C.G., Snider, A.R., Katz, S.M., Peabody, J.L., Brady, J.P. (1982) 'Abnormal cerebral blood flow patterns in preterm infants with a large patent ductus arteriosus.' *Journal of Pediatrics*, **101**, 587–593.

—— Hansen, T.N., Goddard-Finegold, J., Le Blanc, A., Giesler, M.E., Smith, S. (1990) 'Prediction of brain flow using pulsed Doppler ultrasonography in newborn lambs.' *Journal of Clinical Ultrasound*, **18**, 487–495.

Mathew, R.J., Wilson, W.H. (1985) 'Caffeine induced changes in cerebral circulation.' *Stroke*, **16**, 814–817.

Meerman, R.J., van Bel, F., van Zwieten, P.H.T., Oepkes, D., den Ouden, A.L. (1990) 'Fetal and neonatal cerebral blood velocity in the normal fetus and neonate: a longitudinal Doppler ultrasound study.' *Early Human Development*, **24**, 209–216.

Ment, L.R., Oh, W., Ehrenkranz, R.A., Philip, A.G.S., Vohr, B., Allan, W., Duncan, C.C., Scott, D.T., Taylor, K.J.W., Katz, K.H., Schneider, K.C., Makuch, R.W. (1994) 'Low-dose indomethacin and prevention of intraventricular hemorrhage: a multicenter randomized trial.' *Pediatrics*, **93**, 543–550.

Mitchell, D.G., Merton, D., Needleman, L., Kurtz, A.B., Goldberg, B.B., Levy, D., Rifkin, M.D., Pennell, R.G., Vilaro, M., *et al.* (1988) 'Neonatal brain: color Doppler imaging. Part 1. Technique and vascular anatomy.' *Radiology*, **167**, 303–306.

Molicki, J,. Dekker, I., De Groot, Y., Benitez, O., Van Bel, F. (1995) 'Blood velocity wave form of the internal carotid artery as a left ventricle function indicator.' *Pediatric Research*, **38**, 445(A). *(Abstract.)*

Niijima, S., Shortland, D.B., Levene, M.I., Evans, D.H. (1988) 'Transient hyperoxia and cerebral blood flow velocity in infants born prematurely and at full term.' *Archives of Disease of Childhood*, **63**, 1126–1130.

O'Brien, W.D., Brady, J.K., Dunn, F. (1979) 'Morphological changes to mouse testicular tissue from in vivo ultrasonic irradiation (preliminary report).' *Ultrasound in Medicine and Biology*, **5**, 35–43.

Ohlsson, A., Bottu, J., Govan, J.J., Ryan, M.L., Myhr, T., Fong, K. (1994) 'Dexamethasone (DEX) decreases time averaged mean velocity (TAV) in the middle cerebral artery (MCA) in preterm infants.' *Pediatric Research*, **35**, 244A. *(Abstract.)*

Pellicer, A., Gaya, F., Valverde, E., Quero, J., Stiris, T.A., Cabanas, F. (1995) 'Effects of dexamethasone therapy on cerebral haemodynamics studied by colour Doppler flow imaging and near-infrared spectro-photometry.' *Pediatric Research*, **38**, 449(A). *(Abstract.)*

Perlman, J.M., Hill, A., Volpe, J.J. (1981) 'The effect of patent ductus arteriosus on flow velocity in the anterior cerebral arteries: ductal steal in the premature newborn infant.' *Journal of Pediatrics*, **99**, 767–771.

—— McMenamin, J.B., Volpe, J.J. (1983) 'Fluctuating cerebral blood-flow velocity in respiratory-distress syndrome. Relation to the development of intraventricular hemorrhage.' *New England Journal of Medicine*, **309**, 204–209.

—— Goodman, S., Kreusser, K.L., Volpe, J.J. (1985*a*) 'Reduction in intraventricular hemorrhage by elimination of fluctuating cerebral blood-flow velocity in preterm infants with respiratory distress syndrome.' *New England Journal of Medicine*, **312**, 1353–1357.

—— Herscovitch, P., Corriveau, S., Raichle, M.E., Volpe, J.J. (1985*b*) 'Cerebral blood flow velocity as determined by Doppler is related to regional cerebral blood flow as determined by positron emission tomography.' *Annals of Neurology*, **18**, 407. *(Abstract.)*

Pourcelot, L. (1975) 'Application clinique de l'examen Doppler transcutané.' *In:* Peronneau, P. (Ed.) *Vélocimetrie Ultrasonore Doppler.* Paris: INSERM, p. 123.

Pryds, O., Greisen, G., Lou, H., Friis-Hansen, B. (1989) 'Heterogeneity of cerebral vasoreactivity in preterm infants supported by mechanical ventilation.' *Journal of Pediatrics*, **115**, 638–645.

Raju, T.N.K. (1991) 'Cerebral Doppler studies in the fetus and newborn infant.' *Journal of Pediatrics*, **119**, 165–174.

—— Kim, S.Y. (1991) 'The effect of hematocrit alterations on cerebral vascular CO_2 reactivity in newborn baboons.' *Pediatric Research*, **29**, 385–390.

—— Zikos, E. (1987) 'Regional cerebral blood velocity in infants. A real-time transcranial and fontanellar pulsed Doppler study.' *Journal of Ultrasound Medicine*, **6**, 497–507.

Ramaekers, V.T., Casaer, P., Daniels, H., Smet, M., Marchal, G. (1989) 'The influence of behavioural states on cerebral blood flow velocity patterns in stable preterm infants.' *Early Human Development*, **20**, 229–246.

Rennie, J.M. (1989) 'Cerebral blood flow velocity variability after cardiovascular support in premature babies.' *Archives of Disease in Childhood*, **64**, 897–901.

Risberg, J., Smith, P. '1980) 'Prediction of hemispheric blood flow from carotid velocity measurements. A study with the Doppler and ^{133}Xe inhalation techniques.' *Stroke*, **11**, 399–404.

Rosenberg, A.A., Narayanan, V., Jones, M.D. (1985) 'Comparison of anterior cerebral artery blood flow velocity and cerebral blood flow during hypoxia.' *Pediatric Research*, **19**, 67–70.

Rosenkrantz, T.S., Oh, W. (1982) 'Cerebral blood flow velocity in infants with polycythemia and hyperviscosity: effects of partial exchange transfusion with Plasmanate.' *Journal of Pediatrics*, **101**, 94–98.

—— —— (1984) 'Aminophylline reduces cerebral blood flow velocity in low-birth-weight infants.' *American Journal of Diseases of Children*, **138**, 489–491.

Saliba, E., Santini, J.J., Arbeille, A., Chergui, A., Gold, F., Pourcelot, L., Laugier, J. (1985) 'Mesure non invasive du flux sanguin cérébral chez le nourrisson hydrocéphale.' *Archives Françaises de Pédiatrie*, **42**, 97–102.

—— Autret, E., Gold, F., Bloc, D., Pourcelot, L., Laugier, J. (1989) 'Effect of caffeine on cerebral blood flow velocity in preterm infants.' *Biology of the Neonate*, **56**, 198–203.

Sirry, H.W., Anthony, M.Y., Whittle, M.J. (1995) 'Doppler assessment of the fetal and neonatal brain.' *In:* Levene, M.I., Lilford, R.J. (Eds.) *Fetal and Neonatal Neurology and Neurosurgery.* London: Churchill Livingstone, pp. 129–144.

Sonesson, S-E., Herin, P. (1988) 'Intracranial arterial blood flow velocity and brain blood flow during hypocarbia and hypercarbia in newborn lambs: a validation of range-gated Doppler ultrasound flow velocimetry.' *Pediatric Research*, **24**, 423–426.

Ter Haar, G., Duck, F., Starritt, H., Daniels, S. (1989) 'Biophysical characterisation of diagnostic ultrasound equipment—preliminary results.' *Physics in Medicine and Biology*, **34**, 1533–1542.

Tessler, F., Rifkin, M. (1994) 'Color Doppler Energy Imaging.' *Administrative Radiology*, May 1994.

—— Dion, J., Viñuela, F., Perrella, R.R., Duckwiler, G., Hall, T., Boechat, M.I., Grant, E.G. (1989) 'Cranial arteriovenous malformations in neonates: color Doppler imaging with angiographic correlation.' *American Journal of Roentgenology*, **153**, 1027–1030.

Van Bel, F., van de Bor, M. (1985) 'Cerebral edema caused by perinatal asphyxia. Detection and follow-up.' *Helvetica Paediatrica Acta*, **40**, 361–369.

—— Hirasing, R.A., Grimberg, M.T.T. (1984) 'Can perinatal asphyxia cause cerebral edema and affect cerebral blood flow velocity ?' *European Journal of Pediatrics*, **142**, 29–32.

—— Van De Bor, M., Stijnen, T., Ruys, J.H. (1986) 'Decreased cerebrovascular resistance in small for gestational age infants.' *European Journal of Obstetrics and Gynecology and Reproductive Biology*, **23**, 137–144.

—— —— Buis-Liem, T.N., Stijnen, T., Baan, J., Ruys, J.H. (1987*a*) 'The relation between left-to-right shunt due to patent ductus arteriosus and cerebral blood flow velocity in preterm infants.' *Journal of Cardiovascular Ultrasonography*, **6**, 19–25.

—— —— Stijnen, T., Baan, J., Ruys, J.H. (1987*b*) 'The aetiological role of cerebral blood flow alterations in the development and extension of peri-intraventicular haemorrhage.' *Developmental Medicine and Child Neurology*, **19**, 601–614.

—— —— —— —— —— (1987*c*) 'Cerebral blood flow velocity pattern in healthy and asphyxiated newborns: a controlled study.' *European Journal of Pediatrics*, **146**, 461–467.

—— —— Baan, J., Stijnen, T., Ruys, J.H. (1988*a*) 'Blood flow velocity pattern of the anterior cerebral arteries. Before and after drainage of posthemorrhagic hydrocephalus in the newborn.' *Journal of Ultrasound Medicine*, **7**, 553–559.

—— —— Stijnen, T., Baan, J., Ruys, J.H. (1988*b*) 'The influence of abnormal blood gases on cerebral blood flow velocity in the preterm newborn.' *Neuropediatrics*, **19**, 27–32.

—— den Ouden, L., van de Bor, M., Stijnen, T., Baan, J., Ruys, J.H. (1989*a*) 'Cerebral blood flow velocity during the first week of life of preterm infants and neurodevelopment at two years.' *Developmental Medicine and Child Neurology*, **31**, 320–328.

—— van de Bor, M., Stijnen, T., Baan, J., Ruys, J.H. (1989*b*) 'Does caffeine affect cerebral blood flow in the preterm infant?' *Acta Paediatrica*, **78**, 205–209.

—— —— —— —— —— (1989*c*) 'Cerebral blood flow velocity changes in preterm infants after a single dose of indomethacin: duration of its effect.' *Pediatrics*, **84**, 802–807.

—— van Zwieten, P.H.T., Guit, G.L., Schipper, J. (1990) 'Superior mesenteric artery blood flow velocity and estimated volume flow: duplex Doppler US study of preterm and term neonates.' *Radiology*, **174**, 165–169.

—— Schipper, I.B., Klautz, R.J.M., Teitel, D.F., Steendijk, P., Baan, J. (1991) 'Acceleration of blood flow velocity in the carotid artery and myocardial contractility in the newborn lamb.' *Pediatric Research*, **30**, 375–380.

—— de Winter, P.J., Wijnands, H.B.G., van de Bor, M., Egberts, J. (1992*a*) 'Cerebral and aortic blood flow velocity patterns in preterm infants receiving prophylactic surfactant treatment.' *Acta Paediatrica*, **81**, 504–510.

—— Steendijk, P., Teitel, D.F., de Winter, J.P., van der Velde, E.T., Baan, J. (1992*b*) 'Cerebral blood flow velocity: the influence of myocardial contractility on the velocity waveform of brain supplying arteries.' *Ultrasound in Medicine and Biology*, **18**, 441–449.

—— Schipper, J., Guit, G.L., Visser, M.O.J.M. (1993) 'The contribution of colour Doppler flow imaging to the study of cerebral haemodynamics in the neonate.' *Neuroradiology*, **35**, 300–306.

—— —— —— van de Bor, M. (1995) 'Blood velocity wave form characteristics of superior mesenteric artery and anterior cerebral artery before and after ductus arteriosus closure.' *European Journal of Ultrasound*, **2**, 183–189.

Van de Bor, M., Walther, F.J., Sims, M.E. (1990) 'Increased cerebral blood flow velocity in infants of mothers who abuse cocaine.' *Pediatrics*, **85**, 733–736.

—— Ma, E.J., Walther, F.J. (1991) 'Cerebral blood flow velocity after surfactant instillation in preterm infants.' *Journal of Pediatrics*, **118**, 285–287.

Wigglesworth, J.S. (1989) 'Current problems in brain pathology in the perinatal period.' *In:* Pape, K.E., Wigglesworth, J.S. (Eds.) *Perinatal Brain Lesions.* Boston: Blackwell, pp. 1–23.

Winkler, P., Helmke, K. (1989) 'Duplex-scanning of the deep venous drainage in the evaluation of blood flow velocity of the cerebral vascular system in infants.' *Pediatric Radiology*, **19**, 79–90.

—— —— (1990) 'Major pitfalls in Doppler investigations with particular reference to the cerebral vascular system. Part I. Sources of error, resulting pitfalls and measures to prevent errors.' *Pediatric Radiology*, **20**, 219–228.

Wladimiroff, J.W., van Bel, F. (1987) 'Fetal and neonatal cerebral blood flow.' *Seminars in Perinatology*, **11**, 335–346.

—— Noordam, M.J., Van Den Wijngaard, J.A.G.W., Hop, W.C.L. (1988) 'Fetal internal carotid and umbilical artery blood flow velocity waveforms as a measure of fetal well-being in uterine growth retardation.' *Pediatric Research*, **24**, 609–613.

363

NOTES

NOTES

NOTES